THE ENTRY LEVEL
Occupational Therapy Doctoral Capstone

The second edition of *The Entry Level Occupational Therapy Doctoral Capstone* is an essential resource to guide both students and educators through every phase of the doctoral capstone, from development to dissemination.

Fully revised to align with the latest ACOTE accreditation standards and terminology, each chapter of the book is divided into two sections: one for students and one for educators. This updated edition includes new chapters on mentorship and how to build collaborative skills, conducting a literature review, and performing a needs assessment and program evaluation. Student learning activities are redesigned around design thinking principles, such as empathy and identity mapping, and personal mission statements to promote student self-exploration and alignment with capstone sites and populations. Mezirow's transformational learning theory is threaded throughout the content designed for the educator.

Additional guidance for faculty and capstone coordinators includes exemplar assignments, rubrics, and relevant topics, such as artificial intelligence and intellectual property in relation to capstone deliverables. A chapter on post-professional capstones has also been added.

Well-organized and full of practical examples of capstone experiences and projects, this book is a vital tool for students in entry-level or post-professional OTD programs, as well as their educators and mentors.

Elizabeth D. DeIuliis is Clinical Associate Professor at Duquesne University in Pittsburgh, Pennsylvania. She is currently the Program Director and served as the Academic Fieldwork Coordinator from 2010 to 2021. She has been a practicing acute-care practitioner for over 21 years. DeIuliis has published several textbooks and numerous peer-reviewed publications and has presented at state, national, and international conferences on topics related to professionalism, interprofessional education, and experiential learning.

Julie A. Bednarski is the Program Director of Occupational Therapy at Indiana University in Indianapolis. Throughout her career in education, she has gained significant expertise in curriculum design and guiding doctoral students through their capstone experiences and projects. Bednarski is motivated by the transformation seen in students after completion of their doctoral capstone experiences and the impact seen in the lives of those they served.

THE ENTRY LEVEL

Occupational Therapy Doctoral Capstone

A Framework for the Experience and the Project

Second Edition

Edited by Elizabeth D. DeIuliis and Julie A. Bednarski

Routledge
Taylor & Francis Group

NEW YORK AND LONDON

Designed cover image: Getty Images

Second edition published 2026
by Routledge
605 Third Avenue, New York, NY 10158

and by Routledge
4 Park Square, Milton Park, Abingdon, Oxon, OX14 4RN

Routledge is an imprint of the Taylor & Francis Group, an informa business

First edition published by SLACK Incorporated 2019

ISBN: 978-1-032-89222-1 (hbk)
ISBN: 978-1-032-89220-7 (pbk)
ISBN: 978-1-003-54181-3 (ebk)

DOI: 10.4324/9781003541813

Typeset in Minion Pro
by Apex CoVantage, LLC

Contents

Acknowledgments

I would like to express my heartfelt gratitude to my family, colleagues, and students who have contributed to and inspired this second edition book project. My deepest thanks go to my husband, Alessio, and children, Grace and Enzo, for their unwavering support of my "wild-hair" ideas and professional pursuits as an occupational therapist, educator, and academic leader. I am also profoundly grateful to my exceptional faculty team and my "occupational therapy family" at Duquesne University, including Dr. Amy Mattila, Dr. Jeryl Benson, Dr. Meghan Blaskowitz, Dr. Elena V. Donoso Brown, Dr. Retta Martin, Dr. Michelle McCann, Dr. Richard Simpson, Dr. Ann Stuart, Dr. Kim Szucs, and Dr. Kasey Stepansky, and our remarkable administrative duo, Ms. Kelly Kovalsky and Ms. Melissa Blake, for their encouragement, support, and inspiration.

A special note of thanks to the contributing authors in this second edition, whose expertise and insights on several important topics have greatly enriched this work. I am also incredibly appreciative of all the occupational therapy doctoral students and alumni who have generously shared their personal experiences and reflections from their own doctoral capstone experience and projects, which have added valuable depth to this endeavor.

–Elizabeth D. DeIuliis, OTD, MOT, OTR/L, CLA, FNAP, FAOTA

I would like to express my deepest thanks to my family – my son, Connor; daughter-in-law, Sam; Mom and Dad; and sister, Pam, for their love, encouragement, and support. A special thank-you to my husband, James, who is always my sounding board and gives me the strength to believe in myself. Your support has been a constant source of strength throughout this second edition book journey.

For giving me my first job in academia and the inspiration to look through the lens of human-centered design, I thank Dr. Penelope A. Moyers. A very special thank-you to Dr. Becky Barton, who taught me the value of occupational therapy in community-based practice and whose friendship I have valued for over 30 years. Thank you to my students and alumni who offered their insights and reflections. I am grateful to the following students, Dara Grove, IU OTD class of 2026, and Jillian Hiatt, IU OTD class of 2027, for their work on this second edition, providing formatting and reviewing of the chapters. It has been wonderful working with the contributing authors on this second book edition, and I so appreciate their insights, collaboration, and expertise.

Finally, I thank my colleagues at Indiana University OTD, Dr. Jennifer Piatt, Dr. Megan Albright, Dr. Chang Dae Lee, Dr. Tony Chase, Dr. Annie L. DeRolf, Dr. Kristin Hull, Dr. Melinda Kurrus, Dr. Leah Van Antwerp, Dr. Sally Wasmuth, Dr. Victoria Wilburn, Nicole Vicars, and Suzanne Pritchard, for their collaboration, support, and most of all, friendship!

–Julie A. Bednarski, OTD, MHS, OTR

ABOUT THE EDITORS

Elizabeth D. DeIuliis, OTD, OTR/L, CLA, FNAP, FAOTA, has been an occupational therapist for over 21 years. She is a clinical associate professor and currently serves as a program director at Duquesne University in Pittsburgh, Pennsylvania. She previously served as an academic fieldwork coordinator and has nearly two decades of experience in developing fieldwork education programs. Dr. DeIuliis has earned degrees from Duquesne University and Chatham University and completed the American Occupational Therapy Association's Academic Leadership Institute, earning the credential academic leader. She is a distinguished fellow in the National Academies of Practice Occupational Therapy Academy (FNAP) and was inducted to the Roster of Fellows in the American Occupational Therapy Association (FAOTA). She has published several textbooks, numerous peer-reviewed publications, and continued education products and has presented at state, national, and international conferences on topics related to fieldwork education, doctorate capstone, professionalism, interprofessional education, and teaching methodologies. Dr. DeIuliis continues to practice clinically on a per diem basis in the University of Pittsburgh Medical Center (UPMC) Rehabilitation Institute at UPMC Shadyside Hospital.

Julie A. Bednarski, OTD, MHS, OTR, is currently a clinical associate professor and program director at Indiana University in Indianapolis, Indiana. Prior to joining the faculty at Indiana University, she was an associate professor, the doctoral capstone coordinator, and an assistant director of the School of Occupational Therapy at the University of Indianapolis. Dr. Bednarski graduated from Boston University in 1986 with her bachelor of science in occupational therapy. She went on to receive her master's in health science at the University of Indianapolis in 1996. In December 2011, she received her post-professional doctorate in occupational therapy from Chatham University in Pittsburg, Pennsylvania. Dr. Bednarski has more than 35 years of clinical experience and has presented at state and national conferences on topics including occupational justice, teaching methodologies related to the capstone, and community practice, among others. Dr. Bednarski is passionate about the doctoral capstone and the positive impact these experiences have on students, clients, sites, and the profession.

CONTRIBUTOR AUTHORS

Megan Albright, OTD, MS, OTR, CHT (Chapter 13)
Clinical Assistant Professor (Former Post-Professional OTD Program Director)
School of Health and Human Services
Indiana University
Indianapolis, Indiana

Allison Bell, OTD, OTR/L (Chapter 5)
Associate Professor
Jefferson College of Rehabilitation Sciences
Thomas Jefferson University
Philadelphia, Pennsylvania

Ann B. Cook, EdD, OTD, OTR/L, CPAM (Chapter 12)
Clinical Associate Professor (Former Capstone Coordinator)
School of Health and Rehabilitation Sciences
Ohio State University
Columbus, Ohio

Paula J. Costello, OTD, OTR/L (Chapter 6)
Associate Professor and Capstone Coordinator
Quincy University
Quincy, Illinois

Annie L. DeRolf, OTD, OTR (Chapter 4)
Clinical Assistant Professor and Capstone Coordinator
School of Health and Human Services
Indiana University
Indianapolis, Indiana

Elena V. Donoso Brown, PhD, OTR/L (Chapter 8)
Associate Professor and Department Chair
John G. Rangos Sr. School of Health Sciences
Duquesne University
Pittsburgh, Pennsylvania

Erika Kemp, OTD, OTR/L, BCP, FAOTA (Chapter 6)
Clinical Associate Professor and Program Director (Former Capstone Coordinator)
School of Health and Rehabilitation Sciences
Ohio State University
Columbus, Ohio

Amy Mattila, PhD, OTR/L (Chapters 3 and 8)
Associate Professor and Associate Dean for Academic Affairs
John G. Rangos Sr. School of Health Sciences
Duquesne University
Pittsburgh, Pennsylvania

Michelle McCann, OTD, OTR/L, C/NDT, CBIS, PPSC (Chapters 3 and 12)
Clinical Assistant Professor, Capstone Coordinator, and Assistant Dean for Community-Engaged Learning and Service
John G. Rangos Sr. School of Health Sciences
Duquesne University
Pittsburgh, Pennsylvania

Cambey Mikush, OTD, OTR/L (Chapter 9)
Assistant Professor and Capstone Coordinator
School of Medicine
Duke University
Durham, North Carolina

Sara J. Stephenson, OTD, OTR/L, BCPR (Chapter 9)
Clinical Associate Professor and Capstone Coordinator
College of Health and Human Services
Northern Arizona University
Flagstaff, Arizona

Sara Story, OTD, OTR/L, BCG, CAPS (Chapter 13)
Associate Professor and Program Director
College of Nursing and Health Professions
Valparaiso University
Valparaiso, Indiana

Sally Wasmuth, PhD, OTR (Chapter 11)
Assistant Professor
School of Health and Human Services
Indiana University
Indianapolis, Indiana

2nd Edition Book Introduction and Chapters at a Glance

Elizabeth D. DeIuliis, OTD, MOT, OTR/L, FNAP, FAOTA
Julie A. Bednarski, OTD, MHS, OTR

From the inception of this book, which originated in 2018, the purpose has been to provide a step-by-step guide and best practice approaches for the development, planning, implementation, and dissemination of the entry-level occupational therapy doctoral (OTD) capstone experience and project. This 2nd edition is intended for a variety of audiences, yet the primary aim of each chapter is the occupational therapy doctoral student. Each chapter in this new edition is divided into two main sections. The first section is written for direct use by occupational therapy doctoral students to prepare for and throughout the duration of the doctoral capstone. You will notice that the book is written in a style where we speak *directly to you* as the capstone student. The second section of each chapter is written to be used by the educator to showcase recommendations and exemplars for how to integrate the book into the classroom and the occupational therapy doctoral curriculum. This newly defined educator section will be of benefit to the doctoral capstone coordinator as well as occupational therapy faculty members who teach within courses that relate to the doctoral capstone and serve as faculty mentors to capstone projects. The content for the educator will also have strategies and recommendations to translate the knowledge to support the context experts, who are essential members of the capstone team and serve as mentors to the capstone students during their doctoral capstone experience.

The Accreditation Council for Occupational Therapy Education (ACOTE) sets educational standards that must be met and maintained for accreditation for occupational therapy educational programs. The standards established by ACOTE are to serve as the minimum level of expectations for occupational therapy assistant programs, master's-level occupational therapy programs, and entry-level occupational therapy doctorate programs. The curricular standards go through a review, update, and adoption process approximately every five years in response to changes in health care, national educational trends, and other higher education accrediting bodies. Although ACOTE has been regulating entry-level OTD education since 2006, there are few occupational therapy resources to guide faculty, prepare students, and socialize content experts to the capstone experience and project outside of the ACOTE standards. The minimum standards for the capstone curricula in OTD programs are delineated in the D standards (ACOTE, 2023).

The 1st edition of this book, published in 2019, was the first of its kind to provide recommendations to guide the OTD capstone experience and project and was written in alignment with the ACOTE (2018) accreditation standards. This new edition will encompass content and terminology updates that line up to the ACOTE 2023 standards, which went into effect July 31, 2025. Some of the specific terminology and language updates with the shift from the 2018 to the 2023 ACOTE standards are reflected in Table 0-1.

What Is the Occupational Therapy Doctoral Capstone?

A universal requirement for OTD programs is the successful completion of doctoral capstone. A *capstone* (or comprehensive project) is a requirement of many doctoral degree programs. A capstone traditionally represents a culmination of one's doctoral studies with an evidence-based scholarly project. It is an opportunity for doctoral students to translate their acquired knowledge (usually reflecting a specialization or area of interest) into practice and to

Table 0-1. Terminology Updates

2018 ACOTE STANDARDS	2023 ACOTE STANDARDS
Site mentor	Content expert
Memorandum of understanding (MOU)	Experiential plan (EP)
Areas of focus:	Areas of focus:
Clinical practice skills, research skills, administration, leadership, program or policy development, advocacy, education, and theory development	Clinical skills, research skills, administration, program development and evaluation, policy development, advocacy, education, or leadership

potentially lay the groundwork for future scholarship. Although specific requirements will vary among institutions, a capstone typically requires the doctoral student to engage in a self-directed practice experience, with faculty or external advisor/mentor support (or a combination of these), as appropriate. Chapter 1 will be focused on defining and exploring the roles, responsibilities, and general expectations of the capstone team: the occupational therapy doctoral student, doctoral capstone coordinator, content expert, and faculty member.

ACOTE (2023) defines a *doctoral capstone* as

[a]n in-depth exposure to a concentrated area, which is reflective of the program's curriculum design. This in-depth exposure may be in one more of the following areas in occupational therapy: clinical skills, research skills, administration, program development and evaluation, policy development, advocacy, education, or leadership.

(p. 47)

These concentrated areas identified by ACOTE – or as we refer to them in this book, focus areas – ensure that you, the doctoral capstone student, gain comprehensive insight and thoughtful engagement in an area of interest that might live outside "typical generalist" practice and allow you to develop in-depth knowledge and skill. Chapter 2 explores these concentrated focus areas in greater detail.

Tapping into the right area(s) of focus to frame your doctoral capstone might take some self-exploration of your own interests and passions to help identify goodness of fit between a potential capstone site and population. Differing from level II fieldwork, which relies heavily on supervision and instruction, the doctoral capstone requires you to seek out mentorship and initiate and engage in mentoring relationships with individuals that have expertise aligned with your focus area. Chapters 3 and 4 will model important approaches to for you to be introspective as well as self-directed as you begin the doctoral capstone process.

ACOTE (2023) defines the doctoral capstone as consisting of two distinct parts: the capstone **project** and the capstone **experience**. The capstone project is directly aligned with the capstone experience and should be designed to help the doctoral student "relate theory to practice" and synthesize and apply knowledge gained through the capstone experience (ACOTE, 2023, p. 47). In prerequisite didactic curriculum within your occupational therapy program, you, the capstone student, will develop and showcase many talents specific to competencies that help prepare you for the doctoral capstone and related focus areas, including but not limited to the following (ACOTE, 2023):

- Communicate to communities of interest (e.g., consumers, potential employers, colleagues, third-party payers, regulatory boards, policymakers, and the general public) the distinct nature of occupation and the evidence that occupation supports performance, participation, health, wellness, and well-being (Standard B.2.4).

- Identify, analyze, and evaluate the contextual factors, current policy issues, and socioeconomic, political, geographic, and demographic factors on the delivery of occupational therapy services for persons, groups, and populations to promote and advocate for policy development and social systems as they relate to the practice of occupational therapy (Standard B.4.1).

- Design, implement, and disseminate a scholarly study that advances knowledge translation, professional practice, service delivery, or professional issues (e.g., scholarship of integration, scholarship of application, scholarship of teaching and learning) (Standard B.5.2).

- Demonstrate the ability to plan, develop, organize, promote, and support program development and service delivery (Standard B.4.7).

- Demonstrate an understanding of the process of locating and securing grants and how grants can serve as a fiscal resource for evolving service delivery models, professional development, and practice (Standard B.4.7).

There are specific preparatory activities that must occur prior to engaging in the doctoral capstone. First, you will have already completed level II fieldwork. Next, you will work through a process in your OTD coursework that is designed to help you learn more about your doctoral capstone site and population via completing a literature review (Chapter 5), performing a needs assessment (Chapter 6), developing an experiential plan (EP) that identifies your individual goals and objectives (Chapter 7), and preparing a plan to evaluate your capstone project outcomes (Chapter 8). As you can see, this book will truly walk you through the entire process, step-by-step.

Once your preparatory work is complete, you will then formally begin your 14-week doctoral capstone experience (DCE). The DCE is an in-depth mentored and student-driven (or learner-centered) experience. In contrast to level II fieldwork expectations, the capstone experience requires the student to be mentored, rather than supervised, by an individual with documented expertise aligned with the focus of the capstone student's project. *Mentoring* is defined as "a relationship between two people in which one person (the mentor) is dedicated to the personal and professional growth of the other (the mentee)," and the mentor has more experience and knowledge than the mentee (ACOTE, 2023, p. 49). Chapter 9 will provide several best practice approaches and recommendations to guide your attitudes, actions, and behaviors once you are on-site at your DCE and are actually implementing your capstone project. The goal of the 14 weeks is for you to achieve the individual goals and objectives that you established in your experiential plan (EP). These goals and objectives should align with the area(s) of focus you selected. Similar to level II FW, your progress and performance will be evaluated by your content expert. Chapter 10 will provide deeper insights into best practice approaches to guide evaluation during the capstone. This includes your content expert evaluation of you, and you will also most likely have the opportunity to provide feedback and evaluate your content expert and overall experience during the DCE.

During your DCE, in addition to engaging in experiences to accomplish your own individual goals and objectives aligned with your focus area, you will also be implementing a capstone project and then will be expected to disseminate the results or outcomes of your project. This book will integrate a variety of capstone project examples. Capstone projects may take several forms and should ultimately mutually benefit you and the population or site where your capstone takes place. Chapters 11 and 12 will help you think about different levels of impact your capstone project could have, as well as different approaches to disseminate or showcase your findings, which might include a written report, professional presentation, and other scholarly deliverables required by your occupational therapy program or suggested by your capstone site.

Similar to the 1st edition, this book utilizes human-centered design as a conceptual framework to intentionally thread content within the development, planning, implementation, and dissemination of the capstone. Human-centered design (HCD) is a framework designed to help individuals develop a mindset to creatively think through key aspects of innovation, problem-solving, and viability (IDEO.org, 2015). This HCD is frequently used in the startup and technology global market, such as industry located in Silicon Valley, to unlock the creative potential in people and organizations to innovate routinely. This unique framework can be a useful strategy to increase the understanding of all stakeholders involved in the capstone process. See Text Box 1.

TEXT BOX 1

Human-centered design (HCD) and occupational therapy share a common focus on understanding and addressing the needs of individuals, groups, and populations.

Aligned with occupational therapy, human-centered design uses a holistic process that includes three phases: inspiration, ideation, and implementation (IDEO.org, n.d.).

The *inspiration* phase is about "learning on the fly," opening up to creative possibilities, building empathy, and trusting that your ideas will evolve into a creative solution. In the *ideation* phase, individuals come up with ideas, brainstorm possibilities, and refine and improve ideas to build a simple "prototype" that is something tangible. This phase involves getting feedback from those who will benefit from the prototype and integrating their feedback to make it a more client-, group-, and population-centered product (or program). During the *implementation* phase, individuals are building partnerships and getting their idea, product, or prototype into the world. The philosophy of human-centered design complements occupational therapy nicely because it suggests that to build a truly innovative and useful product (or program), one needs to focus on the needs, contexts, behaviors, and emotions of the people that the solutions (program) will serve. Viewing the capstone experience and project through this lens can provide a helpful framework to motivate occupational therapy doctorate students, facilitate engagement with the capstone experience, and enable meaningful collaboration with the capstone coordinator and site mentor. See Figure 0.1 for a schematic illustration of human-centered design as a framework for the doctoral capstone and project.

The student content in each chapter will be in alignment with HCD concepts, while the educator content in each chapter will be rooted in transformational learning theory.

To guide the educator section, each section of every chapter will connect the stage of the capstone process to Mezirow's transformational learning theory (Mezirow, 1997). When you reach the educator section in Chapter 1, we have provided a nice overview of Mezirow's stages and how you can use this theory to guide OTD capstone students through a process of critical reflection, problem-solving, and changes in perspective that are essential constructs that occur throughout the doctoral capstone process.

The content and aim of this book support AOTA's Vision 2025, which challenges the profession to expand our reach and impact, prepare and develop the profession, and advance quality and recognition of occupational therapy practice (AOTA, 2017). Overall, this book, like the 1st edition, will be an essential resource for current, developing, and new OTD programs.

CHAPTERS AT A GLANCE

The concept of critical reflection has been identified as an important part of doctoral education (Brookfield, 2015). To initiate the process and sustain innovation and momentum throughout the capstone experience and project, each

Inspiration/ Development

- Mindsets
- Use of the evidence
- Purpose development
- Interviews
- Development of Goals and Objectives
- Iteration
- Protoyping

Ideation/ Planning

Implementation

- Mindsets
- Iteration
- Integration of the evidence
- Refinement of Goals and Objectives
- Observations
- Outcomes

Sustainability

- Mindsets
- Iteration
- Observations
- Outcomes

Dissemination

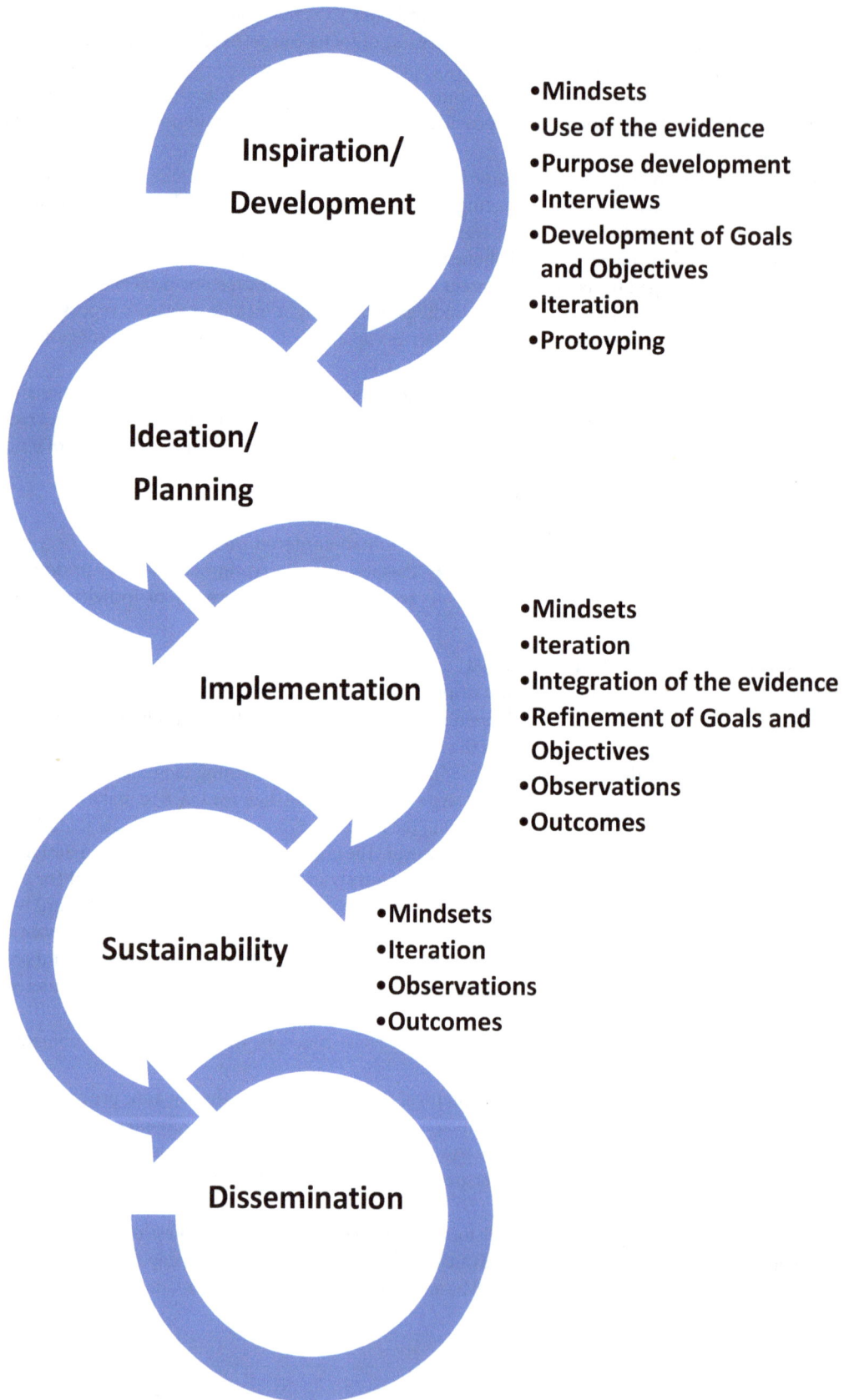

Figure 0-1. Using human-centered design as a framework for the doctoral capstone. *Source:* Adapted from IDEO (2015). *The field guide to human-centered design.* Ideo.org.

chapter begins with reflective questions for the capstone student and the educator that have been intentionally designed to anticipate your learning and stimulate the formation of thoughts and ideas regarding the developmental stage of the capstone process. Conceptual models, human-centered design, and transformational learning are also infused throughout this book as theoretical frameworks.

Part I of this text (Chapters 1 through 4) is the inspiration phase, focusing on the development stage of the capstone process. Building a solid foundational understanding for the overall capstone process is the first focus here, and understanding the ACOTE areas of focus to allow for the brainstorming process of the capstone ideas is the second major focus. Next, a deeper dive on professional identity formation, career-readiness skills, and mentorship relationships is explored to develop skills critical for this self-directed capstone experience and to support collaboration upon the capstone team.

Part II of this text (Chapters 5 through 8) provides an overview of the planning stage (or ideation phase) of the capstone process. The importance of searching and synthesizing the literature to support and develop the purpose for the capstone experience and project is examined first in this section. Coming next, this new edition features a stand-alone chapter that exclusively covers the needs assessment and various ways of how theory can be applied to the needs assessment process. Developing an experiential plan (previously referred to as the memorandum of understanding, MOU), including determining individualized goals and objectives for the capstone project and experience, is an important aspect of the planning stage that is explored. In addition, recommendations for supervision requirements, a plan for mentorship, proposal planning, and developing a project timeline are also discussed. Program evaluation of the impact and outcomes of the project is examined next, including methods to plan, implement, and analyze data/outcomes from the individual capstone project. The importance of a sustainability plan is also explored in this planning stage section.

Part III of this text (Chapters 9 and 10) discusses the implementation stage, which includes the day-to-day happenings of the 14-week doctoral capstone experience. A new, unique focus on utilizing communication and mentoring skills is provided. Implementation of the capstone project is discussed, which might require the student to revisit the prior needs assessment, goals, and objectives. Lastly, methods to evaluate the doctoral capstone experience, including assessing the student and the context expert, are provided.

Part IV (Chapters 11 and 12) discusses various components of the dissemination stage within the capstone process. This final phase involves the production and dissemination of the capstone project. Examples of how to prepare (format) and present scholarly deliverables (such as submissible papers and presentations) and their impact are explored.

Lastly, in this new edition, we have also included an ad hoc chapter at the end of the book that has a unique view on the post-professional OTD degree (PP-OTD) and the scholarly capstone. While the PP-OTD degree is not regulated by occupational therapy accreditors, most post-professional programs in health sciences also have a culminating scholarly project, often named a capstone. Although there are numerous PP-OTD programs that exist across the country, there are very limited resources exclusively available for the PP-OTD realm too. This chapter will compare and contrast doctoral dissertation vs. entry-level capstone projects vs. PP-OTD capstone projects, as well as provide a road map of how this book could be utilized by a PP-OTD student or program.

Each chapter provides sample resources and useful documents appropriate for use with doctoral students, faculty, doctoral capstone coordinators, and those that serve as context experts and mentors. Supplemental materials, including learning activities and resources to enhance teaching and learning regarding the various topics discussed in this text, are also provided in each chapter in the newly organized "Education Section."

REFERENCES

Accreditation Council for Occupational Therapy Education. (2018). *2018 Accreditation Council for Occupational Therapy Education (ACOTE®) standards and interpretive guide.* https://acoteonline.org/accreditation-explained/standards/

Accreditation Council for Occupational Therapy Education. (2023). *2023 Accreditation Council for Occupational Therapy Education (ACOTE®) standards and interpretive guide.* https://acoteonline.org/accreditation-explained/standards/

American Occupational Therapy Association. (2017). Vision 2025. *American Journal of Occupational Therapy, 71*(3), 710342001. https://doi.org/10.5014/ajot.2017.713002

Brookfield, S. (2015). Critical reflection as doctoral education. *New Directions for Adult and Continuing Education, 147*, 15–23.

IDEO. (n.d.). *About IDEO.* https://www.ideo.com/about

IDEO. (2015). *The field guide to human-centered design.* Ideo.org.

Mezirow, J. (1997). Transformative learning: Theory to practice. *New Directions for Adult and Continuing Education*, (74), 5–12. https://doi.org/10.1002/ace.7401

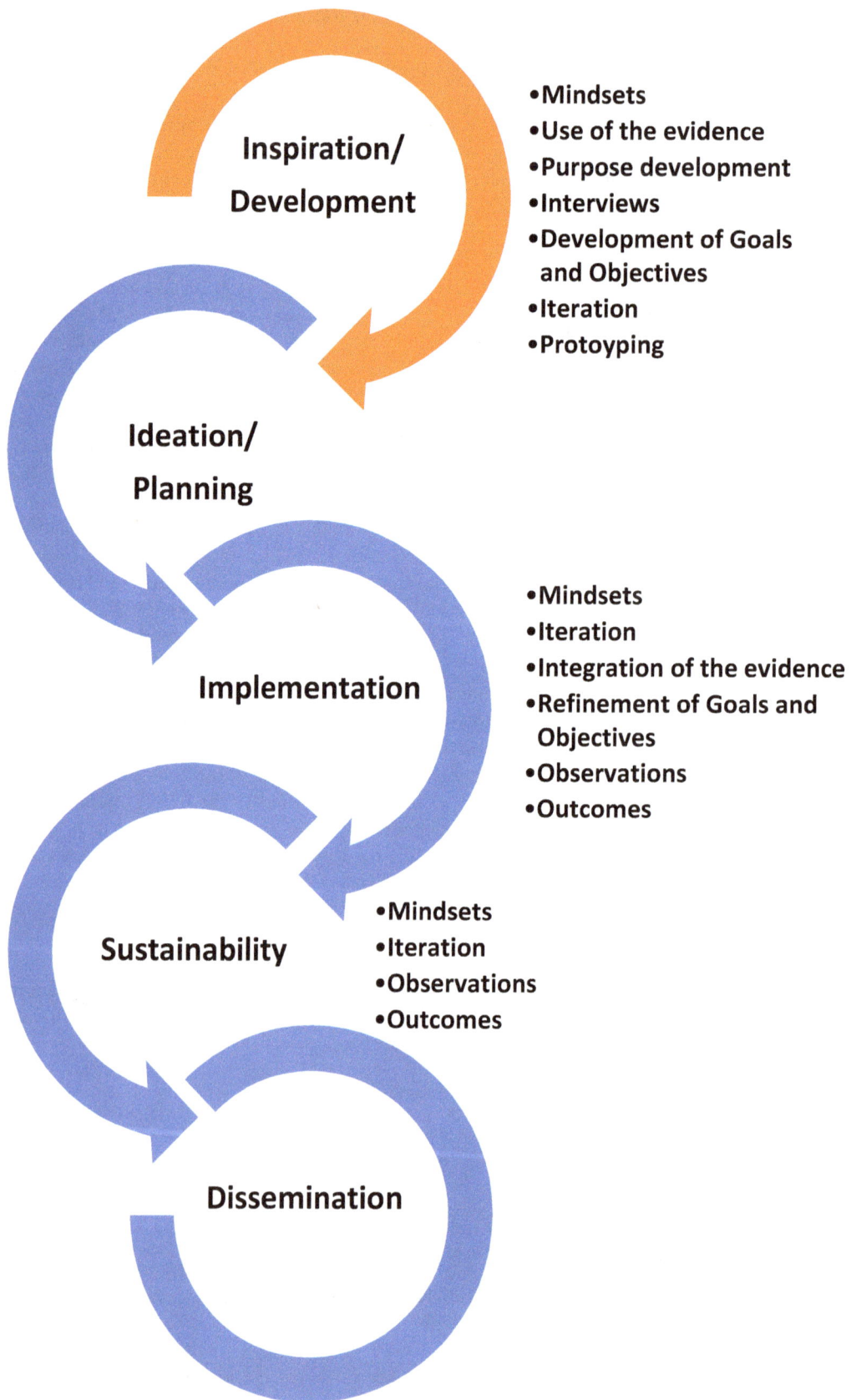

Inspiration/ Development
- Mindsets
- Use of the evidence
- Purpose development
- Interviews
- Development of Goals and Objectives
- Iteration
- Protoyping

Ideation/ Planning

Implementation
- Mindsets
- Iteration
- Integration of the evidence
- Refinement of Goals and Objectives
- Observations
- Outcomes

Sustainability
- Mindsets
- Iteration
- Observations
- Outcomes

Dissemination

PART I. DEVELOPMENT

The first step of the capstone experience and project is **development**, which aligns with the **inspiration** phase of human-centered design. This preparatory phase involves knowledge and skill building. During the inspiration phase, brainstorming is required in order to begin the initial development of the capstone experience and project. Once the inspiration phase has begun, the doctoral student will use evidence, interview potential people that their experience will affect, and frame their design challenge to refine their capstone purpose. Goals and objectives are developed to allow for iteration and prototyping to ensure a client-centered approach to the project.

DOI: 10.4324/9781003541813-1

CHAPTER 1

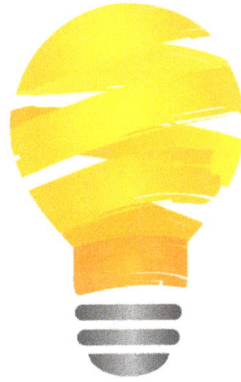

Roles, Responsibilities, and Expectations for the Doctoral Capstone

Elizabeth D. DeIuliis and Julie A. Bednarski

Section 1: Student Focus

Human-Centered Design Mindsets for the Doctoral Student

The human-centered design mindset concepts of optimism and empathy are important for doctoral students to embrace as they begin the initial understanding of the overall capstone experience and project and the roles and responsibilities of the team members.

Optimism. "Optimism is the thing that drives you forward" (John Bielenberg, Founder, Future Partners, IDEO. org, 2015, p. 24). The doctoral capstone requires you to take on a big challenge, and by remaining optimistic, you are able to embrace the possibility of finding solutions to these challenges. Keep your sense of optimism as you begin this initial stage of development. Optimism will drive you forward at a time when you may feel overwhelmed. Optimism will drive you toward solutions, keep you creative, and encourage you to keep moving forward even when things get tough.

Empathy. "Empathy is the capacity to step into other people's shoes, to understand their lives, and start to solve problems from their perspectives" (Emi Kolaswole, IDEO.org, 2015, p. 22). The concept of empathy will be at the forefront of your mind throughout your capstone experience and project. You are designing innovative solutions to problems, but to solve the problems, you must understand your client – which could be an individual, group, community, or population.

INTRODUCTION FOR STUDENTS

It takes a village! This well-known proverb is a good metaphor to describe the development, planning, and implementation of the doctoral capstone. Not unlike fieldwork education, the successful completion of your doctoral capstone requires a sophisticated collaboration among various individuals, both inside and outside the educational program. The capstone is distinct from fieldwork because it is a major aspect of the final preparation of the capstone student for entry-level practice. You, the capstone student; your occupational therapy faculty; the

DOI: 10.4324/9781003541813-2

doctoral capstone coordinator; the academic fieldwork coordinator; and your content expert within your doctoral capstone experience (DCE) each has a significant role and unique responsibilities and expectations for the capstone. This chapter serves as an introduction to the *capstone team*, which includes the aforementioned stakeholders. We will provide a comparison (and contrast) between fieldwork education and the doctoral capstone experience, as well as offer a description of the roles and responsibilities of each capstone team member.

STUDENT REFLECTIVE QUESTIONS

During the development phase of the doctoral capstone, the occupational therapy student may find it helpful to reflect on the following questions:

1. Describe how you feel the roles and expectations of being a capstone student differ from fieldwork.
2. How might the relationship with your content expert differ from that with a traditional fieldwork educator?
3. What initial thoughts do you have about your capstone experience?
4. How do you embrace ambiguity?
5. What plan can you set in motion to keep an optimistic attitude throughout this process?

STUDENT OBJECTIVES

After reading this chapter and completing the learning activities, the reader should be able to:

1. Compare and contrast the curricula and outcomes of occupational therapy fieldwork education and the capstone.
2. Explain the unique expectations of occupational therapy fieldwork students and occupational therapy doctoral (OTD) students in the capstone.
3. Distinguish the roles and responsibilities of the doctoral capstone student, occupational therapy faculty, doctoral capstone coordinator, and content expert.

FIELDWORK EDUCATION VERSUS CAPSTONE

Experiential learning is not unfamiliar to the occupational therapy profession. Like other health-care professions, occupational therapy education requires the component of practical application in the curriculum. Other professions use various terminologies to describe this experiential learning, such as *clinical education*, *residencies*, *externships*, or *internships*. Historically, the occupational therapy profession has primarily identified it as *fieldwork education*. Fieldwork education is often described as a bridge that connects the theoretical didactic classroom instruction to real-world clinical practice and is argued to be the most integral piece of the occupational therapy education process (Aikens et al., 2001; Brandenburger-Shasby et al., 1998; DeIuliis & Hanson, 2023; Hanson & DeIuliis, 2023; Haynes, 2011). Fieldwork is integrated with occupational therapy coursework to apply core values (including professionalism) and curricular threads in practice with supervision and instruction from occupational therapy faculty and fieldwork educators. In occupational therapy education, there are currently two levels of fieldwork education intended to provide students with this opportunity: level I fieldwork and level II fieldwork. In addition, the curriculum for the entry-level doctorate degree requires an in-depth practicum called the capstone (Accreditation Council for Occupational Therapy Education [ACOTE], 2023). Before we take a deep dive into various members of the capstone team, it is important to compare and contrast the capstone with fieldwork.

Level I Fieldwork

According to the 2023 ACOTE standards, the goal of level I fieldwork is "to introduce students to fieldwork, apply knowledge to practice, and develop understanding of the needs of clients" (p. 38). Historically, level I fieldwork is characterized as being designed to reinforce and strengthen the occupational therapy program's didactic coursework through active observation and engagement in aspects of the occupational therapy process. Compared with level II fieldwork, level I fieldwork can be viewed as an introductory experiential clinical learning experience. However, it is still "fieldwork," the first official experiential learning for occupational therapy students and a major stepping stone in the building of their professional identities and clinical skill development. Supervision of a level I fieldwork student requires a qualified professional who may or may not be an occupational therapy practitioner yet affirms their "ability to support the fieldwork experience" and understands the program's curriculum (ACOTE, 2023, p. 38). Examples may include, but are not limited to, currently licensed or otherwise regulated occupational therapists and occupational therapy assistants (OTAs), psychologists, physician assistants, teachers, social workers, nurses, and physical therapists.

Level II Fieldwork

The goal of level II fieldwork is "to develop competent, entry-level, generalist occupational therapists"; to promote clinical reasoning and reflective practice; to transmit the values and beliefs that enable ethical practice; and to develop professionalism and competence in career responsibilities (ACOTE, 2023, p. 39). See Text Box 1-1.

Level II fieldwork is more regulated by ACOTE than level I. ACOTE states that 16 weeks of level II fieldwork are required for occupational therapy assistant (OTA) educational programs, and 24 weeks for occupational therapy programs. The outcome of level II fieldwork student learning is frequently evaluated by the AOTA Fieldwork Performance Evaluation of the Level II Student (AOTA, 2020). Level II fieldwork students are required to be supervised by a currently licensed or otherwise regulated occupational therapist or, for OTA programs, OTA (under the supervision of an occupational therapist) who has a minimum of one-year full-time (or its equivalent) practice experience subsequent to initial certification and who is adequately prepared to serve as a fieldwork educator. The supervising therapist may be engaged by the fieldwork site or by the educational program (ACOTE, 2023).

The level II fieldwork educator is responsible for evaluating if the student's performance demonstrates entry-level competency based on level II fieldwork objectives and a formal evaluation process at the end of the level II fieldwork experience (ACOTE, 2023).

Doctoral Capstone Experience

The entry-level occupational therapy doctorate curriculum differs from the master's level in many ways. One of the most significant differences is the addition of the 14-week capstone experience. This experiential learning requirement for the occupational therapy educational programs is in addition to the existing levels I and II fieldwork education requirements. The goal of the capstone is to provide you, the occupational therapy doctoral student, "an in-depth exposure" to an area of focus (ACOTE, 2023, p. 42). The DCE shall be "an integral part of the [program's] curriculum design" and shall include an in-depth experience in one or more of the following: "clinical skills, research skills, administration, program development and evaluation, policy development, advocacy, education, or leadership" (ACOTE, 2023, p. 42). You will be exposed to these areas of focus for the capstone outlined by ACOTE in greater detail in Chapter 2. You must successfully complete all coursework, level II fieldwork, and preparatory activities (which include a literature review, needs assessment, goals and objectives, and a plan to evaluate project outcomes) before the commencement of the capstone (ACOTE, 2023). To meet these ACOTE standards, you are going to be developing and using a unique set of skills and abilities. Chapter 3 will outline specific "practice-ready" and unique mentorship relationship-building skills that are necessary for the success of the capstone experience and recommendations for occupational therapy programs to facilitate environments or tasks that foster growth in this area.

In contrast to fieldwork educators during fieldwork, the supervising individual during your capstone experience is called a *content expert* (or sometimes also referred to as a site or content mentor). According to the ACOTE standard D.1.2, the doctoral capstone coordinator will ensure documentation and verify that the capstone student is being mentored by an individual with expertise consistent with the student's area of focus (ACOTE, 2023). *Mentoring* is defined as "a relationship between two people in which one person (the mentor) is dedicated to the personal and professional growth of the other (the mentee)" (ACOTE, 2023, p. 49). A *mentor* can be defined as an individual having more experience and knowledge than the mentee. As an occupational therapy doctoral student, you most likely have several "mentors" throughout the doctoral capstone process, which may include faculty at the occupational therapy program, individuals who work at their capstone site, or external mentors who may have subject matter expertise aligned with your capstone's focus area. ACOTE standard D.1.4 states that the doctoral capstone coordinator is responsible for ensuring that there is an experiential plan and written agreement (formerly referred to as a memorandum of understanding, or MOU) which, at a minimum, includes individualized specific objectives; plans for evaluation, supervision, or mentoring; and responsibilities of all parties (ACOTE, 2023, p. 43). The experiential plan and process to develop the individualized learning objectives and plans for supervision and mentorship during the DCE are discussed in greater detail in Chapter 7. Depending on your capstone focus or emphasis, you may have more than one content expert or mentor, but this should be outlined in your experiential plan. (See Table 1-1 for a snapshot of the similarities and differences among level I fieldwork, level II fieldwork, and the DCE.)

"Fieldwork was something necessary for me to practice routine occupational therapy skills and build my competency in becoming a practitioner. The DCE provided me with the opportunity to apply the skills I learned from fieldwork in a non-traditional setting and prompted me to advocate for occupational therapy in a unique way. The DCE also helped me to gain perspective and confidence in my skills through completion of a project on topics that I am deeply passionate about."

– Hanna Davis, OTD, OTR/L,
Duquesne University OTD class of 2024

"From my personal perspective, I felt that the key differences between level II FW and the DCE were the depth of responsibility, autonomy, and the overall emphasis on leadership.

During level II FW, I was primarily building my clinical skills, applying what I had learned during my time at Duquesne into a real-world setting. This experience was very structured and helped me gain competence in delivering OT services while getting feedback from my supervisor.

My DCE experience included taking initiative, being independent, and taking my educational experience into my own hands. While this experience also involved building on and using my skills and knowledge, it also focused on being innovative and creating something that will contribute to the health-care profession in a meaningful way. The DCE helped me to go beyond clinical practice and engage in program development, leadership, and education, all of which required a more advanced level of self-direction

and accountability. This experience felt like a necessary bridge between being a student and an OT practitioner."

– Emma Fitzgerald, OTD, OTR/L,
Duquesne University OTD class of 2024

"I found that I had a lot more responsibility during my DCE as compared to my level II FW. It really took a lot of personal volition for me to fully immerse myself in the DCE and complete my project to the best of my abilities! Whereas during level II FW, I found that I could rely on my FW educator to sort of lessen the workload, my DCE content expert was more of a guiding voice to support the plans that I created independently!"

– Kaitlyn Joyce, OTD, OTR/L,
Duquesne University OTD class of 2023

To ensure a successful collaboration, it is important that all stakeholders involved within your capstone are familiar with one another's roles, responsibilities, and expectations. (See Text Box 1-2.) Now that we have contrasted the different levels of fieldwork education with the capstone experience, let us identify and discuss the key individuals who are involved throughout the planning, execution, and evaluation of your doctoral capstone. These individuals include, obviously, you, the capstone student; your occupational therapy faculty; the doctoral capstone coordinator; and your content expert. We will refer to this collective group as the *capstone team* throughout this book. Although not directly involved with the capstone, the roles, responsibilities, and expectations of the academic fieldwork coordinator are also introduced.

Table 1-1. Similarities and Differences Among Level I Fieldwork, Level II Fieldwork, and Capstone

LEVEL I	
	Length: Not prescribed by ACOTE.
	Supervision requirement: "Ensure that personnel who supervise Level 1 fieldwork are informed of the curriculum and program design and affirm their ability to support the fieldwork experience. Examples include, but are not limited to, currently licensed or otherwise regulated occupational therapists and OTAs, psychologists, physician assistants, teachers, social workers, physicians, speech language pathologists, nurses, and physical therapists" (ACOTE, 2023, p. 38).
	Supervision type: Not prescribed by ACOTE.
	Purpose/goal: "To introduce students to fieldwork, apply knowledge to practice, and develop understanding of the needs of clients" (ACOTE, 2023, p. 38).

continued

Table 1-1. Similarities and Differences Among Level I Fieldwork, Level II Fieldwork, and Capstone (continued)

LEVEL II	**Length:** A minimum of 24 weeks of full-time level II fieldwork. This may be completed on a part-time basis, as defined by the fieldwork placement in accordance with the fieldwork placement.
	Supervision requirement:
	Traditional setting: A minimum of 1-year full-time (or its equivalent) practice experience as a licensed or otherwise regulated occupational therapist before the onset of the level II fieldwork experience (ACOTE, 2023).
	Role-emerging setting: "Document and verify that supervision provided in a setting where no occupational therapy services exist includes a documented plan for provision of occupational therapy services and supervision by a currently licensed otherwise regulated occupational therapist with at least 3 years' full-time or its equivalent of professional experience prior to the Level II fieldwork experience. Supervision must include a minimum of 8 hours of direct supervision each week of the fieldwork experience. An occupational therapy supervisor must be available, via a variety of contact measures, to the student during all working hours. An on-site supervisor designee of another profession must be assigned while the occupational therapy supervisor is off-site" (ACOTE, 2023, p. 41).
	International: Supervised by an occupational therapist who graduated from a program approved by the World Federation of Occupational Therapists and has at least 1 year of experience in practice.
	Supervision type: "Ensure that Level II fieldwork supervision is direct and then decreases to less direct supervision as appropriate for the setting, the severity of the client's condition, and the ability of the student to support progression towards entry-level competence" (ACOTE, 2023, p. 41).
	Purpose/goal: Develop into competent entry-level generalist occupational therapy practitioners (ACOTE, 2023).
DOCTORAL CAPSTONE EXPERIENCE	**Length:** Must be started upon completion of all coursework and level II fieldwork and the completion of preparatory activities, for 14 weeks (and a minimum of 32 hours per week). This may be completed on a part-time basis and must be consistent with the individualized specific objectives and capstone project. Prior fieldwork or work experience may not be substituted for this DCE.
	Supervision requirement: Student is mentored by an individual with expertise consistent with the student's area of focus prior to the initiation onset of the DCE. The content expert does not have to be an occupational therapist.
	Supervision type: Not prescribed by ACOTE.
	Purpose/goal: To provide in-depth exposure to one or more of the following: clinical skills, research skills, administration, program development and evaluation, policy development, advocacy, education, or leadership (ACOTE, 2023, p. 42).

TEXT BOX 1-2

Expectations from individual OTD programs, faculty, and doctoral capstone coordinators may vary, yet the information in this chapter can provide a general framework to help a capstone student understand various components of their role.

THE OCCUPATIONAL THERAPY DOCTORAL CAPSTONE STUDENT

A clear message that you will see throughout this book is that you, the occupational therapy doctoral capstone student, will be expected to play an active role throughout the development, planning, implementation, and evaluation stages of your capstone. The focus and expectations of the capstone differ from those of fieldwork education. Therefore, the responsibilities and skill set required for the capstone also stand apart. Chapter 3 goes into greater detail regarding recommended skills, attitudes, and behaviors that a capstone student should embrace to be successful and effective throughout the capstone process. The following list provides an overview of both general and specific tasks and actions a capstone student can take to ensure preparation and success on the capstone experience and project:

- Understand and abide by your academic program policies and procedures relative to the capstone. This may include a capstone manual or course(s) syllabi.
- Identify personal goals, interests, and appropriate outcomes as bases for planning the capstone experience and project.
- Collaborate to develop and plan your capstone experience with your doctoral capstone coordinator and other faculty as appropriate, including possible settings and populations for the capstone. This may include a *capstone proposal*, which will be discussed in Chapter 7.
- Collaboratively develop the *experiential plan* with your content expert and doctoral capstone coordinator – this includes individualized specific objectives, plan for supervision/mentoring/evaluation, responsibilities of all parties and authorship – and obtain appropriate signatures. This will be discussed further in Chapter 7 as well.
- Obtain evidence of expertise, aligned with your focus area, from your content expert and submit to the doctoral capstone coordinator when required.
- Synthesize knowledge from preparatory coursework in your occupational therapy curriculum to support the development of your capstone project, which may include creating a scholarly question, conducting a needs assessment, identifying a guiding theoretical perspective, developing a searchable question, appraising the literature, and establishing goals and objectives and a plan to evaluate project outcomes. Types of capstone projects and strategies to disseminate are discussed in Chapters 11 and 12.
- Complete the 14-week capstone experience, with at least 32 hours per week. Note that your program will probably ensure a policy that you are responsible to ensure that missed hours are made up for appropriately, at the discretion of your content expert and capstone coordinator. Examples of how to negotiate and structure the weekly schedule are presented in Chapter 9.
- Complete tasks and activities* assigned by your content expert to ensure success of the experience, alignment with chosen focus area(s), and outcome of capstone. (See Text Box 1-3.)

TEXT BOX 1-3

* This may include assigned readings, attending meetings or workshops, and interviewing or meeting with other individuals within your capstone site

to support the development of in-depth knowledge and achievement of the individualized goals and objectives, which you agreed to on the experiential learning plan. Here are a few examples from occupational therapy doctoral students:

"I attended several in-services about different adaptive equipment and got to work closely with several vendors. Some included adapted cars that were brought to the VA for therapists to see; others included different driving-adaptive equipment (hand controls, etc.). Others were just for adaptive equipment or therapy devices, such as devices to help people get off the floor, the Cala Trio representatives, the carbon hand representatives, the Saebo devices, adaptive eating devices, and many more."
– Katelyn Kovalsky, OTD, OTR/L,
Duquesne University OTD class of 2024

"As I did not work under an occupational therapist, I had to find multiple ways to fill my time while also building my understanding of dementia care. I shadowed multiple hospice personnel, which provided insights into end-of-life care, and I attended the Alzheimer's Association International Conference (AAIC) to learn more about the latest research and practices in dementia care. I also created occupational profiles for residents, helping both me and other staff utilizing these to provide more person-centered care. Additionally, I was able to attend daily directive meetings to get a better understanding of the interdisciplinary work within memory care."
– Emma Fitzgerald, OTD, OTR/L,
Duquesne University OTD class of 2024

- Take initiative to communicate with your content expert, occupational therapy faculty, and doctoral capstone coordinator when expected to do so or as needed to ensure success.

"The biggest difference for me was that interacting with my DCE context expert felt more like 'a professional to a professional' relationship rather than 'an educator to a student relationship,' which really prompted me to hold up my end of the bargain and perform to the best of my abilities."
– Kaitlyn Joyce, OTD, OTR/L,
Duquesne University OTD class of 2023

- Demonstrate respectful interaction and communication with your peer student cohort, faculty, mentors, doctoral capstone coordinator, and other individuals who may be a part of your capstone. For example, this may include an individual who is responsible for the institutional review board (IRB) process at your academic institution or capstone site or the health sciences librarian.

- Develop and maintain a structure for working with your capstone team to conduct and complete the capstone experience and project. This should be included in the experiential plan and include clearly delineated responsibilities and timelines, both individual and group.
- Provide appropriate feedback to appropriate stakeholders at your capstone site (and content expert) at the formal midterm and final evaluation to enhance the experience. Although there is not a formal endorsed tool like the AOTA Fieldwork Performance Evaluation to evaluate the capstone, Chapter 10 provides examples of ways to structure evaluation mechanisms for the doctoral capstone.
- Utilize constructive feedback from your faculty, content expert, and doctoral capstone coordinator for your own personal and professional growth. See example that follows:

"Before implementing my project, I spent a lot of time organizing and outlining my timeline. When talking with my faculty mentor, I was able to express that I felt participants may need more time to complete the training modules. My faculty mentor encouraged me to extend the time frame as I had the ability to. This experience showed me how to balance structure with responsiveness, making me realize the importance of flexibility as a leader and adapting to the needs of those around you in an effective way."

– Emma Fitzgerald, OTD, OTR/L,
Duquesne University OTD class of 2024

- Take responsibility of your own skill and professional development. This can include professional writing skills and knowledge of IRB application process, for example. See Text Box 1-4

TEXT BOX 1-4

Know what resources are available to you! Does your academic institution offer a writing center? Do they provide virtual support if your capstone is taking place out of the area? Remember, take initiative and ACT!

- Collect, manage, and analyze data for your capstone project as proposed.
- Demonstrate a professional approach to your capstone, including demonstrating effective and appropriate intrinsic and extrinsic aspects of professionalism

(DeIuliis, 2017), including, but not limited to, time management, observing deadlines, initiating, and reading and responding to communications from the capstone team; regular and thorough communication regarding updates/progress with all members of the team is critical. See Text Box 1-5.

TEXT BOX 1-5

Comply with all laws, policies, and procedures for the academic institution and the capstone site (including, but not limited to, the Health Insurance Portability and Accountability Act, the Occupational Safety and Health Administration, client confidentiality, AOTA Code of Ethics, student code of conduct, IRB training certificates, health and security clearances).

- Complete and submit evaluation of your capstone experience form per capstone policy manual or the deadline indicated on your course syllabus. See Text Box 1-6.

TEXT BOX 1-6

Your doctoral capstone coordinator may encourage you to engage in self-assessment using the capstone evaluation. This can be a good strategy to internalize strengths and growth areas and help guide feedback sessions with your context expert and other relevant mentors at your capstone site. Chapter 10 goes into more detail about this.

- **Be self-directed**, and **take an active role in mentorship** throughout your capstone process, including developing, planning, and completing your capstone experience and project. Strategies to foster self-directedness and practice-ready skills are discussed in Chapter 3.
- Take initiative to finalize all documentation with your context expert, faculty mentor (chair), or doctoral capstone coordinator. This may include release of consent forms, IRB requirements, signature for use in academic library's electronic theses and dissertation system, and additional medical/legal documents, for example.
- Complete and disseminate a culminating capstone project in a format and forum, within the time frame determined by your academic program. See Text Box 1-7.

TEXT BOX 1-7

Dissemination could occur at your capstone site, academic institution, community, and other professional organizations. Examples of scholarly dissemination products and approaches will be covered in Chapters 11 and 12.

"I negotiated with my content expert that I would disseminate my capstone findings at a local caregiver support group, as well as to directive staff at my site. Presenting at the caregiver support group allowed me to connect with those who are impacted by dementia and share practical strategies for caregivers to use with their loved ones. This experience allowed for open dialogue about memory care with those who may be headed toward that route while also highlighting the importance of caregiver support. Disseminating to direct staff at Arden Courts allowed me to share my project's findings with those who are directly impacted by the outcomes. I was able to share the positive impact of my project while also presenting areas for future improvement. These experiences strengthened my confidence in my leadership and communication skills, allowing me to carry that confidence over as a future practitioner."

– Emma Fitzgerald, OTD, OTR/L,
Duquesne University OTD class of 2024

THE DOCTORAL CAPSTONE COORDINATOR

The *doctoral capstone coordinator* is a full-time faculty member as defined by ACOTE and is specifically responsible for the occupational therapy program's compliance with the capstone requirements listed in Standards Section D (ACOTE Standard A.2.4). Although the specific responsibilities of the doctoral capstone coordinator may vary by program, the general role of the capstone coordinator is to provide you, the capstone student, with the structure and information to begin the development of your capstone experiences and oversee each phase of the capstone from development to completion and dissemination. See Table 1-2 for a brief overview of the capstone process.

The doctoral capstone coordinator will ensure that your capstone experience is unique and does not duplicate or interfere with your previous fieldwork experiences. Although the doctoral capstone coordinator is typically the primary faculty member responsible for the overall capstone experience, it can be helpful to have a model where other faculty serve as faculty mentors (or chairs) of doctoral students' capstone projects. The doctoral capstone coordinator should not be assumed to be the faculty mentor for each student. In a program with a large student cohort, this would not be possible. Figures 1-1 and 1-2 allow the reader to visualize a structure for the capstone roles and the supportive features of both the doctoral capstone coordinator and the occupational therapy faculty.

The doctoral capstone coordinator may take the lead, possibly working with the program director or department chair, to organize the match process for capstone students and faculty mentors (or capstone chair) and

Table 1-2. Brief Overview of the Capstone Process

PHASE I: DEVELOPMENT	PHASE II: PLANNING PHASE	PHASE III: IMPLEMENTATION PHASE	PHASE IV: DISSEMINATION PHASE
• Understand ACOTE requirements. • Determine ACOTE area of focus for the capstone project and experience. • Complete review of the literature to support project idea. • Define purpose. • Determine potential capstone site and site mentor. • Develop initial goals and objectives.	• Visit with potential sites/content experts. • Complete capstone project proposal. • Determine whether IRB is required; complete IRB if needed. • Finalize site and content expert, and meet with site mentor to complete experiential learning plan. • Complete literature review, needs assessment, and plan to evaluate project outcomes. • Develop timeline for the DCE and project.	• Complete site requirements. • Update literature review needs assessment. • Finalize experiential plan with updated goals and objectives (as needed). • Implement capstone project and experience. • Evaluate impact/outcome. • Develop sustainability plan.	• Plan for dissemination. • Disseminate results to site. • Disseminate results to university/peers. • Disseminate to community as appropriate. • Disseminate to the field of occupational therapy. • Determine future plans.

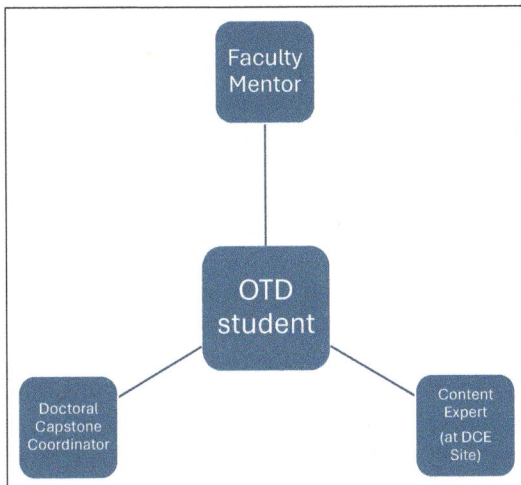

Figure 1-1. Members of the capstone team.

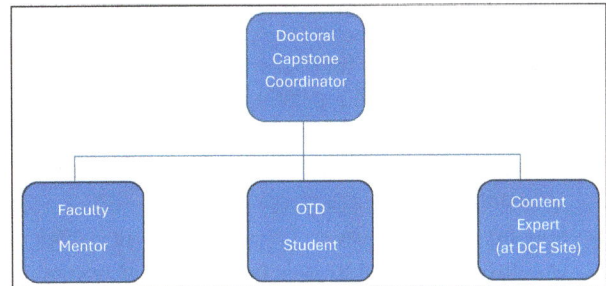

Figure 1-2. Example of an organization chart for the capstone team.

ensure good fit and appropriate mentorship. Depending on the program or school curriculum design and based on the capstone student's goals, interests, and planned focus areas, the doctoral capstone coordinator or assigned faculty mentor will work with each student individually to identify and confirm each capstone site for the capstone experience and project. The doctoral capstone coordinator will also assist the faculty mentors and content experts, as needed, through the planning and execution of the DCEs.

The following list provides an overview of both general and specific tasks and actions the doctoral capstone coordinator can take to ensure preparation and success on the capstone.

- Verify that you, the capstone student, has successfully completed coursework, prior fieldwork experiences, and required preparatory activities defined in ACOTE standard D.1.3.
- Ensure that the DCE and project are consistent with the program's curricular design.
- Instruct you regarding the capstone processes and expectations. This may include orientation sessions, individualized counselling sessions, creation and use of a capstone manual, and course syllabi. (See Appendix 1.A for a sample table of contents for a policy manual.)
- *Collaborate with you and the academic fieldwork* coordinator to identify goals and interests and to ensure no overlap with fieldwork education experiences.
- Educate both capstone students and content experts about the ACOTE focus areas.
- Advise you in determining potential capstone site preferences and project focus ideas.
- Identify and correspond with potential capstone sites and potential site/content experts, establish affiliation agreements, and confirm capstone experience placements.

- Ensure that all policies and procedures are followed according to the academic institution and ACOTE.
- Obtain and disseminate necessary capstone student and site information (including, but not limited to, confirmation letters, student data form, and student health/security clearances, for example.)
- Maintain adequate records of capstone site information, and allow student access.
- Ensure that you, the capstone student, will be mentored by an individual with expertise consistent with the focus area(s) you have identified. (See Text Box 1-8.)

TEXT BOX 1-8

Your doctoral capstone coordinator might request that you obtain your content expert's current résumé, curriculum vitae, or list of specialized training or verify credentials via public domain databases (which may include state licensure board and/or National Board for Certification in Occupational Therapy certification) as evidence to demonstrate content expertise of your content expert is aligned with your area of focus.

- Collaborate with the capstone team and assign faculty mentors (chairs). This can be based on alignment of focus areas, faculty expertise and training, and so on.
- Ensure and verify length and hours of the experience (14 weeks, at least 32 hours per week). This might occur by a time log built into your school's learning management system (LMS) or even an experiential learning database like EXXAT or CORE.
- Ensure all students and content experts have signed the experiential plan, which must include individualized specific objectives, plan for supervisor/mentoring/evaluation, and responsibilities of all parties, and that you, the student, obtain appropriate

collaboration and signatures. The experiential plan must be completed before the commencement of the capstone experience and according to the standards and regulations of all regulating bodies.

- Correspond professionally with capstone student and content expert via electronic communication, phone calls, and site visits, as appropriate.
- Support your progress as a capstone student, which, in some cases, might include remediation as needed.
- Ensure that an objective formal evaluation of your performance as the capstone student is completed. This may include a midterm and a final evaluation. Chapter 10 provides different strategies to structure and design an evaluation of the doctoral occupational therapy student and evaluation of the capstone experience.
- Be available as a resource and consultant for the capstone team before and during the doctoral capstone process.
- Evaluate (including data collection and analysis) the capstone experience to ensure that the program complies with ACOTE D standards and meets academic institution–specific student outcomes and goals.
- Record and assign grades for the capstone experience. The capstone coordinator or faculty mentor could assign grade(s) for the capstone project.
- Ensure that formal letters or certificates are provided to content expert after completion of the DCE, acknowledging the mentorship provided.
- Collaborate or coordinate the capstone proposal and dissemination, and invite various stakeholders.

ACADEMIC FIELDWORK COORDINATOR

Depending on the faculty infrastructure at your educational program, the academic fieldwork coordinator can be an important support system for both you and the doctoral capstone coordinator. The academic fieldwork coordinator can be involved in reviewing student capstone proposals and provide appropriate feedback, as warranted. This level of review by the academic fieldwork coordinator can ensure that your proposed capstone experience is above and beyond your fieldwork experiences and does not duplicate or conflict with any fieldwork experiences. Prior fieldwork or work experience may not substitute for the capstone.

ROLE OF THE OCCUPATIONAL THERAPY FACULTY MENTOR

Although the doctoral capstone coordinator is identified by ACOTE as being the primary faculty member

responsible for the program's compliance with the capstone requirements of standards section D.1.0, other faculty in the OTD program play an important role in the capstone team. Your program might also identify this faculty mentor role as a capstone chair or capstone advisor. ACOTE standards indicate that the capstone coordinator must have sufficient release time and support to ensure that the needs of the capstone program are being met. In addition to administrative staff to assist with clerical tasks, other occupational therapy faculty members can serve as a faculty mentor or capstone chair to OTD student's capstone projects.

The following list provides an overview of both general and specific tasks and actions the occupational therapy faculty can take to ensure preparation and success on the capstone.

- Collaborate with you, the capstone student, on individualized specific objectives for the experience that coincides with your chosen focus area(s).
- Be available to you, the capstone student, as a resource and consultant.
- Notify your doctoral capstone coordinator if problems arise, and collaborate with you, the capstone student, and the content expert on an action or plan for remediation.
- Provide meaningful feedback on drafts of the capstone project and related scholarly deliverables, as appropriate.
- Assign and submit grades for related capstone project assignment as prescribed by the doctoral capstone coordinator.

CONTENT EXPERT

ACOTE (2023) standards define that the individual directly working with the capstone student during the capstone as "a content expert" (p. 42). An important quality of the content expert is to ensure a concentrated experience in the designed area of interest or focus area. Therefore, the content expert should have expertise consistent with the capstone student's area of focus (ACOTE, 2023). Many professionals are qualified to "mentor" capstone students as they learn and carry out in-depth skills in one or more of the eight focus areas specific to their doctoral pursuit. Furthermore, the content expert does not have to be an occupational therapist, which affords the opportunity for interprofessional supervision and mentorship. The content expert does not have to have a doctoral degree. The primary requirement for content experts is the foundation of the expertise they can provide capstone students through mentorship, which coincides with their focus area(s) and capstone project.

Table 1-3 depicts examples of types of site content expert at various settings and sites.

"During my level II experience, my fieldwork educators were occupational therapists who were there to provide clinical supervision, ensuring that I was developing the necessary clinical skills needed for entry-level practice. In contrast, my content expert during my DCE was not an occupational therapist. Her role as my mentor was to guide me in understanding the facility and helping navigate the dynamics of the organization rather than helping build my clinical skills. My mentor helped me understand the needs of the staff and residents without an OT background, giving me a more holistic perspective.

Without constant supervision during my DCE, I had to become more autonomous and self-directed. This higher level of independence allowed me to become more comfortable with my OT knowledge and trusting my own professional judgment. This experience also required embracing a leadership mindset. With my mentor's guidance, I was able to step into a leadership role by taking responsibility with planning and implementing my project. By taking accountability for my own education, I was able to become more confident in my decision-making."

– Emma Fitzgerald, OTD, OTR/L,
Duquesne University OTD class of 2024

The content expert is typically the on-site person who will provide instruction, support, supervision (if needed), evaluation, and mentorship to you, the capstone student, in applying knowledge to practical situations, developing problem-solving skills, and learning practical competencies within the chosen focus area(s). The level and type of supervision are customized to the type of setting, the capstone student's learning objectives, and the focus of the capstone. The doctoral capstone coordinator will collaborate with the content expert and the capstone student to declare supervision responsibilities and mentorship plan in the experiential learning plan before the beginning of the capstone. **Any clinical practice activities you are planning to engage in during your doctoral capstone experience should be supervised by a qualified professional who meets the state and national requirements to perform in the area of practice**. See Table 1-4 for an overview of formal supervision levels.

The following list provides an overview of both general and specific tasks and actions the content expert can take to ensure preparation and success on the capstone:

- Instruct and orient the capstone student as needed to perform specific negotiated learning activities consistent with your individual learning objectives and goals.

Table 1-3. Examples of Types of Site Content Experts

FOCUS AREA	TYPE OF SETTING/SITE	EXAMPLE OF CONTENT EXPERT
Clinical skills	Medical setting	Any individual with expertise aligned with the capstone focus (e.g., nurse, physician, respiratory therapist)
Clinical skills	School setting	Teacher, director of special education
Program development	Not-for-profit agency	Executive director of programming
Program evaluation	Medical setting	Unit manager, corporate compliance officer
Leadership	Professional association (e.g., AOTA, state organization, National Board for Certification in Occupational Therapy)	Executive director, conference committee staff
Policy development	State or local office	Councilman, legislator, individual on a political action committee (PAC)
Administration	Private practice	Owner/sole proprietor, finance officer, department head or director
Research	Health-care or academic setting	Principal investigator
Education	Academia (higher education)	Occupational therapist or OTA faculty member, center of teaching excellence faculty or staff
	Publishing company	Academic publisher, senior editor
Advocacy	National or local association (e.g., local chapter for cystic fibrosis)	Executive director, fundraising chair, volunteer organizer

Table 1-4. Overview of Supervision Levels

TYPES OF FORMAL SUPERVISION LEVELS	DESCRIPTION
Close	Daily, direct contact
Routine	Direct contact at least every 2 weeks, interim supervision by other methods (phone/written)
General	At least monthly direct contact, supervision available as needed by other methods
Minimal	Only on as-needed basis

Source: Adapted from American Occupational Therapy Association (1993). Occupational therapy roles. *American Journal of Occupational Therapy, 47,* 1087–1099.

- Demonstrate willingness and the ability to provide evidence of expertise. This could include documented evidence of terminal degree, current curriculum vitae, or résumé; verification of completed specialty training; and certification or advanced trainings, for example.
- Collaborate with capstone team to delineate mentorship responsibility.
- Provide supervision, mentorship, and evaluation throughout the duration of the capstone according to the agreed-on experiential learning plan.
- Develop (in collaboration with the doctoral capstone coordinator) and maintain a system for documenting your experiential hours on-site and the tasks and activities accomplished during those hours (as identified in the experiential plan). (See Appendix 1.C for a sample time log template.)
- Provide you, the capstone student, an orientation to the site, other personnel, and stakeholders.
- Collaborate with the faculty mentor to guide you, the capstone student, through the needs assessment component of the project proposal.
- Provide guidance on the logistics of completing the capstone at the site, which could include greater detail on workflow at site, general hours of operation, and access to workspaces.
- Proactively correspond with capstone team regarding any potential concerns.
- Evaluate your performance formally during the doctoral capstone experience (may include a midterm and final formal evaluation).
- Actively participate in regular communication with the capstone team in person, virtually (via Skype, Zoom, Teams, Adobe Connect, etc.), by email, or through other means, including giving both verbal and written feedback on implementation and documentation.

STUDENT SECTION CHAPTER SUMMARY

It is evident that the capstone differs from fieldwork education in many ways. Because of this, expectations of the occupational therapy doctoral student and occupational therapy faculty differ. This chapter has provided recommendations of tasks, actions, and responsibilities of the entire capstone team. The concept of mentorship (vs. fieldwork supervision) was also introduced and will be expanded upon throughout the book. Ensuring that the capstone team members understand their role throughout the duration of the capstone process is also critical.

STUDENT LEARNING ACTIVITIES

1. A Venn diagram is a diagram that shows all possible logical relations between variables (see illustration in Figure 1.3). Review Table 1.1 in this chapter. Create a Venn diagram comparing and contrasting the capstone and fieldwork education.

2. Think about your current (or previous) fieldwork educators. Identify one quality or area of expertise that this individual has that could align with one of the ACOTE focus areas.

3. Create a list of your responsibilities for the doctoral capstone.

4. Brainstorm with members of your occupational therapy faculty who could serve as your capstone chair based on your initial interests and focus area.

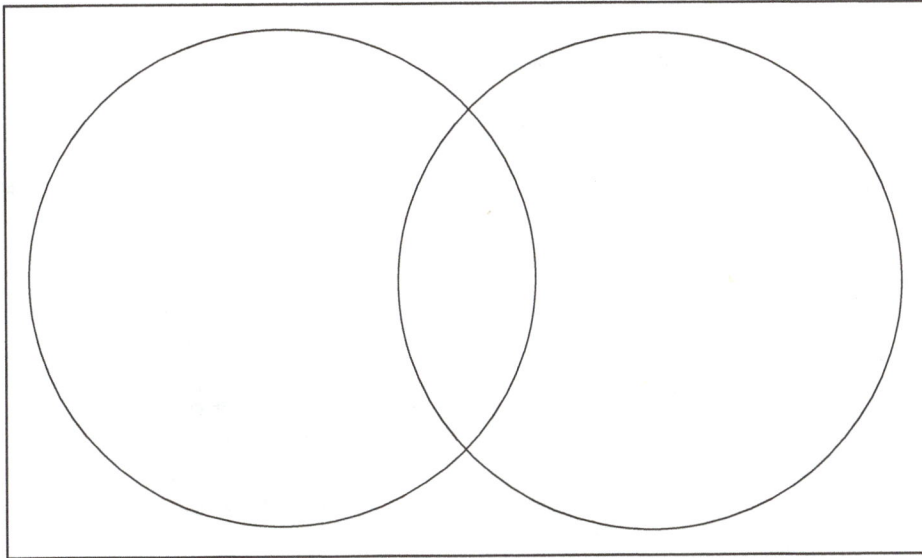

Figure 1-3. Content Experts. *Source:* American Occupational Therapy Association (AOTA), 1993, pp. 1,087–1,099.

Section 2: Educator Focus

Transformational Learning Phases and Framework for the Educator

As an occupational therapy educator, or maybe even as a doctoral capstone coordinator (DCC), you may be reading this book and utilizing it to give some guidance in the development of your capstone curriculum or best practices of how to support and mentor occupational therapy doctoral students during the capstone process. The approach utilized to frame each student section of each chapter is rooted in human-centered design to foster innovation, inspiration, and iteration within the doctoral student. For the educator section, we will be aligning our suggestions to you based upon transformational learning theory. As an educator in a graduate-level program, it is very likely that you have already developed course curriculum to encourage self-directed behaviors within the students and a decreased dependency on the educator. The self-directed approach facilitates an understanding of how to utilize resources and creates an environment in which the student determines their own learning needs, critical judgment, and moral decision-making. These are concepts that line up nicely to Mezirow's transformational learning theory to facilitate adult learning, in addition to personal and professional transformation (Mezirow, 1997). These phases guide learners through a process of critical reflection, problem-solving, and changes in perspective that are often seen as part of the doctoral capstone process.

As this book progresses, you may find it helpful to try to operationalize how students move through Mezirow's ten phases of transformational learning during the doctoral capstone process. To do this, let us briefly look at the stages and how they align with the upcoming chapters you will be reading.

Disorienting dilemma (Chapters 1–2). This phase can occur at the beginning of the doctoral capstone process when students encounter a complex clinical, educational, or organizational problem. They may feel challenged by the scope and demands of the capstone, which pushes them out of their comfort zones and forces them to confront their current knowledge and skills.

Self-examination (Chapters 3–4). As students reflect on their abilities and potential, they may experience self-doubt or guilt about their readiness or capacity to successfully complete their capstone project. The realization that they must apply theory to real-life situations may raise feelings of inadequacy or fear of failure, such as finding an occupational or social injustice or realizing current knowledge is not where it needs to be to find a solution. In this phase, students are examining their own beliefs and feelings in order to develop a meaningful doctoral capstone.

Critical assessment (Chapter 5). During this preparatory phase of the capstone process, students begin to critically examine their existing knowledge, assumptions, and perspectives. This can happen as they conduct a literature review,

(continued)

engage with supervisors or stakeholders, or implement interventions. The students at this point are going to the literature to critically assess evidence to support their experiences and projects.

Recognition of shared experiences (Chapter 6). As students collaborate with peers, mentors, or professional communities, they come to recognize that their struggles and transformative experiences are not isolated. They begin to see that others are going through similar growth processes. As the students work with the site on a needs assessment, they begin to gain insights, and an understanding of new perspectives will begin to transform the way they are thinking.

Exploring options for new behavior (Chapter 6–7). In this phase, students begin to brainstorm and explore different approaches to address the issues identified in the needs assessment as a basis for their capstone project. They consider alternative therapeutic strategies, new methods of collaboration, or innovative solutions. This is the phase in which goals and objectives are developed for their capstone experiences and projects. Students are exploring how they will gain knowledge and synthesize that knowledge.

Planning a course of action (Chapter 7–8). After students identify potential solutions and new perspectives, students begin to plan concrete actions. They develop a strategy for implementing their proposed interventions, collecting data, or analyzing outcomes. Students work with content experts and faculty mentors to develop their experiential plan as they get closer to moving on-site for the doctoral capstone experience.

Acquisition of knowledge, trying new roles, and building confidence (Chapter 9). As students engage with their doctoral capstone experience and project, they acquire new skills and knowledge necessary for implementation. This can involve learning new methods, adapting to unfamiliar clinical environments, or refining communication skills to engage stakeholders. This is now the time when students implement their experiential plans while out on their 14-week experiences. As students successfully implement their experiential plans, they begin to develop competence and confidence in their new roles and skills. They might receive positive feedback from content experts, faculty mentors, colleagues, or participants in their project, reinforcing their growth. They are gaining self-efficacy as they try on new roles and are actively experiencing new things that are shaping their beliefs and understanding.

Reintegration (Chapters 10, 11, 12). In the final stage of transformational learning, students reflect on how the capstone process has transformed them both professionally and personally. As students evaluate and disseminate their project outcomes, integration happens as the students synthesize the knowledge gained and grow in their beliefs and transform as they transition from student to practitioner (Mezirow, 1997).

Mezirow's phases of transformational learning can be a powerful framework for understanding the doctoral capstone process on a pedagogical level as an educator. The capstone is not just an academic project; it is a comprehensive learning experience that fosters deep personal and professional growth in our occupational therapy students. By viewing the capstone through the lens of Mezirow's transformational learning phases, you can better support students in navigating the complex challenges of the doctoral process and ultimately contribute to the field with greater expertise, confidence, and leadership.

CHAPTER INTRODUCTION FOR THE EDUCATOR

This first educator chapter will be purposefully brief. The student portion of this chapter provided you, the educator, a broad description of the roles, responsibilities, and general expectations among the capstone team. As an educator in an occupational therapy doctoral program, you are encouraged to adapt and expand upon these role guidelines and recommendations in your own program handbooks or manuals to align closely to your program mission, curricular design, and overall faculty workload framework regarding how faculty are integrated to support the doctoral capstone. In addition, this educator section will suggest guidelines of how to envision release time and designated clerical support to support the doctoral capstone process. Even for established doctoral programs, with the adoption of new ACOTE standards, all OTD programs are challenged to review, modify, and/or affirm their curriculum, including D.1.0 standards. This chapter will also help promote thinking around how to ensure that the doctoral capstone is "an integral part" of your curricular design and specifically reflects the mission and philosophy of your program.

EDUCATOR REFLECTIVE QUESTIONS

1. What is your program's mission and program philosophy?
2. Does the design of the doctoral capstone in your curriculum reflect this mission and philosophy?
3. What release time are you provided as a capstone coordinator?
4. What type of designated clerical support is provided in your program for the doctoral capstone?
5. How do, or how will, faculty mentors who help design and implement the doctoral capstone project in collaboration with doctoral students receive workload?

EDUCATOR OBJECTIVES

By the end of reading this chapter, the educator will be able to apply principles of transformational learning theory to structure learning activities, assignments, and/or assessments in order to promote the capstone student's ability to:

1. Understand strategies to ensure that the doctoral capstone is integral to your program's curriculum design.
2. Illustrate roles of the doctoral capstone team that align with your institution and program.
3. Identify mechanisms to use required clerical support to streamline doctoral capstone processes.

CONSIDERATIONS TO ENSURE THE DOCTORAL CAPSTONE IS INTEGRAL TO YOUR CURRICULUM DESIGN

There are a few best practice resources to consider when designing or modifying your curriculum. First, of course, is ensuring that you are aligning with current ACOTE accreditation standards. In addition to reviewing the published standards and interpretative guide, do not forget to refer to and use the glossary at the end of the document to help get further definitions and examples of key constructs and terminology. Especially with the recent transition from the 2018 to 2023 ACOTE standards, the published standards document provides clickable hyperlinks to easily access the updated or newer glossary terms.

As a new educator or doctoral capstone coordinator, or even if you are a seasoned educator or capstone coordinator, attending an ACOTE self-study workshop can be a very valuable professional development opportunity and can improve your program's understanding and adherence to the accreditation process. While a primary goal of these workshops is to assist educators and administrators in developing a comprehensive and effective self-study document for initial or renewal accreditation, these workshops also provide an in-depth review of the ACOTE standards, which are essential for maintaining program accreditation. This helps ensure that your curriculum meets the required educational criteria and helps you align your program with best practices in occupational therapy education. This, in turn, helps clarify expectations as to what ACOTE expects from your program during the accreditation process, reducing confusion and guiding you on how you meet certain requirements. Attending the workshop allows you to collaborate with colleagues from other institutions, share experiences, and learn from their challenges and successes in the accreditation process. You can access resources, templates, and examples of successful self-studies, which can be used to improve your own program. ACOTE's accreditation process is not just about meeting minimum standards but also about promoting continuous program development. By attending the workshop, you will gain insights into how to create a culture of ongoing assessment and improvement within your educational program. Overall, attending an ACOTE self-study workshop can provide occupational therapy educators with the knowledge, tools, and strategies needed to successfully navigate the accreditation process. It is an opportunity for professional growth, program enhancement, and networking, ultimately benefiting both educators and students.

Another best practice resource to tap into is the *Occupational Therapy Curriculum Design Framework* (OTCDF), which provides educators an easy-to-follow four-step process for curriculum design, which includes eight essential influential factors (AOTA, 2021).

The four steps of the framework include thus:

1. Establish program philosophy, mission, vision, goals, and threads.
2. Determine and sequence content.
3. Design assessment methods and learning activities.
4. Re-evaluate curriculum on an ongoing basis.

(AOTA, 2021, p. 2)

Aligned with the occupational therapy cornerstone of holism, the OTCDF promotes a holistic and inclusive curriculum design process, due to the influential factors that should be considered throughout each of the four steps. Influential factors include profession, institution, accreditation, teaching and learning, students, community partnerships, clinical practice, and society (AOTA, 2021).

Using these influential factors and the OTCDF framework can be very useful to educators and administrators within an occupational therapy doctoral program, specifically referring to updating or affirming the doctoral capstone. (See Text Box 1-9.)

TEXT BOX 1-9

- What learning outcomes do you have for the doctoral capstone in your program?
- How does the doctoral capstone fit into a curriculum thread in your program?
- What is the sequence of the doctoral capstone courses in your program?
- What learning activities will you have in these courses, as well as overall assessment methods?
- How does your program routinely evaluate the doctoral capstone – including curriculum, support and personnel involved, and overall quality?

While you can access the OTCDF publication, free as an AOTA member, AOTA also hosts and facilitates workshops for educators and administrators which allow attendees to learn more about the process and engage in reflection and application of curriculum design principles to influence the overall curriculum design process at your institution. You can look into upcoming courses on AOTA's website. (See Text Box 1-10.)

TEXT BOX 1-10

As an occupational therapy educator, specifically a doctoral capstone coordinator, you are in an academic leadership position. As members of a profession that embraces (and requires) lifelong learning, engaging in ongoing professional development relative to your role in accreditation and curriculum design is essential. Be sure that you engage in regular discussions with your direct supervisor at your institution regarding support to regularly attend relevant training, such as self-study and curriculum design workshops.

Now, it is one thing to have a curriculum design statement, but especially when accreditation is involved, specifically standard D.1.3, how do you document HOW your program ensures that your capstone is integral to your curriculum design? Here are a few considerations:

- You can include a direct link to your program's curriculum design on every course syllabus, including doctoral capstone courses.
- Explicitly include your program mission and philosophy in your doctoral capstone handbook or manual.
- Provide faculty mentors and content experts a copy of program mission, philosophy, and curriculum design at the very start of the doctoral capstone process, and request their acknowledgment.
- Include your program mission, philosophy, and curricular threads on the student's experiential plan,

which is reviewed and signed by the capstone student, faculty mentor, and content expert.
- Establish a student learning activity where the OTD students write a reflection assignment, or create a discussion board post, where they demonstrate how their doctoral capstone aligns with the program mission, philosophy, and curricular design.

When in doubt, specifically, in vetting how your own program is in alignment and compliance with ACOTE standards, always be sure to contact them directly to share your individual circumstances.

CLARIFYING ROLES OF THE CAPSTONE TEAM AT YOUR INSTITUTION

While ACOTE provides information and language that identify key players that are to be involved with the doctoral capstone, to demonstrate alignment with your own curriculum design and program makeup, it might be necessary to clarify terminology and role names for your own program.

For instance, what term does your program use to describe the individual that is on-site at the doctoral capstone experience site that is providing direct mentorship and supervision to your student? Do you use content expert, site supervisor, or site mentor? Ensure that all parties are speaking the same language and that you are referring to these consistently in program manuals, program webpages, syllabi, and other materials that are provided to the OTD student and capstone sites. (See Text Box 1-11.)

TEXT BOX 1-11

Speaking of the content expert, with you as the doctoral capstone coordinator, it will be important to demonstrate a mechanism to provide them recognition of their role in mentoring the doctoral student during their DCE. If the content expert is an occupational therapy practitioner, they can obtain professional development units (PDUs) for entry-level OTD capstone mentorship. The DCC can prepare a formal letter or certificate on behalf of the OTD program, and it should include the dates of the mentorship experience and hours of supervision provided. The context expert should also maintain copy of the student's experiential plan, which provides a description of the capstone experience plan and objectives. Per National Board for Certification in Occupational Therapy guidelines, each week of mentorship is worth one professional development unit. (See sample template in Appendix 1.B.)

Clarifying role names also goes for the faculty member that is directly involved in supporting the student's doctoral capstone project. Does your program use faculty mentor? Faculty chair? Faculty advisor? Particularly, as occupational therapy programs might use the term faculty mentor and/or advisor to fulfil other required programmatic obligations (such as to address ACOTE A.3.5), it is important that there is a clear distinction so that the students are clear in roles/responsibilities among their faculty support team.

IDEAS FOR CONSIDERATION OF DISTRIBUTING FACULTY MENTOR WORKLOAD FOR THE CAPSTONE PROJECT

Faculty workload has been a recent hot topic in higher education across disciplines. Workload is a key factor in the functioning of academic institutions, and its importance is multifaceted, impacting both the quality of education and the well-being and satisfaction of the faculty.

Assigning workload for mentoring and advising an OTD capstone student requires careful consideration of the time, effort, and expertise required for **each phase** of the capstone process. As this book will reveal, the OTD doctoral capstone is a comprehensive, individualized project that demands ongoing guidance, support, and evaluation from faculty members. Determining the workload of the faculty mentors will be specific to each program and dependent on several factors, such as the number of students in the program, as well as the number of faculty who are able to support this scholarly endeavor. Students can be assigned to a faculty member to "chair" or "mentor" capstone students throughout the DCE or capstone project. One recommendation for the division of workload is to have one faculty member assigned to four or five capstone students during their capstone experience and project. Therefore, if the class size is composed of 30 students, at least six faculty members would need to be assigned load credit for taking a group of four to five students each.

Other considerations for workload allocation might include thus:

Capstone project complexity. The level of complexity in the capstone project may affect the amount of time required for mentoring and advising. More complex projects or those that involve more robust research methods or extensive community or interdisciplinary collaboration might require more faculty time.

Student needs. Different students will have varying levels of need for guidance, which can affect the total workload. Some students may require more frequent meetings or more in-depth feedback, while others may need less.

Multiple students. Faculty mentoring multiple students simultaneously will need to balance their time and prioritize effectively. For example, a faculty member mentoring several OTD capstone students may allocate specific days or hours each week to meet with different students or to review materials.

The doctoral capstone coordinator is responsible for the overall capstone experience; however, they could also take on the role of faculty mentor with a small group of students if their workload and release time allow this.

The program or school curriculum structure will determine when the faculty mentors are assigned and how much their load credit is.

For instance, does the department chair or program director manage faculty workload at your program? Does the DCC weigh in on faculty mentor assignments?

Examples of workload models relative to mentoring doctoral capstone student projects include:

- A 0.5–1 credit/contact hour per capstone student per capstone course/semester.
- A set credit release per academic year to mentor up to a set number of capstone students (e.g., 3 credit release each year to mentor up to four capstone students).
- The doctoral capstone coordinator* might serve as the formal faculty mentor to each student in the OTD cohort.
- Some programs might have an overload stipend model built in to provide faculty mentors an extra salary bump based upon the number of capstone students they mentor each academic year if it is outside their contracted teaching load (e.g., $250 faculty stipend per student per semester).

* **In this scenario, this might be permissible only if sufficient release time is allocated to the DCC.**

IMPORTANCE OF RELEASE TIME AND CLERICAL SUPPORT

Although not explicitly mentioned in the student section of the chapter, dedicated release time and clerical support are essential components to the success of your doctoral capstone program.

ACOTE (2023) standard A.2.4 describes that the doctoral capstone coordinator must have sufficient release time and support (to be provided and documented) to ensure that the needs of the capstone program are being met. Harris et al. (2023) identified several administrative components of the DCC role that support having sufficient release, including establishing and maintaining sites, providing ongoing education to members among the capstone team, creating and enhancing capstone curriculum and ongoing responsiveness to accreditation, and other institutional requirements that indicate management of policies, handbooks, manuals, etc.

As a doctoral capstone coordinator, your release time should specify an actual numerical release and can be formally documented in several ways, such as a formal letter from administration (such as your dean), your employment contract, job description, etc. ACOTE does not provide any suggestions or parameters of what is considered a sufficient release time. Programs need to articulate what is sufficient based upon their institution, program, and curriculum design.

For example, if the doctoral capstone coordinator role is a non-tenure-stream clinical faculty position and the institutional requirement for non-tenure track faculty is to teach 24 "credits" or "contact hours" per academic year.

Based upon the cohort size, etc., a doctoral capstone coordinator might be provided 30% release time from teaching in order to sufficiently support the doctoral capstone program. Therefore, this doctoral capstone coordinator would receive approximately a 7-credit release and only teach 17 credits. This scenario could get more complex if there is no consensus or discussion in advance whether those credits associated with the doctoral capstone program count toward those 17 credits. For example, most OTD programs have designated doctoral capstone courses that directly work on the required preparatory activities (e.g., literature review, needs assessment, program evaluation, etc.) or provide designated space for the doctoral capstone coordinator to directly work with students to develop and plan their DCE and collaborate on the experiential plan, etc.

In the case where a doctoral capstone coordinator is managing the doctoral capstone experience as well as serving as the faculty mentor to all the students in the cohort, they might not have any other didactic teaching requirements in the OTD program, as they are fully released from other teaching in order to manage and oversee the entire doctoral capstone process.

In addition to being mindful of release time from teaching, programs should also be mindful of how other typical academic roles are delegated (or not) to the DCC, such as service and scholarship expectations, or other administrative responsibilities, such as recruitment, etc. (See Text Box 1-12.)

TEXT BOX 1-12

To ensure fairness and equitable practice, doctoral capstone coordinators are encouraged to seek out release time models throughout their school or institution. What is the release time of the academic fieldwork coordinator in your program? What is the release time of the director of clinical education if you have a physical therapy program at your institution?

ACOTE (2023) also stipulates that the OTD program must provide clerical and support staff to meet doctoral capstone requirements per standard A.2.8. While there is no national data that is available to allow programs to

benchmark or compare for the doctoral capstone and specific to the doctoral capstone coordinator, DeIuliis et al. (2021) completed a nationwide descriptive study that investigated the academic fieldwork coordinator role and related supports and barriers. In their study, only 50% of AFWC participants reported received clerical or administrative support from an actual staff member. Other AFWC participants reported receiving support from a graduate student worker (12%). An alarming 12% of the respondents reported that they did not receive any clerical or administrative assistance for fieldwork duties (DeIuliis et al., 2021).

This is another place to dig into institutional practice relative to designated clerical support. What do the other programs in your school or college have relative to staff support, specifically for experiential learning, like fieldwork, or the doctoral capstone?

Advocating for the purchase and use of a clinical database might also be a way to demonstrate a particular aspect of clerical support for the doctoral capstone. Although this data was specific to managing fieldwork duties, DeIuliis and colleagues (2021) shared that nearly 68% of AFWC respondents used a clinical education software. Programs that utilize a platform to support fieldwork are well suited to also integrate the same system for the doctoral capstone. The use of a software system or virtual platform can help operationalize several aspects of the DCC role, including:

- To organize and maintain student, site, and content expert data
- To streamline communication between the OTD program and community/clinical sites
- To reduce redundancy and help contribute to program evaluation approaches

With designated clerical and support staff in place within your program, the doctoral capstone coordinator can delegate a variety of tasks to help contribute to release time, which could include thus:

- Manage capstone site database. This might include commercially available platforms, such as EXXAT, eValue or CORE, etc.
- Create and manage capstone site correspondence using letter template(s).
- Collate and store doctoral capstone site information.
- Assist doctoral capstone coordinator in deploying program evaluation measures, such as the doctoral capstone student/site evaluations and programmatic exit surveys (see Chapter 10).
- Create mentorship certificates to recognize content experts.

An example job description of an administrative support personnel job description dedicated to fieldwork and doctoral capstone programmatic tasks can be found in Appendix D.

EDUCATOR SECTION CHAPTER SUMMARY

This first chapter hopefully set the stage with some important concepts that will be built upon further as this book unfolds. It is so important for all occupational therapy faculty members, not just the doctoral capstone coordinator, to understand the doctoral capstone and be able to articulate how it is integrated into your program's curriculum design, as well as have clarity in individual faculty roles and responsibilities in regard to mentoring and supporting the capstone project. As the book progresses, we will be providing you additional recommendations, suggestions, and exemplars that you can build (or adapt) right into your own doctoral capstone program and courses.

APPENDICES

Appendix 1-A Sample Fieldwork and Doctoral Capstone Policy Manual Table of Contents

Appendix 1-B Sample NBCOT Certificate for Context Expert/Mentor

Appendix 1-C Sample Template for Time Log

Appendix 1-D Sample Administrative or Clerical Support Position Job Description

CHAPTER REFERENCES

Accreditation Council for Occupational Therapy Education. (2023). *Standards and interpretive guide* [PDF]. https://acoteonline.org/accreditation-explained/standards/

Aikens, F., Menaker, L., & Barsky, L. (2001). Fieldwork education: The future of occupational therapy depends on it. *Occupational Therapy International, 8*(2), 86–95.

American Occupational Therapy Association. (1993). Occupational therapy roles. *American Journal of Occupational Therapy, 47,* 1087–1099.

American Occupational Therapy Association. (2020). *Fieldwork performance evaluation (FWPE_ for the occupational therapy student) revised in 2020.* https://www.aota.org/-/media/corporate/files/educationcareers/fieldwork/fieldwork-performance-evaluation-occupational-therapy-student.pdf

American Occupational Therapy Association. (2021). Occupational therapy curriculum design framework. *American Journal of Occupational Therapy, 75*(Supplement_3), 7513420020. https://doi.org/10.5014/ajot.2021.75S3008

Brandenburger-Shasby, S., Hills, L., Huie, C., Jansen, K., Johnson, L., & Josey-Lamont, A. (1998). Fieldwork: The critical link. *Education Special Interest Section Quarterly, 8*(3), 1–3.

DeIuliis, E. D. (2017). *Professionalism across occupational therapy clinical practice.* SLACK Incorporated.

DeIuliis, E., & Hanson, D. (2023). *Fieldwork educator's guide to level II fieldwork.* SLACK Incorporated. ISBN 10: 1630919659

DeIuliis, E. D., Persons, K., Laverdure, P., & LeQuieu, E. D. (2021). A nationwide descriptive study: Understanding roles, expectations, and supports of academic fieldwork coordinators in occupational therapy programs. *Journal of Occupational Therapy Education, 5*(4). https://doi.org/10.26681/jote.2021.050415

Hanson, D., & DeIuliis, E. (2023). *Fieldwork educator's guide to level I fieldwork.* SLACK Incorporated. ISBN 10: 1630919624

Harris, H. L., Kiraly-Alvarez, A. F., Costello, P. J., & Schmeltz, B. (2023). Understanding the doctoral capstone coordinator position: A unique faculty role in occupational therapy education. *The Open Journal of Occupational Therapy, 11*(2), 1–14. https://doi.org/10.15453/2168-6408.2039

Haynes, C. J. (2011). Active participation in fieldwork level I: Fieldwork educator and student perceptions. *Occupational Therapy in Health Care, 25,* 257–269. https://doi.org/10.3109/07380577.2011.595477

IDEO. (2015). *The field guide to human-centered design.* Ideo.org.

Mezirow, J. (1997). Transformative learning: Theory to practice. *New Directions for Adult and Continuing Education,* (74), 5–12. https://doi.org/10.1002/ace.7401

Appendix 1-A

SAMPLE FIELDWORK AND DOCTORAL CAPSTONE EXPERIENCE POLICY MANUAL TABLE OF CONTENTS

CRITICAL INCIDENTS
CONFLICT OF INTEREST
STUDENT HEALTH REPORTS/CLEARANCES
      CRIMINAL BACKGROUND CHECK
      FBI FINGERPRINTING
      DRUG TESTING
PROFESSIONAL BEHAVIOR EXPECTATIONS
      CELL PHONE AND ELECTRONIC DEVICE USE
      COMPUTER USE, SOCIAL MEDIA, AND NETWORKING
      USE OF PHOTO OR VIDEO
      DRESS CODE
      TARDINESS/ABSENTEEISM
            HOLIDAYS
            INCLEMENT WEATHER
      CONFIDENTIALITY, PRIVACY, AND HIPAA
AFWC AND CAPSTONE COORDINATOR MONITORING AND SITE VISITS
POST-GRADUATION INFORMATION
REQUESTING PROFESSIONAL REFERENCE
      FACULTY
      FIELDWORK EDUCATOR
CONTENT EXPERT
GUIDELINES FOR NATIONAL AND STATE CREDENTIALING

Appendix 1-B

SAMPLE CERTIFICATE FOR MENTORING DOCTORAL CAPSTONE STUDENT

Certificate of Completion

THIS IS TO CERTIFY THAT

(insert name of content expert or mentor)

Has earned _____ PDUs for successfully mentoring an OTD student during the doctoral capstone.

Insert program or institution logo or crest here

(insert dates of the DCE)

Awarded insert date here

_____

Name/Signature of the Capstone Coordinator

Appendix 1-C

SAMPLE TEMPLATE FOR TIME LOG

Appendix C Sample Template for Time Long

DCE Log of Hours

Overall total hours must equal 560 hours with at least 80% occurring on-site. Periodic site mentor signature required.

Week 1	On Site	Off Site	Accomplished
Sunday			
Monday			
Tuesday			
Wednesday			
Thursday			
Friday			
Saturday			
Total			
Site Mentor Signature			

Week 9	On Site	Off Site	Accomplished
Sunday			
Monday			
Tuesday			
Wednesday			
Thursday			
Friday			
Saturday			
Total			
Site Mentor Signature			

Week 2	On Site	Off Site	Accomplished
Sunday			
Monday			
Tuesday			
Wednesday			
Thursday			
Friday			
Saturday			
Total			
Site Mentor Signature			

Week 10	On Site	Off Site	Accomplished
Sunday			
Monday			
Tuesday			
Wednesday			
Thursday			
Friday			
Saturday			
Total			
Site Mentor Signature			

Week 3	On Site	Off Site	Accomplished
Sunday			
Monday			
Tuesday			
Wednesday			
Thursday			
Friday			
Saturday			
Total			
Site Mentor Signature			

Week 11	On Site	Off Site	Accomplished
Sunday			
Monday			
Tuesday			
Wednesday			
Thursday			
Friday			
Saturday			
Total			
Site Mentor Signature			

Week 4	On Site	Off Site	Accomplished
Sunday			
Monday			
Tuesday			
Wednesday			
Thursday			
Friday			
Saturday			
Total			
Site Mentor Signature			

Week 12	On Site	Off Site	Accomplished
Sunday			
Monday			
Tuesday			
Wednesday			
Thursday			
Friday			
Saturday			
Total			
Site Mentor Signature			

Week 5	On Site	Off Site	Accomplished
Sunday			
Monday			
Tuesday			
Wednesday			
Thursday			
Friday			
Saturday			
Total			
Site Mentor Signature			

Week 13	On Site	Off Site	Accomplished
Sunday			
Monday			
Tuesday			
Wednesday			
Thursday			
Friday			
Saturday			
Total			
Site Mentor Signature			

Week 6	On Site	Off Site	Accomplished
Sunday			
Monday			
Tuesday			
Wednesday			
Thursday			
Friday			
Saturday			
Total			
Site Mentor Signature			

Week 14	On Site	Off Site	Accomplished
Sunday			
Monday			
Tuesday			
Wednesday			
Thursday			
Friday			
Saturday			
Total			
Site Mentor Signature			

Week 7	On Site	Off Site	Accomplished
Sunday			
Monday			
Tuesday			
Wednesday			
Thursday			
Friday			
Saturday			
Total			
Site Mentor Signature			

Week 8	On Site	Off Site	Accomplished
Sunday			
Monday			
Tuesday			
Wednesday			
Thursday			
Friday			
Saturday			
Total			
Site Mentor Signature			

Overall Total	On Site	Off Site

Appendix 1-D

SAMPLE ADMINISTRATIVE ASSISTANT JOB DESCRIPTION

Location: Occupational Therapy–School of Health Sciences
Position Status: Full-time (35 hours/week)
Hours: M–F, 8:30 a.m.–4:30 p.m.
FLSA Status: Non-exempt

NATURE OF WORK

The administrative assistant will assist the department chair (DC), program director (PD), academic fieldwork coordinator (AFWC), and doctoral capstone coordinator (DCC) with curricular, clinical, and community education management, which requires an extreme amount of detail-oriented work. The administrative assistant will also assist the PD with program evaluation in preparation for accreditation studies. This is a complex and responsible clerical position which involves the performance of high-level secretarial work. Strong, consumer-oriented interpersonal skills and database management experience are essential, as this position requires extensive contact with staff, faculty, students, and prospective students/families. The typical work hours are from 8:30 a.m. to 4:30 p.m., Monday through Friday. However, these times are expanded as necessary to meet departmental needs. (Examples: proctoring exams, virtual Q&A recruitment sessions, weekend open house, evening/weekend seminar/conference/reception, school graduations, continuing education programs.)

ILLUSTRATIVE EXAMPLES OF WORK

1. Maintains the full range of the Exxat database, as detailed in the following.
2. Maintains Exxat fieldwork database with information relating to individual site requirements and personnel changes. Runs reports related to clinical/community education for PD/DC as requested.
3. Is responsible for all correspondence between AFWC and students and clinical/community sites through email and Exxat (i.e., managing fieldwork slot requests; setting up student placement wish lists and placement sessions; sending placement notifications, student profiles, and required documents to sites and students; sending letters for NBCOT PDUs; etc.)
4. Maintains fieldwork, community, and DCE site contact info for each fieldwork placement in Excel or OneDrive (FWED contact information, fieldwork educator/site mentor demographic, site contact information, site-specific paperwork, etc.).
5. Assists AFWC in training and orientation of Exxat Approve to students.
6. Manages Exxat Approve, which includes correspondence with account managers, answering student inquiries regarding health requirements and clearances, updating OT department Canvas page.
7. Maintains departmental records for the ongoing accreditation through ACOTE. Assists in preparing accreditation materials as needed.
8. Deploys surveys utilizing Qualtrics surveys to students after level II FW and DCE, and assists AFWC/DCC and PD in analyzing results.
9. Coordinates experiential learning CECQs and SPOT needs with clinical contracts manager, department instructors, and educational technology.
10. Assists PD/AFWC with program evaluation tasks, such as sending out exit, alumni, and employer surveys and analyzing results for annual reports and accreditation studies.
11. Maintains student records to indicate academic progress and program completion.
12. Prepares credentialing paperwork for graduates for completion by the PD.
13. Composes a yearly spreadsheet of all adjunct clinical instructors (fieldwork educators, DCE site mentor/CEL site supervisors), including additional clinicians that have worked with students during their clinical rotations.
14. Processes all fieldwork education, community, and DCE paperwork received following each FW experience (i.e., evaluations, outcomes entered into spreadsheet, strengths and weaknesses summarized and entered into a Word document).

15. Is responsible for updating FW/DCE manual and uploading to website and OT department Canvas site, under direction of AFWC/DCC.

16. Follows purchasing procedures for FWEd appreciation gifts, which includes maintaining inventory, obtaining quotes, preparing purchase requisitions, and handling shipping needs.

17. Follows purchasing procedures for prospective and current student merchandise, which includes maintaining inventory, obtaining quotes, preparing purchase requisitions, and handling shipping needs.

18. Assists OT faculty members with the following: correspondence, proofreading, copying, equipment needs, etc.

19. Supports student workers and graduate assistants, which includes determining if they are working efficiently and effectively.

REQUIREMENTS OF WORK

The successful candidate will have a minimum of high school diploma and associate's degree and 2–4 years of progressively more responsible and related support experience. A bachelor's degree in business or closely related field of study is preferred and highly desirable, or any equivalent combination of experience and training which provides the knowledge, skills, and abilities required to perform the essential job functions. This includes, but is not limited to, the following: knowledge of basic marketing skills, including use of social media, database management, and the ability to work both independently and as part of a team; excellent interpersonal skills, with a customer service orientation; ability to communicate effectively, both orally and in writing; excellent organizational skills, with the ability to be attentive to the details; ability to work a flexible schedule as needed in order to attend department, school, and university events; thorough knowledge of and proficiency in using the current Microsoft Office Suite: Word, Excel, PowerPoint, and Access; willingness to learn new technologies relevant to the position; ability and willingness to assist with other tasks in the office as needed; enthusiasm in seeking out work and new assignments; interest and initiative in taking on new and challenging assignments; good problem-solving skills, with a can-do approach; ability to work independently on complex and confidential issues related to the day-to-day operations of the department; effective organizational and administrative skills; ability to initiate and follow through with work responsibilities and to meet deadlines; ability to establish and maintain effective working relationships with the university community; ability and willingness to contribute actively to the mission and to respect the Spiritan Catholic identity of Duquesne University. The mission is implemented through a commitment to academic excellence, a spirit of service, moral and spiritual values, sensitivity to world concerns, and an ecumenical campus community.

CHAPTER 2

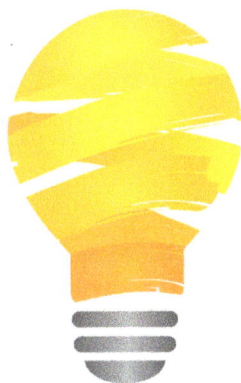

Understanding the ACOTE Areas of Focus for the Capstone

Julie A. Bednarski and Elizabeth D. DeIuliis

Section 1: Student Focus

Human-Centered Design Mindsets for the Doctoral Student

Human-centered design mindset concepts of creative confidence, embracing ambiguity, and optimism are important for the doctoral student to adopt as they begin to explore and develop their capstone area of focus.

Creative confidence. "Creative confidence is the belief that everyone is creative, and that creativity isn't the capacity to draw or compose or sculpt, but a way of understanding the world" (IDEO.org, 2015, p. 19). This is a time to learn, understand, and digest the areas of potential focus for your capstone and begin to think creatively about problems in these areas and problems you might want to solve.

Embrace ambiguity. Remember, ambiguity can lead to creativity. The process of the capstone experience and project is not linear. It is a fluid process and will continue to be so. Take the time to explore and embrace the ambiguity!

Optimism. This will continue to be an important mindset throughout your capstone experience and project. Your journey is in the initial stages; be patient, stay positive, and enjoy the learning!

INTRODUCTION FOR STUDENTS

As the initial process of inspiration and development begins, it is important to understand the Accreditation Council for Occupational Therapy Education (ACOTE) areas of focus. The focus areas help determine what area of occupational therapy you will gain in-depth exposure to to design a capstone project that will allow you to demonstrate a synthesis and application of the knowledge gained on your capstone experience (ACOTE, Standard D.1.0,

2023). The focus area that you ultimately choose will guide the development of your doctoral capstone experience (DCE) and project. This chapter defines and describes the ACOTE areas of focus for the DCE and will assist you, the doctoral student, to become inspired through brainstorming potential populations, potential areas of practice, and/or sites for your 14-week capstone experience and ideas for the types of capstone projects that can be completed in a 14-week period to demonstrate the knowledge gained during your experience.

DOI: 10.4324/9781003541813-3

STUDENT REFLECTIVE QUESTIONS

When developing the doctoral capstone, you may find it helpful to reflect on the following questions:

1. What is your inspiration for your capstone?
2. How does your plan for your capstone compare or contrast with your planned or completed fieldwork experiences?
3. What area of focus is most important to you as you think about your capstone?
4. What type of sites are you interested in exploring?
5. What type of individuals can you see yourself being mentored by, based on your planned focus area?

STUDENT OBJECTIVES

By the end of reading the student portion of this chapter and completing the learning activities, the reader should be able to:

1. Describe each of the eight ACOTE areas of focus.
2. Compare and contrast the areas of focus across different types of settings.
3. Formulate general ideas for a capstone project within each of the areas of focus.

FRAMING THE ACOTE AREAS OF FOCUS

With mentorship from your faculty mentor and doctoral capstone coordinator, you will first need to develop a clear understanding of what the focus areas are and how they complement your previous fieldwork experiences and overall professional development plan as a future occupational therapy practitioner. Your doctoral capstone should be directly aligned with one or a combination of focus areas. Although this list is not exhaustive, this chapter illustrates examples and strategies to help you, the doctoral student, increase your understanding of the focus areas. The areas of focus include:

- Clinical skills
- Research skills
- Administration
- Program development and evaluation
- Policy development
- Advocacy
- Education
- Leadership

Although ACOTE indicates that the doctoral capstone should be a collaborative process designed by the student and a faculty mentor and provided in a setting consistent with the program's curriculum design, the capstone should be developed to mutually benefit the doctoral student and the capstone site. Note that the full basis for your capstone project will not be fully developed until you seek guidance and mentorship from your content expert (see Chapter 3), dive into the literature (see Chapter 5), and perform a formal needs assessment (see Chapter 6). This chapter is meant to provide ideas to get your thoughts flowing. Designing your capstone experience and project is a process. Know that there will be many iterations to your capstone experience and project, and this is what needs to happen. As you read through these examples, just keep an open mind and keep that creative confidence.

CLINICAL SKILLS

If you are seeking to complete a DCE in the area of clinical skills, you will want to identify a site or setting where more advanced (or a narrower focus of) occupational therapy practice is utilized. You may find clinical skills as a focus area which could also satisfy components of your experience by pursuing and completing continuing education courses, advanced trainings, certificates, and so on.

- For example, if you are interested in advancing your knowledge and skill set (beyond the generalist level) on sensory integration as a clinical practice, focus area could pursue getting formally trained to administer the Sensory Integration and Praxis Test (SIPT) as a portion of your capstone experience.
- In contrast, those who want to become competent in lymphedema management to deepen their knowledge and practice skills among the oncology population may register for formal training courses (such as the Norton School or Academy of Lymphatic Studies) to develop an in-depth skill area in managing this chronic state of edema as a component of their capstone experience.

Types of Sites and Settings

A starting inspiration point to brainstorm potential doctoral capstone experience (DCE) sites within this focus area could be to review the American Occupational Therapy Association (AOTA) clinical practice topics on the AOTA website. Featured clinical topics include sex as an activity of daily living (ADL), women's health, stroke, trauma and post-traumatic stress disorder, functional cognition in OT, mental health and well-being, musculoskeletal conditions, and driving and community mobility (AOTA.org, 2024). Spend some time on the AOTA website or even on the CommunOT discussion forums reading through topic areas that interest you and spark some passion. Based on the type of knowledge you would like to gain, some ideas of site and/or specialty services or programs include:

- Dysphagia
- Pelvic health
- Hippotherapy
- Low vision
- Ergonomic assessment

- Driver rehabilitation
- NICU
- Hand therapy
- Primary care

This is by no means an exhaustive list but, rather, a list to promote idea generation. With clinical skills as your chosen area of focus, think about the overall experience you want to have during the 14 weeks at the site and then your project, remembering that they are two distinct entities. Oftentimes, as a doctoral student wanting clinical skills as your focus area, you might first design your experience and then work with the site to develop an initial idea for the project that will meet the needs of the site. For example, your capstone experience may be to work under the supervision of a registered occupational therapist (OTR) to gain skills in working in a primary care setting and understanding in-depth knowledge on the role of occupational therapy. Your project may then be to design evidence-based group protocols for the OTR utilizing the constructs and concepts of lifestyle medicine (lifestylemedicine.org, 2024). Or you might have interest in driving rehabilitation, and you collaborate with an OTR who is a certified driver rehabilitation specialist (CDRS) to develop a 14-week experience in which you will gain skills in this area of practice and begin to work toward your own CDRS. To give you another idea, you might seek out and plan to use national best practice standards, such as the National Association of Neonatal Therapists (NANT) Core Competencies as a guideline to track your progress during a capstone experience in the neonatal intensive care unit (NICU), to demonstrate you have achieved an understanding of in-depth neonatal topics (de Castro Mehrkens et al., 2024).

Capstone Projects Ideas Within the Clinical Skills Focus Area

Remember that with every capstone experience, a student is developing and implementing an individual capstone project. The capstone project can take many forms,

depending on the clinical practice area. Examples might include:

- Developing (or refining) a practice guideline, pathway, clinical protocol, or best evidence statement. (See Text Box 2-1.)

TEXT BOX 2-1

For example, a capstone student could develop and implement an evidence-based bowel bladder management protocol for individuals with neurodegenerative disorders, refine the critical pathway used in a NICU that triggers a lactation consultant for premature babies, or develop and implement an evidence-based clinical practice care guideline to assist in assessing driver readiness amongst novice drivers with an autism spectrum disorder (ASD).

- Developing an evidence-based intervention guide for a specific area of practice. (See Text Box 2-2.)

TEXT BOX 2-2

A capstone student focused on clinical hand therapy skills for their experience. To demonstrate and apply knowledge, the student created and implemented an evidence-based orthosis guidebook to aid clinicians and students with selecting, fabricating, and modifying orthoses as their project (Sweeney, 2024).

Each of these examples provides you the opportunity to be mentored by an individual inside or outside the field of occupational therapy. (See Text Box 2-3.) Using the previous example regarding a focus on developing in-depth skills in sensory integration and getting SIPT-trained, the capstone project could involve helping a pediatric site develop an intense multi-sensory (IMS) stimulation program or a formalized non-invasive stimulation program. Other innovative ideas for a capstone project designed to advance in-depth clinical skills are depicted in Table 2-1.

Table 2-1. Examples of Practice Areas

AOTA PRACTICE AREA	DCE AND CAPSTONE PROJECT EXAMPLES
Children and youth	Explore the impact of hippotherapy on children with autism spectrum disorder (ASD).
Health and wellness	Understand the benefits of kangaroo-care protocol in the NICU.
Mental health	A wellness exploration group for women with substance use disorder (Mathieu, 2024).
Productive aging	Understand how sensory stimulation programs can be used with elderly adults diagnosed with dementia.
Rehabilitation, disability, and participation	Create a practice guideline to address sexuality with individuals who have a spinal cord injury.
Work and industry	Create a clinical pathway rooted in the biopsychosocial model to address chronic pain among individuals who have sustained a work-related injury.

RESEARCH

A capstone focus area on research is an experience that involves participating, collaborating, and learning from recognized individuals who are actively engaged in projects that include research design and planning, data collection, analyzing and effecting evidence-based practice, and disseminating results. Although the B standards in ACOTE do stipulate required learning objectives in this realm, a capstone experience would involve an in-depth exposure to the researcher role and more advanced research skills.

Your OTD program may allow for an opportunity for doctoral students to participate in faculty research opportunities. As a doctoral student, you may have the opportunity to serve as an apprentice to a faculty member if your area of focus is research. You will work with the faculty member to establish your role and your specific goals and objectives on the research team so that you can meet the requirements of the overall doctoral capstone.

Types of Sites and Settings

A focus area in research could take place anywhere: in the clinic, in the community, or within academia.

Capstone Projects Ideas Within the Research Focus Area

A capstone project with a focus area of research can take many forms. Examples include the following:

- An outcome study (e.g., determining the outcome of smartphone training and use as an intervention and cognitive aid for individuals with mild traumatic brain injury).
- A rapid systematic review of evidence related to an occupational therapy program or intervention of interest (e.g., systematic review of literature pertaining to a sensory integration intervention for children with ASD).
- Retrospective research study, such as looking at how many children with intensive feeding issues had NICU stays as infants. What can be done to improve current treatment in an outpatient setting with these children?
- A scoping literature review of an emerging practice focus.
- A critically appraised topic.
- A meta-analysis of evidence regarding a specific intervention or approach.

- An example of a student working alongside a faculty researcher is a 2024 project completed with the Skills on Wheels Program at Indiana University Indianapolis. Hadley (2024) developed and implemented a protocol to increase the reliability and validity of wheelchair skills testing with the Skills on Wheels program.
- Understanding the experiences of occupational therapists' burnout at a large trauma hospital through a mixed-method phenomenological approach and utilizing the outcomes to assist with programmatic health and wellness needs of therapists at the facility (Brooks, 2024).

ADMINISTRATION

If you choose an administration focus area, you will be responsible for developing in-depth knowledge and skills in systems of practice, administrative, or management function in traditional or role-emerging practice settings.

Types of Sites and Settings

Examples can include working with distinguished, expert administrators, entrepreneurs, managers, and supervisors who may or may not be an occupational therapy practitioner. Settings could include private practices, managed care organizations, health systems, and community sites.

Capstone Project Ideas Within the Administration Focus Areas

An administrative capstone project requires active skill building and collaboration in administration, management, and supervision, outside of the generalist expectations that can be found in ACOTE standard B 4.4, which aligns with the business aspects of practice. Examples could include the following:

- Conduct a financial analysis to compare care models and potential cost savings or return on investment (ROI).
- Develop and/or evaluate care models or service delivery models (e.g., implement and evaluate the effectiveness of an evidence-based teamwork program, such as TeamSTEPPS 3.0 [Agency for Healthcare Research and Quality, 2023]).
- Complete a workflow analysis on the use of transport in a health-care facility, and evaluate the impact on employee productivity.
- Write a strategic business plan to initiate a new program or entrepreneur effort.
- Create a grant proposal to secure funding for an occupational therapist 8 hours per week at an adult day center to provide consultative services.

- Develop a system based on evidence for a program evaluation process for merit and promotion of employees.
- Revamp the administrative onboarding process for volunteers and students at a clinical site.
- Create a system-wide approach for the adoption and integration of a new electronic medical record (EMR) system.
- Create an evidence-based proposal to increase the retention of occupational therapy personnel.
- Evaluate and refine processes and systems to measure patient/client satisfaction.
- Standardizing an organizational approach to hospital accreditation for an inpatient rehabilitation unit (Pridemore, 2021)
- Measuring the impact of "xyz" variables on reducing readmission rates. (See Text Box 2-4.)

TEXT BOX 2-4

A study published in *Medical Care Research and Review* found that "occupational therapy is the only spending category where additional hospital spending has a statistically significant association with lower readmission rates" for the three health conditions studied: heart failure, pneumonia, and acute myocardial infarction (Rogers et al., 2016, p. 668). How can this monumental research study provide inspiration for the capstone to demonstrate the distinct value of occupation from an administrative lens (e.g., reduce costs, lower readmission rates, improve client outcomes, and increase consumer satisfaction)?

PROGRAM DEVELOPMENT AND EVALUATION

Program development refers to the systematic process of identifying the needs of a group of individuals, community, or organization and designing evidence-based programs to meet the needs that have been identified (Centers for Disease Control and Prevention [CDC], 2024). "Program evaluation can help clarify how to improve programs and organizations and produce findings and recommendations for decision-making" (CDC, 2024, n.p.). A capstone with this focus would include approaches, principles, and methods for developing and evaluating occupation-based programs and interventions for individuals, groups, and populations. An essential component of this process is to evaluate the effectiveness and outcomes of the program once it has been implemented. This type of capstone project may address needs assessment, program planning, proposal writing, and measurement of program outcomes on a deeper level. Program development could take place in clinical and/or community (role-emerging) settings.

Furthermore, as health-care policy is continually evolving, greater emphasis is being placed on chronic disease management, care coordination, wellness, and prevention, which provide opportunities for program development for the capstone student. Although the focus areas stipulated by ACOTE do not specifically distinguish program development into clinical and community settings, recommendations for both are provided separately in these next sections.

CLINICAL PROGRAM DEVELOPMENT

Developing and testing outcomes of occupational therapy programs in clinical settings and determining how to evaluate the outcomes of the program developed. This could include any type of occupational therapy setting, such as inpatient or outpatient rehabilitation, medical, or mental health facilities.

Types of Sites and Settings

Examples include hand therapy, geriatrics, pediatrics, mental health, rehabilitation, and school-based occupational therapy, among others.

Capstone Project Ideas Within the Clinical Program Development and Evaluation Focus Area

The capstone project with a program development focus can take many forms. A few examples include the following:

- Development and implementation of a sensory diet for children with ASD in a school setting
- Creation of a bedside cognitive rehabilitation program for adults with chemotherapy cognitive-induced impairment in an acute-care hospital
- Development of an aquatic therapy safety awareness program for children who have ASD and their parents.
- Creation of a Snoezelen room or space in a dementia-care unit to manage agitation (Berkheimer et al., 2017).
- Creation of a "reverse" activities of daily living program on an inpatient rehabilitation unit to address sleep routine and sleep hygiene.
- Establishment of an occupational therapy–based program to address postpartum/perinatal depression within a behavioral health unit.

COMMUNITY PROGRAM DEVELOPMENT

Program development focus areas could also occur in the community at role-emerging sites. If you choose this focus area, you may be responsible for developing a program or product idea and operationalizing it based on a specific need in the community, site, or population. Part of program development is evaluating outcomes of your program, as this is an important component of program development and is included within this focus area. Depending on the needs, this may also entail seeking grant funding to address sustainability.

Types of Sites and Settings

Examples of sites can include homeless shelters, programs for at-risk youth, long-term structured residence (LTSR), veteran programs, inner-city outreach programs, criminal justice settings, foster care, adult day-care facilities, or psychosocial clubhouses, to name a few possibilities.

Capstone Project Ideas Within the Community Program Development and Evaluation Focus Area

The capstone project with a focus on program development can also include the following examples of capstone projects:

- Development and implementation of a community wellness program for individuals who have a history of polysubstance use in a halfway house.
- Creation and execution of a sleep hygiene program in a day program for veterans with posttraumatic stress disorder.
- Creation of sensory-friendly programs at a museum (Fletcher et al., 2018) or other public spaces, such as a sports arena, zoo, or theater. (See Text Box 2-5.)
- Implementation of an evidence-based program for self-management of chronic disease (e.g., diabetes mellitus) in a primary care setting.
- Development of a university therapeutic sensory garden to enhance student, faculty, and staff sense of well-being and quality of life (Stepansky et al., 2023).
- Initiate and implement a medication management program for individuals with intellectual disabilities in an adult day program.

TEXT BOX 2-5

Through assessment and evidence from the literature, one capstone student developed an accessibility report for a children's museum to provide strategies and guidelines to improve accessibility for children to engage with the exhibits (Sharlow, 2024). In this example, the student evaluated the effectiveness of the program by obtaining feedback from the staff and those who participated in the training and carried out the strategies recommended.

POLICY DEVELOPMENT

A policy development focus area for a capstone could include working and collaborating with recognized individuals who are engaged at federal, state, or regional legislative levels to develop and implement innovative programs or to create evidence-based health and social policy.

Types of Sites and Settings

Examples can include local, regional, state, or national offices. This can include using a state organization or a national organization such as AOTA as a capstone site.

Capstone Projects Within the Policy Development Focus Area

The capstone project with a focus on policy can take many forms. Examples include, but are not limited to, the following:

- Analyze a local, state, or national health-care policy, and propose a change in the policy and implementation of the policy.
- Work with a legislator to propose policy changes related to access to and reimbursement for occupational therapy.
- Create and implement a professional development plan indicating that you will run for an elected position related to advocacy and legislation.
- Seek out and engage in lobbying efforts with national interest groups, such as the Disability and Rehabilitation Research Coalition (DRRC), as it urges Congress to fully support disability, independent living, and rehabilitation research through a variety of federal agencies.
- Build and participate in a campaign with an elected official that aligns with important issues that matter to the occupational therapy profession.
- Establish a framework to propose justice, equity, diversity, inclusion, and belonging (JEDIB) policies within a school or college of health sciences.

(See Text Box 2-6.)

TEXT BOX 2-6

A capstone student analyzed current DEI practice standards within an OTD program and student and faculty perception of diffusion into the classroom setting to evaluate and make future recommendations to increase the understanding and real-life application of DEI to further our profession (Smith, 2022).

ADVOCACY

A focus area in advocacy could include working and collaborating with recognized individuals that are engaged at the federal and state legislative levels regarding issues that affect our practice (such as reimbursement and scope of practice guidelines). (See Text Box 2-7.)

Types of Sites and Settings

Examples can include community organizations, state and national organizations, and offices of legislators.

Capstone Project Ideas Within the Advocacy Practice Area

The capstone project with a focus on advocacy can take many forms. Some examples include the following:

- Develop and test a program that improves consumers' abilities to navigate health systems to improve access to, delivery of, or outcomes of health care.
- Create a referral pathway for occupational therapy in a primary care setting.
- Generate and implement an advocacy project to help promote CarFit with local offices, such as the American Automobile Association (AAA) and the American Association for Retired Persons (AARP).
- Plan and implement an advocacy project, such as AOTA's Capitol Hill Day.
- Create and implement a community occupational therapy advocacy project, such as backpack awareness in a public school district or fall prevention initiative in a retirement community.
- Complete an in-depth analysis and policy statement regarding a particular practice issue.
- Work with an advocacy special interest group within a state organization to lobby for critical scope of practice issues, such as encroachment.

TEXT BOX 2-7

One capstone student advocated for the integration of occupational therapy services in the transplant continuum of care through collection of data from clinicians and patients to define the need for OT services (Koppen, 2024).

EDUCATION

A focus area in education would explore the role of the occupational therapist as educator, which could include various communities of learners, such as clients, staff, and students in community, clinical, and classroom settings. Understanding adult learning theory, comparing and contrasting pedagogy and andragogy, creating a teaching philosophy statement, addressing learning styles and other essential aspects of being an educator (such as student assessment and instructional design), and curriculum development are examples of individualized learning objectives that may be used to guide a capstone student to engage in in-depth learning in a focus area of education. Collaborating and working with individuals who are actively pursuing an academic career or who have expertise in education, which can also include individuals that may have expertise in developing continuing education modules, programs, or academic publishers. Examples include understanding academic institution culture and policies; attending academic meetings; performing literature reviews to learn more about pedagogy, andragogy, and curriculum design; and assisting in teaching and mentoring students. Clair et al. (2022) developed a process framework to assist capstone students who are developing a focus area in education which you may find beneficial if education will be your focus area.

Types of Sites and Settings

Examples can include school systems; higher education settings, including occupational therapy assistant and occupational therapy degree levels; and other sites that have employees/staff who require annual training/learning.

Capstone Project Ideas Within the Education Focus Area

The capstone project with an education focus area can take many forms depending on the student's interest. Examples include, but are not limited to, the following:

- Academic or elective course development
- Curricular development and testing of learning outcomes of coursework in traditional and/or online educational environments with occupational therapy or occupational therapy assistant students
- Development and implementation of a hybrid (face-to-face and online) occupational therapy course
- Development and implementation of a continuing education course or instructional webinar
- Client/family education program
- Curricular development and testing of learning outcomes of coursework in traditional and/or online educational environments with clients and/or their families and caregivers
- Development of an educational program at a local pool geared toward promoting water safety among the ASD population
- Staff development program (i.e., creating a staff development training program at a local recreation center on best practice approaches to work with children with disabilities)
- Education and training on sexuality and intimacy in rehabilitation to promote occupational justice and holistic health care (Spencer, 2022)
- Development of a training module for staff in a disaster relief organization (such as American Red Cross, FEMA, and UNICEF) on cultural humility concepts
- Development of training modules for staff in a hospice facility on end-of-care occupational engagement
- Consultation with a school system bus service to create an evidence-based child-passenger safety protocol

- Textbook or instructional technology development
- Development of publishable teaching materials or instructional technology designed for occupational therapy or other health professional, non-health professionals, consumer, or family audiences
- Development of a systematic review of best practice guidelines and an outcome product, such as clinical guidelines, a tool kit, or a video that can be used for educational purposes, manuscript for children's book on disabilities awareness, resource manual for parents of children with special needs
- Creation of a professional development course for OT practitioners covering the social determinants of health (Clair et al., 2022)
- Identify technology supports for individuals with IDD living within a supportive apartment community, and provide the site with educational resources, technology supports based on assessment outcomes, and in-service training (Harris, 2023).

LEADERSHIP

Leadership is noted as an essential theoretical perspective and tenet of the occupational therapy profession, and therefore, all occupational therapy students are exposed to leadership styles in their didactic education via ACOTE B.2.11. A capstone focus area of leadership can involve working and collaborating with recognized individuals who are involved in exercising influence and representing different areas of the profession regionally, nationally, and internationally. This may involve you stepping out of your "comfort zone" to engage in effective and meaningful collaboration with clients, other professionals, and key stakeholders and not only to adapt and adjust to changing systems and practices but to become transformational in leadership outcomes. Individualized learning objectives within this focus area may include exploration of personal styles of leadership, re-examination of leadership theories, and thorough assessment and critique of a leadership project.

Types of Sites and Settings

Examples include a mentored experience at the World Health Organization, National Institutes of Health, other national volunteer organizations (such as the AOTA), the National Board Certification for Occupational Therapy, state organizations, and other not-for-profit organizations.

Capstone Project Ideas Within the Leadership Focus Area

The capstone project with a leadership focus area can take many forms. Examples include the following:
- Create and implement a leadership development project, such as leadership training, with your state

occupational therapy association or licensure board related to occupational therapy practice and policy.
- Create and implement a leadership project within your student organization, such as Student Occupational Therapy Association (SOTA) or Coalition of Occupational Therapy Advocates for Diversity (COTAD).
- Create and implement a leadership initiative within your state organization to increase membership.
- Develop and administer staff instruction and training to create a culture of safety through education by teaching other disciplines about patient handling (Copolillo et al., 2010).

ROLES AND FUNCTIONS OF AN OCCUPATIONAL THERAPY PRACTITIONER

The ACOTE focus areas for the capstone provide a framework to propel you to develop and synthesize in-depth knowledge. Depending on the focus area you choose, this could (potentially) move you beyond a generalist level in a concentrated area. In layperson terms, a *generalist* can be described as a "jack-of-all-trades, a master of none." Occupational therapy generalists are expected to have comprehensive skills and knowledge from a set of core knowledge that is essential for all occupational therapy practitioners (established by ACOTE) and deliver care across a spectrum of ages, conditions, and practice settings. The role of an occupational therapy practitioner has long been referred to as multifaceted (see Figure 2-1) even at the generalist level and demands a vast set of responsibilities, functions, and performance areas (American Occupational Therapy Association [AOTA], 1993).

In contrast, specialists acquire a deeper understanding of specific areas of practice, a particular aspect of occupational therapy, or knowledge of impairments (Foto, 1996). If you take a moment to review the basic role descriptors in Table 2-2, you may become inspired as you think about your potential individuals to serve as content experts.

It can be difficult for you at the beginning of your capstone journey as you grapple with feeling like you might not yet have the skills or knowledge to understand what you want to do or how you will be able to obtain the skills necessary to prove competency in one of the focus areas. If you are feeling this way, you are not alone. Just keep moving forward and know this process is iterative and not a straight-line trajectory; you will be moving through stages as you gain the skills you desire.

Benner's (1984) model, which appeared in *From Novice to Expert: Promoting Excellence and Power in Clinical Nursing Practice*, frames skill acquisition as moving through various stages. The five stages are (1) novice, (2) advanced beginner, (3) competent, (4) proficient, and (5) expert. (See Table 2-3.)

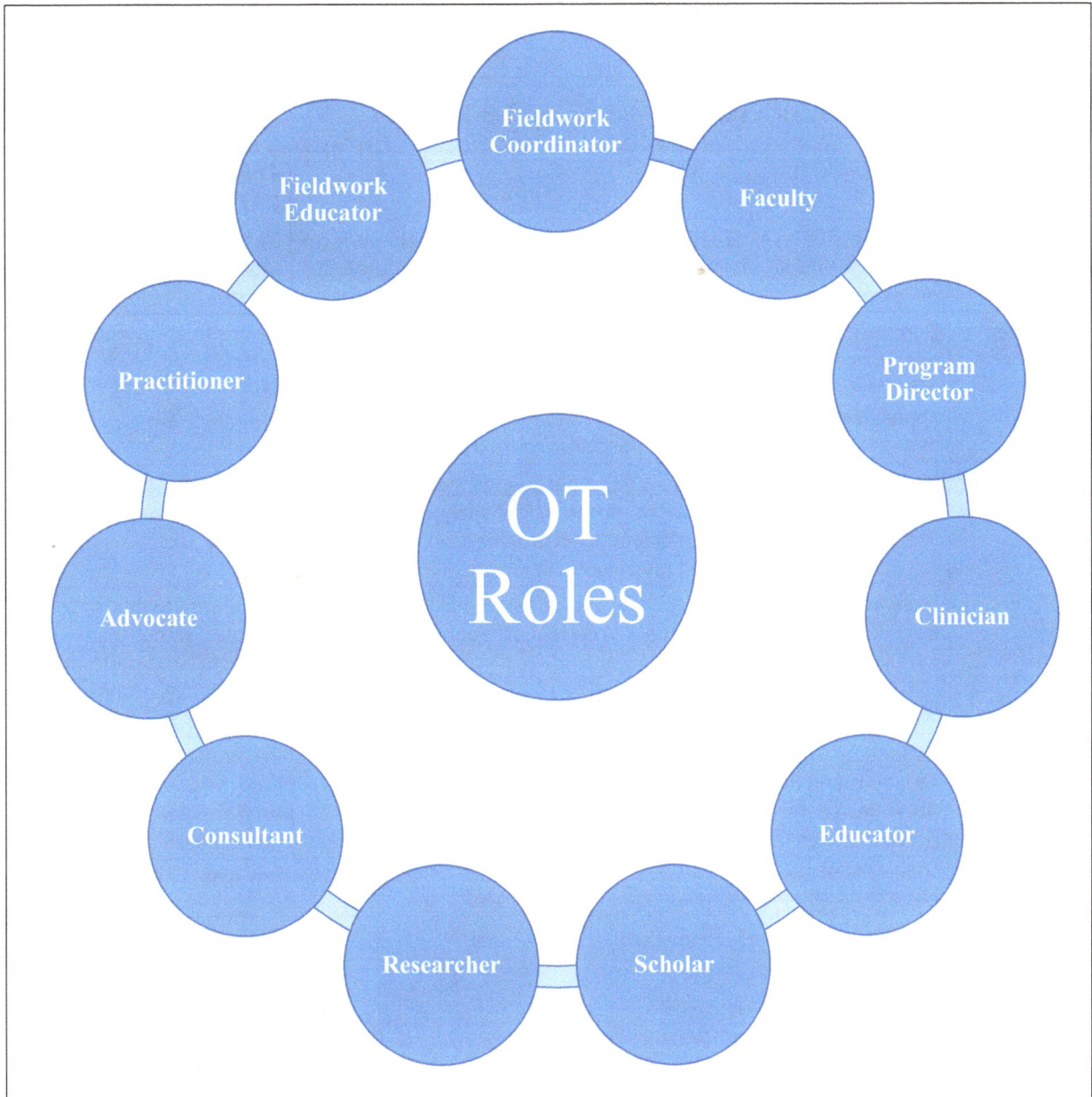

Figure 2-1. OT Roles. *Source:* Adapted from American Occupational Therapy Association (1993). Occupational therapy roles. *American Journal of Occupational Therapy, 47,* pp. 1087–1099. https://doi.org/10.5014/ajot.47.12.1087.

Table 2-2. Occupational Therapist Roles and Functions

OCCUPATIONAL THERAPIST ROLE	MAJOR FUNCTION
Practitioner	Provide assessment, intervention, and program planning and implement discharge planning.
Educator	Develop and provide educational offerings and trainings.
Fieldwork educator	Manage level I or level II fieldwork in practice setting while providing opportunities for students to fulfill practitioner competencies.
Supervisor	Manage overall daily operations of occupational therapy services.
Administrator	Manage department, program, services, or agency providing occupational therapy services.
Researcher/scholar	Examine, develop, refine, and evaluate the profession's body of knowledge and theoretical and philosophical foundations.

Source: Adapted from American Occupational Therapy Association (1993). Occupational therapy roles. *American Journal of Occupational Therapy, 47,* pp. 1087–1099. https://doi.org/10.5014/ajot.47.12.1087.

Table 2-3. Benner's Model of Skill Development

STAGE	DESCRIPTION	APPLICATION TO THE CAPSTONE
Novice	Beginner with no experience; taught general rules to help perform tasks, for example, "Tell me what to do and I'll do it"; learners focus on learning the rules of a particular skill.	Needs constant guidance; seeks affirmation regularly.
Advanced beginner	Demonstrates acceptable performance; has gained prior experience in actual situations to recognize recurring components; principles are based more on experience. Learners focus on applying the rules of a skill in specific situations that become increasingly dependent on the particular context of the situation.	Begins to apply knowledge and skills.
Competent	More aware of long-term goals, gains perspective from planning own actions based on conscious, abstract, and analytical thinking, and helps achieve greater efficiency and organization. Learners see actions in terms of long-range goals or plans.	Consciously aware of their skills.
Proficient	More holistic understanding; improved decision-making. Learns from experiences what to expect in certain situations and how to modify plans.	Perceives situations as "wholes" rather than "aspects," and performance is guided by intuitive behavior.
Expert	No longer relies on principles, rules, or guidance to connect situations and determine actions; has an intuitive grasp of situations. Learners integrate mastered skills with their own personal styles	Performance is now fluid, flexible, and highly proficient (within their focus area).

Source: Adapted from Benner, P. (1984). From novice to expert: Excellence and power in clinical nursing practice. Addison-Wesley and Deluliis, E. D. (2017). Professionalism across occupational therapy clinical practice. SLACK Incorporated.

As you begin your capstone journey, you are naturally a novice, requiring guidance and focusing on all the required components of the doctoral capstone. So at this point in time, if you feel like a novice, you are completely on track and are starting at the point that all students begin. It will take time to move into the next stages, but by the end of your 14-week capstone experience and the completion of your capstone project, you will feel proficient or even an expert within your focus area and your specific capstone project. Through the doctoral capstone process, you will develop competency, proficiency, and expertise by knowing "how," not knowing "what." This provides a useful lens for you to view your progression as you move toward and through your capstone experience.

Researchers have demonstrated that it takes time to gain expertise. The capstone is not designed for you to obtain expert-level skills but, instead, to develop an in-depth knowledge and skill set in a focused area that is developed under mentorship over 14 weeks. The ACOTE focus areas provide opportunities for you to learn outside of the traditional scope of practice and develop an in-depth skill(s) and knowledge in the focused area of study.

STUDENT SECTION CHAPTER SUMMARY

As you finish reading this chapter, the hope is you have found some inspiration to initiate and move forward on your capstone journey. You may be finding as you research sites, populations, and the focus areas that you are being challenged in your views, values, or beliefs. You may begin to question your previous understanding of situations, problems, or assumptions you have made, and this is good; learning is occurring as you are questioning the status quo and embracing the ambiguity of the capstone experience and project process. As you move into the next chapters, you will begin to think further about how to match with a site and how to clearly define your population and the experience you would like to achieve. Keep your mind open, and have that creative confidence that you will find the best fit for yourself, your site, and the clients and population you want to serve.

STUDENT LEARNING ACTIVITIES

1. List two or three potential populations with which you would be interested in gaining in-depth knowledge.

a. For each population, identify an occupational therapy–related outcome (using the Occupational Therapy Practice Framework: Domain and Process – Fourth Edition; AOTA, 2020) that you will want to help the participants achieve. (Also, think about how you might measure this outcome – more on that topic is featured in Chapter 12.)

2. List two or three potential settings where you would be interested in gaining in-depth knowledge.

a. Are these traditional or role-emerging settings?

b. How do they complement your planned fieldwork experiences?

Section 2: Educator Focus

Transformational Learning Phases and Framework for the Educator

As an educator, you want to determine how to best move your students through the stages of development, planning, implementation, and dissemination of the doctoral capstone. A way to facilitate doctoral students' understanding of the capstone experience and project is to utilize Mezirow's transformational learning framework (Mattila et al., 2020). This chapter focuses on development and the understanding of the ACOTE areas of focus for the doctoral capstone. When doctoral students are in this initial development phase, they will be challenged with trying to understand the doctoral capstone and how it relates to their learning. Mattila and colleagues (2020) found that students during the development phase of the capstone often experienced challenges that led to a "disorienting dilemma" or "self-examination." Doctoral students, as they begin their capstone journey, are often drawn to a specific population and a setting through a "disorienting dilemma," which is the first step in Mezirow's transformational learning theory (Mattila et al., 2020). This is the first step in the doctoral capstone learning process. This chapter will assist you as the educator to apply principles of transformational learning theory to learning activities to facilitate the students learning of the ACOTE focus areas.

EDUCATOR OBJECTIVES

By the end of reading this chapter, the educator will be able to apply principles of transformational learning theory to structure learning activities, assignments, and/or assessments in order to promote the capstone students' ability to:

1. Describe each of the ACOTE areas of focus.

2. Compare and contrast the areas of focus across different types of settings.

3. Formulate general ideas for a capstone project within each of the areas of focus.

ACOTE AREAS OF FOCUS

The ACOTE standards indicate that the capstone student must demonstrate and synthesize in-depth knowledge and application of knowledge gained through an in-depth experience, where occupational therapy is currently practiced or settings where it is emerging. In-depth practice gives capstone students a greater opportunity to immerse themselves in evidence-based practice and include data collection for interventions (Case-Smith et al., 2014). The capstone must include one or more of the following focus areas: clinical skills, research skills, administration, program development and evaluation, policy development, advocacy, education, or leadership (ACOTE, 2023). Guided by these focus areas, the doctoral capstone will help occupational therapy students address the complexity of client diagnoses, requirements to collect and analyze clinical data, use evidence-based practice, emphasize health promotion programs, and strengthen interprofessional relationships (Case-Smith et al., 2014). The capstone requires students to seek knowledge in practice competencies and service delivery models and be able to synthesize and apply knowledge gained. This will help future occupational therapy practitioners assume advanced roles in practice settings, such as a direct care provider, consultant, educator, manager, leader, researcher, and advocate.

KNOWLEDGE ACQUISITION

To further understand experience and competence continuums, it can be helpful to look toward the Dreyfus and Dreyfus Skill Acquisition Model (Dreyfus & Dreyfus, 1980) and the Benner Stages of Clinical Competence (Benner, 1984). Dreyfus and Dreyfus (1980) developed a framework of skill acquisition that provides developmental stages of competency for the mental processing, logic, and principles that guide reasoning as one advances through the various stages of skill attainment. Dreyfus and Dreyfus propose four stages: (1) novice, (2) competence, (3) proficiency, and (4) expertise (Table 2-2). Patricia Benner, a nursing scholar and theorist, reworked the model created by Dreyfus and Dreyfus (1980) and presented the novice-to-expert continuum to describe the process through which nurses develop skills and understanding, as well as experience, over time. Benner's (1984) model, which appeared in *From Novice to Expert: Promoting Excellence and Power in Clinical Nursing Practice*, also frames skill acquisition as moving through various stages, yet in a more suggestive manner. The five stages are (1) novice, (2) advanced beginner, (3) competent, (4) proficient, and (5) expert (Table 2-3).

A commonality of these frameworks is that feedback and self-monitoring decrease over time and with experience. An individual develops competency, proficiency, and expertise by knowing "how," not knowing "what." This provides a useful lens to view the progression of the capstone student.

Occupational therapy educators can use research-based frameworks in the preparation of capstone students. According to Benner (1984), an expert has a deep connection and understanding of the situation (Table 2-3). Although the language used by ACOTE to describe the capstone does not include *expert*, experience (in conjunction with reflection) is depicted as having a significant impact on the development of professional growth and innovative change and is a prerequisite for expertise. The combination of higher-level learning didactic requirements and in-depth practice and experience (such as the 14-week capstone) can allow the capstone student to move along the continuum of skill development and help better discern the capstone student moving beyond the generalist and developing increased professional maturity in a chosen focus area.

As an educator, you can look to other clinical doctorate degrees for guidance in how they describe practice beyond a generalist or introductory stage. For example, the International Council of Nursing defines *advanced practice* as the demonstration of skills that reflect an expert knowledge base, complex decision-making skills, and clinical competencies for expanded practice, the characteristics of which are shaped by the context in which services are being provided (ICN Nurse Practitioner/Advanced Practice Nursing Network, 2018). Physical therapy organizations in the United Kingdom use the term *advanced practice physiotherapy* (APP) to describe a clinician with advanced skills, knowledge, and attitudes, together with the core set of physiotherapy skills and knowledge, tailored to individual patients and local environments (Chartered Society of Physiotherapy, 2018). Although a different degree level, the American Physical Therapy Association (2017) has an Advanced Proficiency Pathway for physical therapist assistants, which is curricula that include a group of didactic courses and mentored clinical experiences. Pharmacy educational programs are also adopting similar language, such as the advanced practice pharmacist. For example, the University of Southern California's School of Pharmacy offers an advanced practice pharmacy curriculum, which requires a residency training program and at least 1,500 hours of direct patient care services. These examples support the combination of didactic and mentored-experiential learning.

The capstone is not designed to develop practitioners with expert-level skills but instead to develop knowledge and skill set in a focused area that is developed under mentorship over 14 weeks. The ACOTE focus areas provide opportunities for occupational therapy students to learn outside of the traditional scope of practice and apply knowledge gained in the focused area of study.

FRAMING THE ACOTE FOCUS AREAS

With mentorship from their faculty and doctoral capstone coordinator, capstone students need to have a clear understanding of what the focus areas are and how they complement their previous fieldwork experiences and professional development plan. The DCE and project should be directly aligned with one or a combination of focus areas. The student section of this chapter describes each area of focus and gives the student some examples to think about and become inspired through brainstorming. In the educator section, we will give teaching tips to facilitate student learning. Although ACOTE indicates that the capstone should be designed and administered by faculty and provided in setting(s) consistent with the program's curriculum design, the capstone should be a mutual benefit for the student and the site.

Note: Depending on your institution's mission, program philosophy, or curricular design, as an OTD program, you might only offer a select group of the eight focus areas where students can choose from. Refer back to the educator section in Chapter 1, where we discussed strategies to ensure that the doctoral capstone is integral to your curriculum design.

EVOLVING COMPLIANCE FOR ACCREDITATION OF HEALTH-CARE INSTITUTIONS

One vantage point within the brainstorming process can be to increase one's awareness of the needs, expectations, and requirements of potential sites. Changes to health-care service delivery models, reimbursement systems, and compliance agencies are challenging community and clinical sites to measure outcomes and improve quality. The Joint Commission (TJC) and the Commission on Accreditation of Rehabilitation Facilities (CARF) are just two examples of regulatory bodies that require their certificants to collect and analyze data on specific performance measures and operationalize clinical practice guidelines to ensure evidence-based and quality care.

TJC (n.d.a) accredits and certifies nearly 22,000 health-care organizations and programs in the United States. Accreditation and certification are recognized nationwide as symbols of quality that reflects an organization's commitment to meeting certain performance standards. Accreditation can be earned by an entire health-care organization (e.g., hospitals, nursing homes, ambulatory care centers, office-based surgery practices, home care providers, and laboratories). Certification is earned by programs or services that may be based within or associated with a health care organization (TJC, n.d.b). For example, a TJC-accredited medical center can have TJC-certified programs or services for diabetes or heart disease care. These programs could be within the medical center or in the community.

Similar to ACOTE, which has educational standards, TJC has "National Patient Safety Goals," which are specific areas that accredited facilities need to address in regard to patient safety. For hospital facilities, these include things such as correctly identifying patients, using medicine correctly, using alarms safely, preventing infection, identifying patient safety risks (such as falls or suicide risk), addressing health equity, and preventing mistakes in surgery (TJC, 2024). Various work units within the facility are responsible for creating a process, tracking data, and analyzing outcomes to improve patient safety. In regard to the reduction of falls, a capstone student could be involved in various aspects of this quality initiative, such as creating staff education on best practices in fall prevention, reviewing retrospective data to look for trends among falls, and designing and measuring the impact of activities or interventions to reduce the rate of falls. For instance, outcome measures, such as the Berg Balance Scale (Berg et al., 1989), Functional Reach Test (Duncan et al., 1990), Physical Performance Test (Delbaere et al., 2006), and Timed Up and Go (Podsiadlo & Richardson, 1991), can be used to measure fall risk. When fall risk is high, occupation-based intervention activities to address aspects of dynamic balance can be developed, and these tools can then be used to show improvement during the clients' stay and a reduction in the overall fall rate.

For TJC, reporting requirements include non-standardized measures (stage I) and standardized measures (stage II). These performance measurements require the collection of monthly data points as an indication of the organization's performance in relation to a specific process or outcome. Table 2-4 provides an overview of the types of performance measures.

CARF is an independent, international, nonprofit accreditor of health and human services in the following areas: aging services, behavioral health, child and youth services, employment and community services, vision rehabilitation, and medical rehabilitation, among others. CARF accredits more than 50,000 programs and services at 25,000 locations. It is a voluntary accreditation that demonstrates accountability to funding sources and referral agencies (CARF, n.d.). The criteria foci for CARF accreditation are similar to TJC's and include the following:

- Reducing risk
- Addressing health and safety concerns

Specific aspects that CARF certification require facilities to demonstrate compliance with accreditation requirements, including, but not limited to, competency of personnel, that services delivered are person-centered and individualized, and that service delivery and communication are based on an acceptable field practice. A capstone student could create competencies or staff training to ensure that employees in a CARF-accredited setting have the knowledge and skills to work with patients of a specific age-group (e.g., neonatal intensive care unit [NICU]), specific skills involved in using specific equipment in the performance of job duties (e.g., the use of the ArmeoSpring technology in an inpatient rehabilitation unit), or competencies related to specific skill or procedure (e.g., manual lymph drainage and complete decongestive therapy for lymphedema management).

Learning and understanding these two international health-care compliance organizations is just one perspective of how the doctoral capstone coordinator and student can think about existing mechanisms in traditional health-care settings that require data collection, outcome measurement, and quality improvement.

A capstone student has a skill set to support these data collection and interpretation initiatives. ACOTE (2023) requires entry-level occupational therapy doctoral students to learn how to collect, analyze, and report data in a systematic manner for evaluation of client and practice

Table 2-4. Overview of Performance Measures

CATEGORY	PROCESSES OR OUTCOMES OF CARE TO EVALUATE	CAPSTONE PROJECT EXAMPLE
Administrative/ financial	Addressing organizational structure for the coordination and integration of services, functions, and activities	Develop and evaluate facility workflow using a contingency diagram to determine worker efficiency and productivity.
Perception of care/service	Patient/customer satisfaction	Create, implement, and evaluate a model for concierge care to proactively address client concerns.
Participants' health status	Examples: falls, vent-associated pneumonias, urinary tract infection rate, central-line infections, restraint use, and medication errors	Create and implement staff training modules based on current evidence regarding fall prevention.

outcomes. Because the outcome and expectations of the capstone differ from those of fieldwork (as discussed in Chapter 1), it is important for the doctoral capstone coordinator and the capstone student to educate the content expert and other essential personnel at the capstone site.

EVOLVING DYNAMIC OF OUR CONSUMERS

Another critical vantage point to consider when planning and developing the capstone is the dynamic of our consumers, whether at the level of an individual client, groups, communities, or populations. At the individual client level, our current health-care consumers are more sophisticated, educated, technologically savvy, and socially connected (Bachman, n.d.). Some literature labels these individuals as empowered health-care consumers rather than patients, placing government agencies, insurance companies, employers, and private companies under greater scrutiny to collect, analyze, and publish data about their facility (McNamara, 2012) and to develop care models that personalize service. Readily available data on patient engagement, care outcomes, and quality measurement are in the hands of consumers, which challenge health systems to be at the top of their game with high-quality outcomes and strong patient satisfaction. Contemporary examples of consumer-driven health care are depicted using a concierge model, which provides a higher level of personal interaction to the patient. Measures of patient satisfaction (such as the Press Ganey patient satisfaction survey) and other patient-oriented report cards will assume increasing importance in the industry.

Occupational therapy doctoral students could work directly with a site to develop their capstone project and improve the patient experience, based on outcomes of a satisfaction survey, such as Press Ganey (2018). For example, after interpreting feedback received from a Press Ganey survey, a site may desire to improve its process in integrating the client and family into a care plan. Capstone students could immerse themselves in the literature surrounding improving the patient experience; interview various health-care providers, clients, and family members; then develop, pilot, and measure the impact of a new procedure to increase client and family involvement in care planning.

HEALTH CARE INDUSTRY ADOPTING PERSON-CENTERED AND TEAM-BASED CULTURE

Although certainly not new to the occupational therapy profession, we are in an era of health systems adopting patient-centeredness, which provides a clear opportunity for occupational therapy practitioners, who have long proclaimed a commitment to embracing a person-centered approach (Law et al., 1995; Tickle-Degnen, 2002). Primary care has been a buzzword among the health-care industry, legislation and policy, and service delivery models. An important aspect of primary care is the integration (and collaboration) of the health-care team and a consumer-centered model. *Team-based care* is defined by the National Academy of Medicine (formerly known as the Institute of Medicine) as

the provision of health services to individuals, families, and/or their communities by at least two health providers who work collaboratively with patients and their caregivers – to the extent preferred by each patient – to accomplish shared goals within and across settings to achieve coordinated, high-quality care.

(Babiker et al., 2014, p. 9)

Interprofessional education, interprofessional collaboration, and interprofessional practice are also well-known concepts used in health science education to better prepare allied health-care students for the evolving demands of the industry.

Across the globe, health-care systems have been adopting person-centered culture and putting importance in the delivery of care that is whole-person oriented, coordinated, and personal (Coulter & Oldham, 2016). A specific aspect of the Patient Protection and Affordable Care Act of 2010, the patient-centered medical home is just one approach designed to facilitate higher-quality care because it is more integrated and personalized. This shift in culture has provided unique and novel opportunities for the discipline of occupational therapy (Dahl-Popolizio & Rogers, 2017), which is rooted in holism, person-centeredness, and inclusion. On behalf of the AOTA, Metzler et al. (2012) discuss implications for the occupational therapy profession in primary care and identify that "developing sustained relationships" is an important aspect of person-centered care that occupational therapy should fully adopt and use. Roberts et al. (2014) built upon this work and further outlined the unique role that the occupational therapy profession plays in primary care. More recently, the white paper "Role of Occupational Therapy in Primary Care" was published (AOTA, 2020). These papers can provide inspiration for both the doctoral capstone coordinator and the student on ideas for the DCE and project.

An important element of the capstone is that it is a clear win–win situation – both for the capstone student's learning and for the growth and sustainability of the capstone site. Increasing quality measures and available evidence will demonstrate a capstone site's commitment to high standards of practice and provide a more competitive edge in the current health-care arena. It is beneficial for the capstone student and doctoral capstone coordinator to be aware of setting or site compliance initiatives and strategic goals during the developing process of the capstone. Appendix 2.A provides a framework of how to brainstorm capstone fit and focus area alignment with sites. (More on this is discussed in Chapters 4 and 6.) Our professional organization, AOTA, also provides some guidance to help understand the rationale of the focus areas.

Vision 2025

A *vision statement* is a public way in which an organization indicates who or what they want to become. It indicates transformation, direction, and growth. Vision 2025 is the transformational roadmap for the future of the AOTA.

> As an inclusive profession, occupational therapy maximizes health, well-being, and quality of life for all people, populations, and communities through effective solutions that facilitate participation in everyday living.
> (AOTA, 2018)

The AOTA further narrows the scope of the organization's future vision by articulating five pillars. Vision 2025 and these five pillars (see Table 2-5) can be used to help explain and understand the value, purpose, and rationale for the purpose of the capstone and more specifically the focus areas.

As part of the capstone development process, the doctoral capstone coordinator and faculty need to empower the capstone student (who is also the next generation of practitioners) to see themselves as leaders and agents of change. The capstone experience provides additional learning opportunities to nurture leadership, communication, and systems skills, which society and our consumers are demanding. Now that we have discussed overarching influences on the ACOTE focus areas and systems and organizations that could be used as inspirational guides for the development of the capstone, let us review how to assist doctoral students in determining which focus area will best meet their needs and the needs of their clients. You may review the specifics of each individual focus area and ideas in the student section of this chapter. What will be presented in this educator section will be ideas to assist with student learning and ideas for learning activities.

Teaching Tip

Organize a panel of former OTD students to talk with students who are engaging in the initial stages of capstone development can be very helpful. These areas of focus can be quite daunting to students as they embark on their capstone journeys, so the more they hear about what others have done and their stories, the more it seems to help the students identify their own focus areas.

Clinical Skills

This focus area is for a student who wants to gain higher-level skills in a particular area of occupational therapy practice. What is difficult with this focus area

Table 2-5. The Five Pillars

PILLAR	DESCRIPTORS/RATIONALE
Effective	• Evidence-based • Client-centered • Profitable or cost-effective • Capstone focus area example: research, clinical practice, administration
Leaders	• Influential • Change agent • Catalysts • Capstone focus area example:
Collaborative	• Teamwork • Systems approach • Outcome-oriented • Capstone focus area example: administration, program development
Accessible	• Responsive • Customized • Capstone focus area example: program development, advocacy, policy
Equity, inclusion, and diversity	• Inclusive • Equitable • Capstone focus area example: advocacy, policy, education

is how it is different from a level II fieldwork experience. As the educator, you will need to facilitate the student's ability to determine how and why the capstone will differ from fieldwork. What will the student utilize to demonstrate the synthesis of their in-depth knowledge related to clinical skills? It may be the completion of an in-depth case study or the completion of a certification course, for example. A student wanting to gain in-depth knowledge and skill within the Parkinson's disease population may get certified in Lee Silverman Voice Treatment (LSVT) BIG during their capstone experience. (See Text Box 2-8 and Text Box 2-9.)

TEXT BOX 2-8

As discussed in Chapter 1, it is essential to collaborate with the academic fieldwork coordinator during the development and planning phase. During their preparation for level II fieldwork, students often have specific ideas or interests that they originally intend to pursue for fieldwork yet are not provided the generalist training that is required. Settings or sites that offer very narrow, more specialized training most likely are not appropriate for level II fieldwork yet offer a great potential capstone experience (more on this collaboration is discussed in Chapter 4).

TEXT BOX 2-9

If the capstone experience requires any direct care or service delivery, it is important for the doctoral capstone coordinator to vet supervision requirements per the site and/or state regulatory board and communicate proactively with the capstone student and site mentor.

Research Skills

This area of focus can allow for students to work alongside faculty on their research agendas and gain skills as a researcher. (See Text Box 2-10.)

TEXT BOX 2-10

Many occupational therapy programs already have a model in their curriculum that includes faculty–student research opportunities, in which students have the opportunity to serve as an apprentice to a faculty member. A capstone focus on research could involve a continuation of this project, yet with greater responsibilities and expectations for the student.

Administration

Aspects of an administration focus area may include a deeper understanding of systems theory to develop system-thinking skills such as a focus on interactions, relationships, and adaptation (Mele et al., 2010). The importance of occupational therapy educators to use systems theory as a structure or framework for learning was noted by occupational therapy pioneer and scholar Mary Reilly (Schemm et al., 1993). Students may work in areas of hospital administration or nonprofit administration. If a student is interested in administration, you may want to connect with hospital administrators or rehabilitation department managers you know to discuss potential ideas to bring back to students. Oftentimes, having community and clinical site partners come to class with ideas for projects will start the discussion of this area of focus and how a student could develop a capstone experience and project around administration.

Program Development and Evaluation

For this practice area, it is important for the student to understand what program development is and the process of program evaluation. Your program may have a specific course focused on program development or it may be a part of a course within the capstone course curriculum. Either way, it is an important educational component of the capstone process. (See Text Box 2-11.)

TEXT BOX 2-11

Oftentimes, program development is a focus area that students tend to gravitate toward. It is helpful for the students to reference other student experiences and projects to gain inspiration. OT practice is a great starting point to identify possible populations and programs that may be a fit, and spending time on the AOTA website in the practice areas can give inspiration.

Policy Development

A capstone student can seek to further explore the distinct value of occupational therapy and health-care reform. Lamb and Metzler (2014) provide a useful framework to inspire capstone projects that may align with initiatives from the Center for Medicare and Medicaid or Primary Care. *Primary care* is defined as care provided by physicians trained for comprehensive first contact, that is, the patient's first entry into the health-care system. Primary care is performed by a physician who often collaborates with other health-care professionals to provide sufficient patient advocacy (American Academy of Family Physicians, 2016). As an educator, you may be able to connect students who want to engage in policy development to organizations working on policies at the local, state, or national level, such as the American Occupational Therapy Political Action Committee. AOTPAC is a voluntary, nonprofit, nonpartisan, unincorporated committee associated with AOTA. The purpose of AOTPAC is to further the legislative aims of the Association by influencing or attempting to influence the selection, nomination, election, or appointment of any individual to any Federal public office, and of any occupational therapist, occupational therapy assistant, or occupational therapy student member of AOTA seeking election to public office at any level.

Advocacy

Oftentimes the student may want to work in the political arena to advocate for occupational therapy services in a state or work with their state OT associations, AOTA, or COTAD. For example, in the state of Pennsylvania, there has been recent, ongoing advocacy initiated by the Board of Directors of the Pennsylvania Occupational Therapy Association and the Pennsylvania Occupational Therapy Political Action Committee (PAC) as the discipline of recreational therapy has sought Pennsylvania state licensure. Language in the proposed scope of practice, from recreational therapy directly encroaches on the existing Pennsylvania Practice Act of Occupational Therapy. A capstone student could be mentored by an individual on the PAC or the state licensing board to build an awareness campaign and launch a statewide initiative.

Education

Students often want to focus on educating others in health care, whether it be clients, families, or health-care workers. Some students may have an interest in working with a faculty member to address a curricular need and/or gain some experience in academia. (See Text Box 2-11.)

TEXT BOX 2-11

I had a student who was interested in education and wanted to work with the older adult population. Since I teach the OT practice course on productive aging in our program, I asked if she had an interest in working alongside me to integrate CarFit into the course and determine the impact on second-year OTD students. The student determined this was a good fit and developed the following capstone purpose:

The purpose of this project was to understand OTD students' perceived experiences of a CarFit training program and to determine if CarFit should be added to the OTD curriculum. Through this exploration, the project aim was to provide insight and guidance to older adults attending a CarFit event and to provide experiential learning for IU OTD students who will prepare for and execute their evaluation skills with older adults.

(Instenes, 2024, pp. 4–5)

After completion of the capstone project, the student determined that adding CarFit in the OTD curriculum could make a positive impact on second-year OTD students and align with the curriculum by

---

TEXT BOX 12-3 (continued)

providing the students with a socially responsive health-care experience and education on productive ageing (Instenes, 2024, p. 12).

Julie A. Bednarski, OTD, MHS, OTR, OT,
Program Director and Clinical Associate Faculty,
Indiana University Indianapolis

Leadership

Examples of leadership theories that may be beneficial for a capstone student to engage in a self-study to support in-depth learning and exposure to this focus area could include completion of the Six Sigma Leadership certifications (Atmaca & Girenes, 2011).

Occupational Therapy Leaders and Legacies Society is a member organization that is made up of a community of occupational therapy leaders who have demonstrated expertise in leadership abilities and skills. Members of the society design and lead projects that honor occupational therapy history and social contributions, as well as recognize and engage those individuals whose contributions have sustained and enriched the profession (Kolodner, 2018).

Doctoral capstone coordinators and doctoral students can explore existing leadership projects and/or promote the idea of a leadership project with Occupational Therapy Leaders and Legacies Society to support a focus area in leadership for the capstone. (See Text Box 2-12.)

TEXT BOX 2-12

Teaching Tip: To start the inspiration process for the students, having program graduates come to class to discuss their capstone experiences and projects will help. If you set up a panel of recent graduates who can speak on the different focus areas, it will help reduce the ambiguity of these focus areas. The students are at the point in the process where they need to hear concrete examples and hear from students who went through the process and were successful. Another idea is to have a panel of potential content experts come in to discuss their site and the needs of the site and project ideas. It is important to provide examples to the students and provide connections for the students so they can begin to create a vision for what they want to do for their individualized experiences. It is also helpful to continue to build on the relationships with the sites and build upon previous capstone projects to work toward sustainability. Students often think they have to come up with a totally "new" idea for a capstone, so it is important that they begin to understand the idea that their experience can build upon a previous student's experience.

EDUCATOR CHAPTER SUMMARY

Vision 2025 and other influences in health care, community practice, and society are all sculpting the occupational therapy profession to pursue advanced roles in diverse settings. The growing focus on the provision of high-quality health care has significantly altered occupational therapy service delivery in the spectrum of health-care settings. The occupational therapy profession continues to make the necessary adaptations in response to these challenges. Through the focus areas and doctorate capstone experience, occupational therapy doctoral students can develop knowledge and refine skills in practice areas, such as consultant, educator, manager, leader, researcher, and advocate for the profession and the consumer, to meet the unique demands of the time (Molitor & Nissen, 2018). The capstone creates meaningful opportunities that can have a positive impact on individuals, groups, and populations and, at the same time, offer the capstone student opportunities for professional growth in an identified focus area. It is because of this that the capstone should be viewed (and marketed to potential DCE sites) as a win–win scenario. The capstone allows the development of forward-thinking students who, through mentorship, have the opportunity to design, evaluate, educate, and lead. A critical element to support success of the development of the capstone is rooting the capstone in evidence and collaboration and communication among the capstone team. The authors build on this foundation in subsequent chapters.

REFERENCES

Accreditation Council for Occupational Therapy Education. (2023). *2023 Accreditation Council for Occupational Therapy Education (ACOTE®) standards and interpretive guide.* https://acoteonline.org/accreditation-explained/standards/

Agency for Healthcare Research and Quality. (2023). *TeamSTEPPS 2.0.* https://www.ahrq.gov/teamstepps/instructor/index.html

American Academy of Family Physicians. (2016). *Primary care.* https://www.aafp.org/about/policies/all/primary-care.html

American Occupational Therapy Association. (1993). Occupational therapy roles. *American Journal of Occupational Therapy, 47,* 1087–1099. https://doi.org/10.5014/ajot.47.12.1087

American Occupational Therapy Association. (2018). *Vision 2025.* https://www.aota.org/Publications-News/AOTANews/2018/AOTA-Board-Expands-Vision-2025.aspx

American Occupational Therapy Association. (2020). Role of occupational therapy in primary care. *The American Journal of Occupational Therapy, 74*(Suppl. 3). https://doi.org/10.5014/ajot.2020.74S3001

American Occupational Therapy Association. (2024). *AOTA.* https://www.aota.org

American Physical Therapy Association. (2017). *About the PTA advanced proficiency pathways (APP) program.* http://www.apta.org/APP/About

Atmaca, E., & Girenes, S. S. (2011). Lean six sigma methodology and application. *Quality & Quantity, 47,* 2107–2127.

Babiker, A., El Husseini, M., Al Nemri, A., Al Frayh, A., Al Juryyan, N., Faki, M. O., Assiri, A., Al Saadi, M., Shaikh, F., & Al Zamil, F. (2014). Health care professional development: Working as a team to improve patient care. *Sudanese Journal of Paediatrics, 14*(2), 9–16.

Bachman, R. E. (n.d.). *The future of healthcare consumerism: Empowering consumers through new medical delivery models.* http://www.theihcc.com/en/communities/health_access_alternatives/the-future-of-health-care-consumerism-empowering-htln3omt.html

Benner, P. (1984). *From novice to expert: Excellence and power in clinical nursing practice.* Addison-Wesley.

Berg, K., Wood-Dauphinee, S., Williams, J. I., & Gayton, D. (1989). Measuring balance in the elderly: Preliminary development of an instrument. *Physiotherapy, 41,* 304–311. https://doi.org/10.3138/ptc.41.6.304

Berkheimer, S. D., Qian, C., & Malmstrom, T. K. (2017). Snoezelen therapy as an intervention to reduce agitation in nursing home patients with dementia: A pilot study. *Journal of American Medical Directors Association, 18,* 1089–1091.

Brooks, E. (2024). *The phenomenon of burnout among occupational therapists: A phenomenological mixed methods study* [Doctoral capstone, Indiana University]. ScholarWorks Indianapolis. https://scholarworks.indianapolis.iu.edu/items/b34c4e6b-3cf2-434f-a977-9d02a8180002

Case-Smith, J., Page, S. J., Darragh, A., Rybski, M., & Cleary, D. (2014). The professional occupational therapy doctoral degree: Why do it? *American Journal of Occupational Therapy, 68,* e55–e60. https://doi.org/10.5014/ajot.2014.008805protection/fetp/training_modules/15/community-needs_pw_final_9252013.pdf

Centers for Disease Control and Prevention. (2024). *CDC program evaluation framework 2024.* https://www.cdc.gov/globalhealth/health-protection/fetp/training_modules/15/community-needs_pw_final_9252013.pdf

Chartered Society of Physiotherapy. (2018). *Advanced practice in physiotherapy.* http://www.csp.org.uk/publications/advanced-practice-physiotherapy

Clair, S., Corcoran, S., Bubel, E., & Amini, D. (2022). A process framework for the education-focused capstone: Supporting expansion and sustainable outcomes. *Journal of Occupational Therapy Education, 6*(4). https://doi.org/10.26681/jote.2022.060412

Commission on Accreditation of Rehabilitation Facilities (CARF). (n.d.). *CARF international.* https://carf.org/

Copolillo, A., Shepherd, J., Anzalone, M., & Lane, S. J. (2010). Taking on the challenge of the centennial vision: Transforming the passion for occupational therapy into a passion for leadership. *Occupational Therapy in Health Care, 24,* 7–22. https://doi.org/10.3109/07380570903304209

Coulter, A., & Oldham, J. (2016). Person-centred care: What is it and how do we get there? *Future Hospital Journal, 3*(2), 114–116. https://doi.org/10.7861/futurehosp.3-2-114

Dahl-Popolizio, S., & Rogers, O. (2017). Interprofessional primary care: The value of occupational therapy. *Open Journal of Occupational Therapy, 5*(11), 1–10. https://doi.org/10.15453/2168–6408.1363

de Castro Mehrkens, K. N., & Bateman, T. N. (2024). Utilizing the NANT core competencies to guide the occupational therapy doctoral capstone experience and project in the NICU. *Journal of Occupational Therapy Education, 8*(2). https://encompass.eku.edu/jote/vol8/iss2/19

Delbaere, K., Van den Noortgate, N., Bourgois, J., Vanderstraeten, G., Tine, W., & Cambier, D. (2006). The physical performance test as a predictor of frequent fallers: A prospective community-based cohort study. *Clinical Rehabilitation, 20,* 83–90. https://doi.org/10.1191/0269215506cr885oa

Dreyfus, H., & Dreyfus, S. (1980). *A five-stage model of mental activities involved in directed skill acquisition.* Operations Research Center, University of California.

Duncan, P. W., Weiner, D. K., Chandler, J., & Studenski, S. (1990). Function reach: A new clinical measure of balance. *Journal of Gerontology, 45*(6), 192–197.

Fletcher, T. S., Blake, A. B., & Shelffo, K. E. (2018). Can sensory gallery guides for children with sensory processing challenges improve their museum experience? *Journal of Museum Education, 43,* 66–77. https://doi.org/10.1080/10598650.2017.1407915

Foto, M. (1996). Generalist versus specialist occupational therapists. *American Journal of Occupational Therapy, 50*, 771–774. https://doi.org/10.5014/ajot.50.10.771

Hadley, R. (2024). *Skills on wheels: Program evaluation and modifications to increase the reliability and validity of the wheelchair skills test* [Doctoral capstone, Indiana University]. ScholarWorks Indianapolis. https://scholarworks.indianapolis.iu.edu/items/df7e5a03-a8db-4597-af6d-caa07e958c9b

Harris, B. (2023). *Increasing technology supports for individuals with disabilities* [Doctoral capstone, Indiana University]. ScholarWorks Indianapolis. https://scholarworks.indianapolis.iu.edu/items/569378ff-df4b-4ea3-a198-280ad0c729a8

ICN Nurse Practitioner/Advanced Practice Nursing Network. (2018). *Definition and characteristics of the role.* https://international.aanp.org/Practice/APNRoles

IDEO. (2015). *The field guide to human-centered design.* Ideo.org.

Instenes, H. (2024). *IU occupational therapy doctorate students' perceived experiences on CarFit training* [Doctoral capstone, Indiana University]. ScholarWorks, Indianapolis. https://scholarworks.indianapolis.iu.edu/items/a769402e-2691-43bc-a67d-40c3bc44e2ec

The Joint Commission (TJC). (n.d.a). *Facts about the joint commission.* https://www.jointcommission.org/who-we-are/facts-about-the-joint-commission/#:~:text=The%20Joint%20Commission%20accredits%20and,programs%20in%20the%20United%20States

The Joint Commission (TJC). (n.d.b). *What is certification?* https://www.jointcommission.org/what-we-offer/certification/what-is-certification/

Kolodner, E. (2018). *OT leaders & legacies society.* http://www.otleaders.org/

Koppen, A. (2024). *Advocating for the role of occupational therapy in the transplant continuum of care* [Doctoral capstone, Indiana University]. ScholarWorks Indianapolis. https://scholarworks.indianapolis.iu.edu/items/3767e1cd-b260-4f9b-9c0b-89a7c068d719

Lamb, A. J., & Metzler, C. A. (2014). Defining the value of occupational therapy: A health policy lens on research and practice. *American Journal of Occupational Therapy, 6*, 9–14. https://doi.org/10.5014/ajot.2014.681001

Law, M., Baptiste, S., & Mills, J. (1995). Client-centred practice: What does it mean and does it make a difference? *Canadian Journal of Occupational Therapy, 62*, 250–257.

Lifestyle Medicine. (2024). *American college of lifestyle medicine.* https://lifestylemedicine.org/

Mathieu, H. (2024). *Implementation of a wellness exploration group for women with substance use disorder* [Doctoral capstone, Indiana University]. ScholarWorks Indianapolis. https://scholarworks.indianapolis.iu.edu/items/48572254-0907-4908-8471-2882b4af6913

Mattila, A., Deiuliis, E., & Cook, A. (2020). Evaluating the professional transformation from a doctoral capstone experience. *Journal of Transformative Learning, 7*, 34–44.

McNamara, S. A. (2012). Hospital report cards: What nurses need to know. *AORN Journal, 95*(3), 395–399. https://doi.org/10.1016/j.aorn.2011.12.016

Mele, C., Pels, J., & Polese, F. (2010). A brief review of system theories and their managerial applications. *Service Science, 2*, 126–135.

Metzler, C. A., Hartmann, K. D., & Lowenthal, L. A. (2012). Defining primary care: Envisioning the roles of occupational therapy. *American Journal of Occupational Therapy, 66*, 266–270. https://doi.org/10.5014/ajot.2010.663001

Molitor, W. L., & Nissen, R. (2018). Clinician, educator and student perceptions of entry-level academic degree requirements in occupational therapy education. *Journal of Occupational Therapy Education, 2*, 1–23.

Occupational therapy practice framework: Domain and process-fourth edition. (2020). *The American Journal of Occupational Therapy, 74*(Suppl. 2), 7412410010p1–7412410010p87. https://doi.org/10.5014/ajot.2020.74S2001

Podsiadlo, D., & Richardson, S. (1991). The timed "Up & Go": A test of basic functional mobility for frail elderly persons. *Journal of the American Geriatrics Society, 39*, 142–148. https://doi.org/10.1111/j.1532-5415.1991.tb01616.x

Press Ganey. (2018). *About the Press Ganey survey.* http://www.pressganey.com/solutions/patient-experience/consumerism-transparency/about-the-press-ganey-survey

Pridemore, A. (2021). *Standardizing and organizational approach to hospital accreditation at an inpatient rehabilitation unit* [Doctoral capstone, Indiana University]. ScholarWorks Indianapolis. https://scholarworks.indianapolis.iu.edu/items/7502b594-8458-40d3-8c75-7821c7bc7e12

Roberts, P., Farmer, M. E., Lamb, A. J., Muir, S., & Siebert, C. (2014). The role of occupational therapy in primary care. *American Journal of Occupational Therapy, 68*(3), S25–S33. https://doi.org/10.5014/ajot.2014.686S06

Rogers, A. T., Bai, G., Lavin, R. A., & Anderson, G. F. (2016). Higher hospital spending on occupational therapy is associated with lower readmission rates. *Medical Care Research, and Review, 74*, 668–686. https://doi.org/10.1177/1077558716666981

Schemm, R. L., Corcoran, M., Kolodner, E., & Schaaf, R. (1993). A curriculum based on systems theory. *American Journal of Occupational Therapy, 47*(7), 625–634. https://doi.org/10.5014/ajot.47.7.625

Sharlow, T. (2024). *Addressing early childhood accessibility at a children's museum: A community based capstone project* [Doctoral capstone, Indiana University]. ScholarWorks Indianapolis. https://scholarworks.indianapolis.iu.edu/items/3f10ff36-57b7-4212-badd-8ce3110d4256

Smith, C. (2022). *Diversity, equity, and inclusion practices: Student and educator perspectives* [Doctoral capstone, Indiana University]. ScholarWorks Indianapolis. https://scholarworks.indianapolis.iu.edu/items/cad13ba7-5d9c-489b-b9f4-2094df1d97e1

Spencer, B. (2022). *Promoting occupational justice and holistic healthcare: Education and training on sexuality and intimacy in rehabilitation* [Doctoral capstone, Indiana University]. ScholarWorks Indianapolis. https://scholarworks.indianapolis.iu.edu/items/aa339acd-42cb-412a-a0c2-608eef8e6a1b

Stepansky, K., Delbert, T., & Bucey, J. C. (2023). *Therapeutic impact of engagement in green spaces.* IntechOpen. https://doi.org/10.5772/intechopen.1001148

Sweeney, K. (2024). *Improving patient and clinician education in upper extremity rehabilitation* [Doctoral capstone, Indiana University]. ScholarWorks Indianapolis. https://scholarworks.indianapolis.iu.edu/server/api/core/bitstreams/33224d30-3de7-49c0-9b4c-e5c2c72af5fa/content

Tickle-Degnen, L. (2002). Client centered practice, therapeutic relationships and the use of research evidence. *American Journal of Occupational Therapy, 56*(4), 470–474.

TJC. (2024). *Hospital: 2024 national patient safety goals.* https://www.jointcommission.org/standards/national-patient-safety-goals/hospital-national-patient-safety-goals/

APPENDICES

Appendix 2-A Framework to Help Guide Brainstorming of Doctoral Capstone Experience Fit at a Site

Appendix 2-A

FRAMEWORK TO HELP GUIDE BRAINSTORMING OF DOCTORAL CAPSTONE EXPERIENCE FIT AT A SITE

Type of site:

Review accreditations/certifications/outcome measures tracked/measured:

LTG of Department/Work Unit: 3 to 5 years

1.

2.

3.

STG of Department/Work Unit (6 months to 3 years):

1.

2.

3.

4.

5.

Individuals with specialty training/expertise (in and outside of your department/work unit):

1.

2.

3.

4.

Brainstorm an idea for a DCE experience/project using the following focus areas:

1. Clinical skills

2. Research skills

3. Administration

4. Program development and evaluation

5. Policy development

6. Advocacy

7. Education

8. Leadership

CHAPTER 3

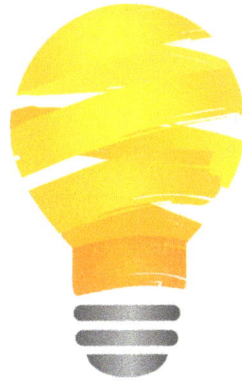

Practice-Ready and Mentorship Skills for the Capstone

Michelle McCann and Amy Mattila

Section 1: Student Focus

Human-centered design mindsets for the doctoral student. The human-centered design mindsets of learning from failure and having optimism are important to reflect on as the capstone student begins to develop self-efficacy and emotional intelligence.

Learning from failure. Do not get down on yourself if something you planned or developed does not work out in the first iteration – this is normal and expected. It is how you react to the failure that can affect change and growth. What is important is that you learn from something that failed, because when you do, you then are failing forward. You are reflecting on what went wrong and then making necessary adjustments; this is moving forward! As painful as it may seem, you grow from failures when you stop and reflect and do not take failures personally.

Optimism. Here is that word again – it must be important! Keep an optimistic mindset, and the entire experience will be much more productive and enjoyable. Find a way to keep your stress under control, which will help you remain optimistic and stay healthy throughout the process.

INTRODUCTION FOR STUDENTS

The descriptor "career-ready" or "practice-ready" has become a buzzword among higher education professional degree programs in depicting desired outcomes and skills sets; however, this may be an unfamiliar concept to you as you consider the transition from student to emerging practitioner. For example, as you move toward careers that need to conform to the health-care organizations requirements, as a novice clinician, you face many clinical challenges as you advance from students to occupational therapy practitioners. For example, in nursing schools across the country, nursing residency programs (NRPs) have been shown to help close the gaps in job-related knowledge, expertise, and attitudes that affect new nurses, health-care organizations, and care quality, by offering real-life instruction and resources for new graduate nurses (Smith, 2021), thereby alleviating some of the practice challenges faced by new graduate nurses (Chant et al., 2019). In addition to business and nursing, allied health-care programs are defining what

DOI: 10.4324/9781003541813-4

it means to be a practice-ready student. Pharmacy and nursing have explored key areas in which their graduates need to develop to be "work-ready" in each of their fields, such as critical thinking, problem-solving, appropriate interprofessional skills, and confidence in autonomous work (Gruenberg et al., 2021; McGarity et al., 2023; Noble et al., 2019). Skill sets of these professionals, and specifically occupational therapy, are often described as either hard skills or soft skills (Hardie et al., 2022; Deepa & Seth, 2013). In many ways, the term *practice-ready* is replacing the commonly used term *soft skills*. In your academic journey so far, you have been exposed to the "hard skills" or competency or technical-based areas of practice. However, concepts such as attitudes and behaviors (soft skills) can be more positively correlated with your success in your fieldwork experiences and beyond (Campbell et al., 2015). In occupational therapy practice, *practice-ready skills* refer to your ability to display competency in entry-level skill – making safe, team-oriented, collaborative, self-directed, professional, and efficient decisions in today's current, productive-driven environment.

In addition to career-readiness preparations, the ACOTE (2023) standards D.1.1 and D.1.6 emphasize how you, as the student, will be collaborative within your capstone team. Cultivating strong relationships with your "team," including the content expert, faculty mentor, and any other key experts, will help enhance your overall capstone experience. Aligned with the American Occupational Therapy Association's (AOTA) Vision 2025, it is essential that you and your capstone team have mutual expectations in establishing a positive mentoring relationship in order that your experience builds the positive attributes and productive behaviors which will be essential in launching your career (Byars-Winston & Dahlberg, 2019). In particular, mentorship is recognized as an integral component of preparing you to be a professional as a whole and is a key aspect in strengthening individual attributes of your professional identity (Henry-Noel et al., 2019; Torres et al., 2021).

As you become more familiar with health-care models and their evolving emphasis on outcome-based and performance-based data to inform care and reimbursement throughout your experiential exposures, you will grow in your proficiency and the ability to demonstrate practice readiness. It is important that you and your content expert form mutual expectations to build a positive relationship early to foster and align learning opportunities together. An essential element in creating this mutual alignment is establishing a communication plan and setting collective goals and expectations from one another (Kroll & Delbert, 2023; Stephenson et al., 2020). When communication plans and expectations are clear between each other, mutual trust is established, and the mentoring relationship benefits (Goodsett, 2021). Collaborative relationships, such as those built through mentorship, will help provide you with essential knowledge and resources for addressing role emerging practice. In short, the end result for you within your occupational therapy educational program

is for graduates to be practice-ready at graduation. This chapter reflects on practice-ready and mentorship skills to facilitate success in your doctoral capstone experience.

STUDENT REFLECTIVE QUESTIONS

1. What challenges or barriers do you anticipate facing during your capstone experience?
2. What type of skills or abilities do you think would be essential to have to overcome these challenges or barriers
3. What action steps can you commit to taking to become "practice-ready" for your capstone?
4. What mentors already exist in your life? How have they contributed to your personal and professional growth?

STUDENT OBJECTIVES

By the end of reading this chapter and completing the learning activities, the reader should be able to:

1. Examine current and potential future challenges and barriers of the capstone experience.
2. Compare and contrast qualities of a successful fieldwork student vs. the expectations of the doctoral student.
3. Compare and contrast mentorship vs. supervision models, and apply best practice to the capstone experience.
4. Identify practice-ready and mentorship skills that are instrumental to the successful completion of the capstone experience.
5. Apply concepts of career readiness through engagement in the capstone experience.

A REVIEW OF ATTRIBUTES OF THE SUCCESSFUL FIELDWORK STUDENT

Traditional fieldwork within occupational therapy has used the apprenticeship model of supervision, in which students are supervised directly on-site by an occupational therapy practitioner (DeIuliis & Hanson, 2022, Chapter 2; Mattila & Dolhi, 2016). Successful placements are often described by having detailed and clear expectations, quality feedback, and a structured learning environment (Rodger et al., 2011). Students at this level of experiential learning are expected to embody the skills and traits of an entry-level practitioner or practice-ready professional at the culmination of the level II fieldwork experiences. As outlined in Chapter 1 of DeIuliis and Hanson (2022), an overview of the traits of a successful fieldwork student is summarized in Table 3-1.

Although these traits will still be essential to your fieldwork education and occupational therapy coursework, additional opportunities and challenges for more autonomy

"When I transitioned from fieldwork to the DCE, there was a shift from depending on my fieldwork educator for direct instruction to becoming the leader of a capstone team. While I felt I had more than adequate supports from faculty and mentors, the DCE curriculum ensures that capstone students learn to take ownership of their projects and have more autonomy than during fieldwork. During my fieldwork, I was provided with daily schedules and structure for student expectations, treatment planning, and evaluations. However, during the DCE, it was expected that I create my own weekly schedule, develop materials and structure for the program, and take initiative to seek out guidance and feedback from mentors.

Some strategies that helped me navigate this transition were keeping a notebook with ongoing questions or ideas to share with the capstone team, proactively reaching out to my mentors with any questions or concerns that arose, and establishing a support network with my peers who were also navigating this transition and developing their capstone projects. I found it beneficial to keep very open communication with all members of the capstone team, to ensure all DCE requirements were being met, and to find a positive peer group who were willing to problem-solve and share resources.

Another aspect of transitioning to the DCE was an emphasis on developing my professional portfolio to prepare starting my career after graduation. During the DCE, I and many peers had opportunities to complete specialized certificates and trainings that were connected to our DCE topic and align with our experiential plan goals. Having these skills and certifications contributed to my practice readiness, stood out to potential employers during interviews, and allowed me and my peers to continue pursuing areas of passion in OT beyond the academic timeline of the DCE.

Completing the DCE offered more flexibility in scheduling than during fieldwork. While this flexibility was an appreciated change from the structured hours of fieldwork, it made me refine skills in time management, prioritizing tasks, anticipating challenges, and proactively communicating to the capstone team. To stay engaged in developing, delivering, and disseminating a capstone project throughout a year, and even beyond, I felt it was important to select a topic that I was passionate to learn more about and motivated to explore.

Some of the skills that helped me expand my knowledge during the DCE was networking with other professionals within my DCE focus area. I found it most helpful to accomplish this through attending conferences, community events, and introductions to individuals with expertise through connections within my capstone team. All these skills have continued to be relevant and useful while beginning my first clinical or role.

During the DCE, it was beneficial to discuss with my capstone team how these skills I was building could be generalized from a specific focus area to an OT role beyond the scope of the capstone. I use the skills I developed during my DCE daily in my clinical role. Completing the DCE gave me the opportunity to refine these skills to develop practice readiness for an OT career."

– Erica Glaneman, OTD, OTR/L,
Duquesne University OTD class of 2023

Table 3-1. Highlights of Traits of Successful Fieldwork Students

A successful fieldwork student:
- Seeks and responds well to feedback
- Is inquisitive and asks questions
- Demonstrates high emotional intelligence and maturity
- Is self-directed and seeks help when necessary
- Builds positive therapeutic relationships
- Demonstrates strong communication and organization skills
- Takes risks
- Collaborates effectively
- Exhibits a commitment to the profession
- Balances productivity, leisure, and rest

Source: Adapted from Deluliis, E., and Hanson, D. (eds.) (2023). *Fieldwork educator's guide to level II fieldwork*. SLACK Incorporated.

and role development may help you identify as a generalist practitioner who now demonstrates in-depth knowledge of delivery models, policies, and systems, as mentioned previously. In addition, due to changes in health-care service delivery, reimbursement demands, and the exponential growth of occupational therapy educational programs across the United States, greater and more diverse opportunities exist for the capstone experience to challenge more traditional models of health care. Attributes that are unique to the successful capstone student are discussed in the next section.

ATTRIBUTES OF A PRACTICE-READY CAPSTONE STUDENT

To meet both the demands of the doctoral capstone experience and current health system needs, a variety of attributes are central to your success as a practice-ready doctoral student, which will help you transition to a mentoring relationship in your capstone. These suggested skills include *confidence* and *perceived self-efficacy*, *high emotional intelligence* and *maturity*, and an *openness to self-directed* and *self-regulated learning*. In addition, the opportunities afforded to you in an intensive mentorship can provide you with team-building capacity to develop a close reciprocal relationship with your content expert within a safe environment to test knowledge and form joint decision-making. In return, building a successful relationship with your content expert can bolster your satisfaction and may provide you with increased confidence, which can lead to greater practice readiness and more team-based work inculturation (Torres et al., 2021). In combination with the curricular structure provided within the scope of your academic program, emphasis on building meaningful connections through mentorship can help you conceptualize your own emerging identity as a professional and the impact on services you wish to embrace. This mentorship approach can prepare you to develop productive, healthy peer relationships, make interprofessional/intraprofessional connections, and advance the quality of recognition of the profession, all with the confidence and maturity of a doctoral graduate. Each of these attributes is explored further in this section of the chapter through a social cognitive approach to learning.

"The doctoral capstone experience has been a pivotal 14-week opportunity. I completed my capstone project and experience that was focused on program development and advanced clinical practice skills on a spinal cord injury unit at an inpatient rehabilitation hospital. During my capstone, I developed a site-specific clinical pathway for interprofessional pressure injury prevention and held weekly educational sessions focused on wound prevention, interprofessional collaboration, and evidence-based practice. Additionally, I was able to work alongside various members of the interdisciplinary team to identify facilitators and barriers to collaboration, which led to effective patient care on-site. I quickly learned how to become comfortable with the uncomfortable.

This process facilitated a self-guided experience where I could be a valued leader amongst a group of interprofessional clinicians. As an occupational therapy student, I find genuine interdisciplinary opportunities to be scarce, especially for those who complete their fieldwork experiences at sites where occupational therapists predominantly work within their own silos. It is only because I completed my doctoral capstone experience that I gained confidence in my ability to advocate for best practice, preventative care, and effective patient-centered care in an interprofessional environment. These opportunities for growth have vastly increased my confidence in myself as an entry-level clinician who desires to spark systemic change within health care. The continuous development of professionalism that is awarded to students who complete the doctoral capstone experience is absolutely unparalleled.

In addition to increasing my confidence and leadership skills, the doctoral capstone experience afforded me the ability to obtain numerous advanced clinical practice skills. To a large degree, clinicians of all backgrounds do not get enough training and exposure to skin health and/or wound care. I was provided with unmatched opportunities to observe and work alongside wound care–certified clinicians in multiple practice settings. Additionally, I learned how to carry out best practices for working with individuals with neurologic, cardiopulmonary, and orthopedic impairments. All patients are unique, and rarely does a patient resemble exactly what you have been taught in your courses. This experience allowed me a safe and facilitated environment to gain comfortability with thinking on my feet and modifying treatment plans to adhere to contraindications and precautions for various patient presentations.

Thanks to the doctoral capstone, I now know the type of occupational therapist that I want to become. I will always be a fierce advocate for patients and my colleagues. I will be an honest and communicative leader in interdisciplinary environments. I will also be confident in developing evidence-based treatment plans for my patients. It is only because I completed the doctoral capstone experience that I can say my hopes and dreams are well within arm's reach."

–_Alicia Colossi, OTD, OTR/L,
Duquesne University OTD class of 2024

A SOCIAL COGNITIVE APPROACH TO THE CAPSTONE EXPERIENCE

As you have progressed through the occupational therapy curriculum within your program, you probably have been introduced to the social cognitive approach to learning and how this approach enhances practice-ready skills in clinical education. This theory assumes that adults, such as graduate students like yourself, have an intrinsic motivation to learn when the activity is meaningful or directly related to their current life roles or they perceive a need for new knowledge and understanding (Bandura, 1977). Through active involvement in your learning, changes in your learning capacity take place, meanings are created, a sense of belonging is developed, and identities are constructed, such as envisioning yourself as a future occupational therapy practitioner (Dall'Alba, 2009). This transformation potentially forms not only the experiences of you as the learner but also the social context, as practice change can occur as a result of the contributions you make, which is one of the key components of adding a capstone experience for occupational therapy doctorate programs (Lave & Wenger, 2003).

Social cognitive theory states four key factors which can create your perceived self-efficacy: (1) enactive mastery experiences, (2) vicarious (observational) experiences, (3) social persuasions, and (4) physiological and psychological states (Bandura, 1997). *Enactive mastery experiences* are authentic in nature and allow you to deal with a situation in a successful manner. This type of mastery experience is considered the most influential in creating strong self-efficacy (Bandura, 1997). Mastery experiences can generally be attributed to one's own effort and skill. For example, you, as a capstone student, can increase your self-efficacy by successfully using therapeutic use of self (an internal skill) to build rapport with clients at your capstone site (Mattila, 2017). As you are able to interpret your own results and outcomes, you can then use those interpretations you have ascertained to develop beliefs about your ability to repeat the task successfully. In these situations, developing strong self-efficacy is not created with easy success but requires persistence and drive in overcoming challenges you encounter. (See Text Box 3-1.)

TEXT BOX 3-1

Read the previous sentence again, specifically: "requires persistence and drive in overcoming challenges." This is an important revelation within the framework of human-centered design – learning from mistakes and failing forward is part of the process. It is from failure that innovation (or reiterations and prototyping) occurs.

Social persuasion, the third source, states that students often receive information or feedback that affirms their ability to complete a task (Schunk, 1989). During difficult situations, you, as a capstone student, can overcome obstacles if you have a significant connection to another individual who can boost or instill confidence through clear communication and evaluative feedback. The importance of evaluation and recommendations to structure informal and formal evaluation of you, as the doctoral student, with your content expert throughout the doctoral capstone experience is discussed in Chapter 10.

Finally, Bandura (1997) states that people draw a sense of self-efficacy from their physiological, emotional, and mood states. Feelings such as anxiety, stress, or tension can allow for interpretation of failure, whereas positive feelings can strengthen overall self-efficacy. (See Text Box 3-2.)

TEXT BOX 3-2

Did you know that professionals outside of academia use Bandura's research and theory? Personal trainers and certified physical conditioning specialists use self-efficacy theory to develop physical fitness.

"A person with high self-efficacy within exercise will feel that they have the ability to be successful in exercise-related activities. Fitness professionals will help clients to be more successful if they can guide clients to higher levels of self-efficacy" (Jackson, 2010, p. 67). Occupational therapy educators can benefit from using Bandura's self-efficacy theory to further enhance the preparation of occupational therapy students for the capstone.

Stress reactions can manifest in various ways, including physiological changes, such as increased heart rate, sweating, hyperventilation, and can produce feelings of anxiety and fear that may negatively affect performance. It is important to keep your awareness of internal stress reactions in check in order to resolve any barriers which may impact your doctoral capstone experience.

The impact of psychosocial stressors on well-being and quality of life is well-known within the discipline of occupational therapy. Specific to higher education, occupational therapy literature has documented students' perceived stressors among their education (Clarke & Foxe, 2017; Everly et al., 1994; Pfeifer et al., 2008) and specifically linked to expectations of fieldwork education (Mitchell & Kampfe, 1990, 1993). More specific to the impact of one's psychological and physiological state, recent studies also have shown that Generation Z, born between 1995 and 2010, face both challenges and opportunities in the workforce (Mahapatra et al., 2022). While Generation Z (Gen Z) have advantages in understanding technology applications and greater diversity in working with community populations, they can face challenges in accepting feedback related to the quality of their work or their perceived value, making them more susceptible to experience perceived stress (Mahapatra et al., 2022). Gen Z may perceive feedback as being hypercritical of their work and may lack essential communication skills by relying on technology to convey their thoughts and attitudes, creating a disconnect between those in other generations (Mahapatra et al., 2022).

This is important to recognize and respond to in advance because anxiety is currently the most common health diagnosis affecting all levels of occupational therapy students (Soja et al., 2016). Depression and stress rank second and third as the most common psychosocial problems in college-age students. (See Text Box 3-3.)

TEXT BOX 3-3

Stress Busters During the Capstone Experience

Managing stress effectively is crucial for not only your learning but also your overall well-being. Evidence-based strategies can make a significant difference (Stillwell et al., 2017).

- Prioritize sleep.
- Practice mindfulness and meditation.
- Stay physically active.
- Maintain social connections.
- Break tasks into smaller steps.
- Practice time management.
- Maintain a balanced diet.
- Focus on self-compassion.

There are strong suggestions that mindful and gratitude-based teachings result in positive outcomes for students. Dr. Robert Emmons has made large contributions to the ever-growing research on the positive impacts of gratitude. In one of his many studies, he found that individuals who kept gratitude journals on a weekly basis were more content with their lives as a whole and were more optimistic about the future than individuals who focused on negative or neutral occurrences of the week (Emmons & McCullough, 2003). (See Text Box 3-4.)

TEXT BOX 3-4

How to Create an Attitude of Gratitude Through Journaling

Consider some of these prompts for your own journaling during your OTD curriculum or capstone experience:

- Who is someone you are thankful for in your educational journal and why?
- What is one thing you love about your school or capstone site?

TEXT BOX 3-4 (continued)

- What is one challenge you faced today, and how did it help you grow?
- Write about a teacher or mentor that has positively impacted you.
- What is a life lesson you have learned from a client at your capstone site?
- What are you looking forward to tomorrow?
- What is a goal you are excited to work on, and why does it matter to you?
- At the end of your capstone experience, imagine writing a thank-you letter to yourself. What would it say?

Studies such as Dr. Emmons's work suggest that there are ways for individuals to cope with stress in a healthy manner and lead more positive and productive lives (2003). By all accounts, aligned with generational theory, the current generation of occupational therapy students are unlike preceding generations. They view the world differently and have redefined the meaning of success, both personally and professionally. A growing movement among occupational therapy educators is needed to create successful, ethical, well-rounded, and practice-ready students in terms of both their content knowledge and their mental well-being.

CONFIDENCE AND PERCEIVED SELF-EFFICACY

The *level of perceived self-efficacy* is defined as the degree to which people believe they can succeed at any given aspect of an activity, varying from total certainty to total uncertainty. The stronger the sense of self-efficacy, the greater the perseverance toward a successful experience. Traits of self-efficacy that align with practice-ready skills include confidence, willingness to take risks, adaptability, innovation, and overall professional competence.

Health science students who reported higher levels of perceived self-efficacy were found to have performed better in clinical rotations, had increased documentation and evaluation skills, and demonstrated increased clinical decision-making skills (Artino, 2012; Cook, 2023). The transition toward greater practice readiness is strengthened through the mentorship component in experiential learning. Aligning with a stakeholder such as a content expert in your selected focus area can provide you with various perspectives on your capstone in a systematic way, which can help you grow in competence and confidence during your doctoral capstone (Kemp et al., 2020). In turn, this mentor alignment can help you build new connections toward creating a rewarding network of colleagues who can help support you in your professional career.

"Completing the doctoral capstone experience left me feeling qualified to enter my career as an entry-level occupational therapist with maturation of skills beyond completing level II fieldwork. Through my capstone project, I was able to discover a passion for supporting individuals in making health- and wellness-related lifestyle changes to best support their occupational engagement and quality of life. Having the opportunity to work within a traditional medical setting where occupational therapy was not an interdisciplinary team member helped improve my comfort and passion for advocating for occupational therapy's distinct value in comprehensive obesity care. Undertaking responsibilities and challenges associated with completing an individualized capstone project helped me prove to myself that I am capable of prioritizing, problem-solving, and creating positive solutions – all of which are skills that can support me in any position I may find myself in as an occupational therapist.

– Mina Stolberg, OTD, OTR/L,
Duquesne University OTD class of 2023

In relationship to experiential learning, perceived self-efficacy can serve as an indicator of the success or failure of a student in a stressful new clinical context, such as a capstone experience (Baird et al., 2015). Students with higher perceived self-efficacy are also more likely to transfer knowledge on a single activity to other similar or different activities. In occupational therapy curriculum, we often refer to this as a core component of clinical or professional reasoning. For example, Baird et al. (2015) evaluated the effects of transfer training in a simulated environment on occupational therapy students' perceived self-efficacy. The authors found that students who were completely confident in the training would have a higher level of perceived self-efficacy than those who were unsure of their skills for transferring patients. This is extremely valuable for the capstone, as doctoral students will continue to practice skills one way in the classroom but need to be able to translate those skills to varying populations and settings, often in a more advanced context, during the capstone experience. Increasing self-efficacy can help the capstone student persevere and fail forward when faced with adversity during the capstone.

One example of this transfer of learning from classroom to capstone application can be drawn from the value of interprofessional education opportunities within academic programs. As a student, you have been immersed in opportunities to increase your awareness of the importance of interprofessional learning to increase your competency and understanding of the roles of other health program disciplines and how you collectively can improve the quality and safety of outcomes for clients (Godwin et al., 2021). As you transfer this basic knowledge of how teams may function into your focused capstone, you begin to simultaneously learn about how the team and system applicable to your own capstone experience can translate into "real-world" outcomes for those which you and your site serve. This lived interprofessional experience can foster your views on teamwork, promote your own confidence and competence, and reinforce how effective provider–provider collaboration can be in solidifying your own practice readiness.

EMOTIONAL INTELLIGENCE

Emotional intelligence (EI) describes how people, such as capstone students, may monitor and manage emotional responses to better communicate with and relate to others (Carmeli & Josman, 2006; Mayer et al., 2008). Both EI theory and the principles of occupational therapy address the importance of relationship-building skills that support the connection between self and others. In contrast to therapeutic use of self, EI is situated within the individual and indirectly influences relationships with others. The focus of the EI theory's process of how emotions influence thinking supports the interactive reasoning process commonly discussed in occupational therapy (McKenna & Mellson, 2013). Collaborative reasoning relies heavily on self-awareness and perception, which inform clinical reasoning, relationship-building, and decision-making – all important practice-ready skills for the capstone student (Cronin & Graebe, 2018). Successful mentor–mentee relationships can foster greater self-awareness and the ability to empathize and influence the interest in promoting others (Byars-Winston & Dahlberg, 2019). Previous studies have also found that fieldwork students with higher EI have demonstrated increased scores in competencies related to patient outcomes, teamwork skills, dealing with stress, and overall patient satisfaction (Andonian, 2013; Gribble et al., 2017). In the capstone process, EI is situated within the capstone student and directly impacts other stakeholders in the capstone process, as shown in Figure 3-1. Through mentorship, a doctoral student can openly share issues, gain direction in different approaches to problem-solving while receiving constructive feedback.

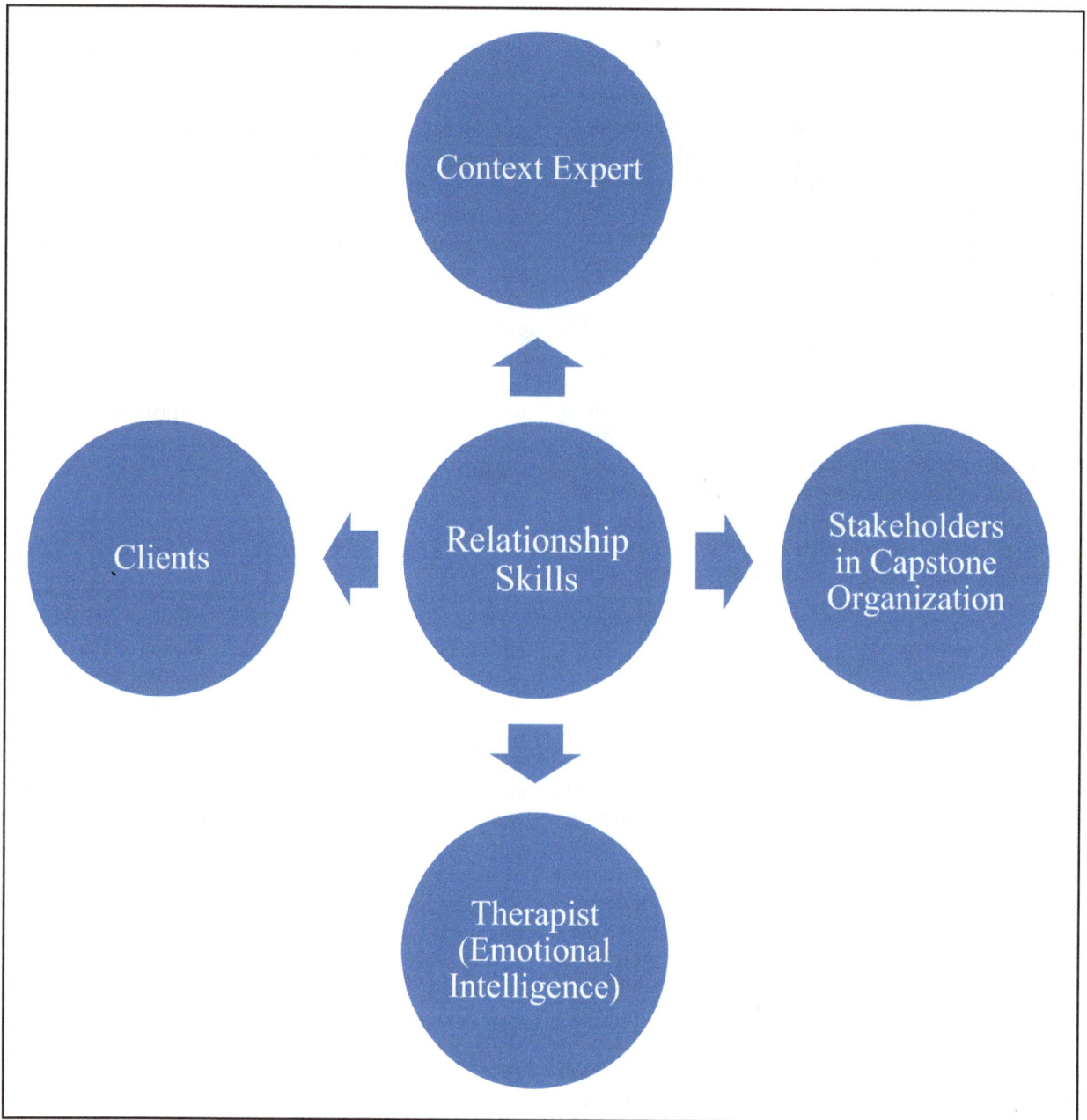

Figure 3-1. EI, situated with the capstone student, informs all relationships in the capstone process.

STRATEGIES TO DEVELOP PRACTICE-READY SKILLS IN THE MENTORED DOCTORAL CAPSTONE RELATIONSHIP

The nature of mentoring relationships can be complex. Each relationship is cultivated differently and varies with the level of activities and purpose of the mentorship between the student and mentor in order that the student refine practice readiness skills to develop into a successful professional. Mentorship styles vary based upon the objectives of the program or project, the goals of the experience, the amount of attention, information onboarding, or advice required by the student. Transitioning from fieldwork experiences where supervision is provided by a fieldwork educator to a content expert who provides mentorship can be daunting. While some students may not find difficulty in transitioning to proactively seeking guidance from a mentor, other students may feel reluctant to reach out or have greater difficulty in knowing what questions to ask or information to seek.

"In transitioning from a fieldwork student to a doctoral student, the biggest changes for a student may be advocating for occupational therapy and being confident in practicing in a more independent way. The DCE provided me with the opportunity to apply the skills I learned from fieldwork in a non-traditional setting and prompted me to advocate for occupational therapy in a unique way. In my experience, my fieldwork educators acted more as hands-on teachers that gradually scaffolded my education and consistently directly observed everything that I was doing onsite. Throughout my DCE, my content expert had more of a guiding role, and while she was always available for support when I needed it, it was ultimately up to me to decide when to seek guidance and when to lead things on my own.

As a capstone student, my biggest attitude shift was in my confidence and knowledge that I had the skills needed to lead others. When completing the DCE, it is important to feel comfortable in leadership roles and trust yourself and your ideas while still being open to feedback and learning from your content expert.

It can feel daunting as a capstone student to ask more administrative or interprofessional questions, but approaching these things with curiosity is what benefited my relationship with my site mentor the most. During my capstone, I made sure to get to know the culture of my site, the relationships between staff, and how certain processes worked before addressing ideas, questions, or concerns with my mentor. This relationship existed because I was sure to be honest and open to new experiences. When asking about funding, systems in place, policies, and areas for growth that the site had, I was sure to offer any insights that I had, in a respectful way that was beneficial to both my learning and the site's growth. The biggest takeaway I had from my experience was learning how to mesh together my passion with what my site's needs were, and in doing that, I was able to foster a working relationship with my content expert."

– Hannah Davis, Duquesne University
Pittsburgh, Pennsylvania, OTD class of 2024

The mentorship relationship may take time to develop within the doctoral capstone. Mentorship is characterized by mutual trust, understanding, and empathy to advance the educational and personal growth of students. Mentorship expectations can be challenging to establish due to the range of capstone settings; diverse areas of focus; complexity of the client, group, or population being addressed; and any number of variable factors. Expectations of the mentorship relationship can be shaped by the mentor's prior exposure

to occupational therapy services or lack of understanding, personal preferences, or general personality, and their additional roles and responsibilities (Pfund et al., 2014).

Capstone students who complete their experience and project in a non-traditional setting or emerging practice area where occupational therapy has not been previously established may face additional challenges of having to explain the role of occupational therapy and the range of services which occupational therapy offers distinct value from other services. It is essential that the capstone student and mentor establish a clear set of expectations early in the relationship to help establish mutual goals within the capstone (Stephenson et al., 2020). Addressing institutional, organizational, and personal barriers early in the capstone mentorship relationship can help align perspectives, which can promote positive experiences for both the student and their mentor (DeIuliis & Hanson, 2022). (See Text Box 3-5.)

TEXT BOX 3-5

Clearly defined expectations should be established for your mentoring relationship to develop. Consider completing the following exercise by answering the questions about your own preferences in establishing a mentorship. You can make this a mutual exercise and coordinate this learning activity with your mentor for them to complete as well.

For mentee: What would you like to get out of this relationship?

For mentor: What would you like for the mentee to get out of this relationship? What would *you* like to get out of this relationship?

Together as mentor and mentee, discuss the following items to further define your personal and relationship expectations as you begin your mentoring relationship.

Both: How often will you meet? In person? By phone or email? Who will make the arrangements for the meetings? How will the agenda be established for each meeting?

Both: What will be your "ground rules" for how the time will be spent? Who runs the meetings? How will you respect one another's time? How will conversations be kept confidential? Are there any topics off-limits?

Adapted from the Mentoring Resource Center, Wake Forest University (2024). *Defining personal and relationship expectations worksheet.* https://mentoring.opcd.wfu.edu/tools-and-resources/.

In addition to clear expectations, establishing a positive pathway for communication is also vital. The capstone student and content expert need to establish a plan for regular and consistent communication, which includes the expected method, manner, and frequency of regular check-ins and updates on progress. When patterns of positive communication are fostered, this can improve the confidence and competency of the capstone student and lead to greater perceived self-assurance and belief in oneself (Keinänen et al., 2023). While not prescriptive or the same across all capstones or capstone teams, weekly meetings may facilitate mutual understanding of performance of one another's ongoing roles, responsibilities, and program effectiveness in "real time," which can help reduce the potential for unexpected outcomes at the end of the capstone experience and project. One way of doing this is through developing a mutual agreement, called a **mentoring compact**.

MENTORING COMPACT

A *mentoring compact* is a written agreement between a mentor and a mentee which serves as a framework for the outline of goals and expectations for the capstone. It can aide in promoting a solid and productive outline for the mentorship relationship. Key elements of a compact include the objectives or goals for the mutual alignment or reason behind the mentorship. It can also provide valuable structure for the commitment and investment of time within the relationship. Throughout the capstone process, a mentor compact can help promote a regular method and mechanism for provision or receipt of feedback too. (See Figure 3-2, which contains an example of such an agreement from a mentee perspective.)

Doctoral Capstone Experience Mentee-Mentor Compact

OTD Mentee: Alicia Colossi, OTS

Faculty Capstone Chair/Mentor: Michelle McCann, OTD, OTR/L, C/NDT, CBIS, PPSC, Assistant Clinical Professor/Capstone Coordinator

Goals of OTD Mentee-Mentor Relationship:

Develop a collaborative learning relationship based on intentionality, responsiveness, reciprocity, and trust.

Foster opportunities to identify potential occupational therapy services in a variety of community settings and/or with underserved population groups within your capstone focus.

Reflect on skills required for effective leadership in developing new practise arenas or services in emerging practise areas utilizing present and past experiences.

Promote diversity, equity, and inclusion of all stakeholders while allowing individuals with a variety of experiences and backgrounds to come together for a common purpose.

Create pathways for dissemination of knowledge and key outcomes of the doctoral capstone experience in order to advance the field of occupational therapy and access to services.

Commitments of Student Mentee (Alicia Colossi)

I acknowledge that I have the primary responsibility for the successful completion of my doctoral capstone experience and all related coursework, assignments, and opportunities.

I will be appreciative and respectful of my mentor's time and investment in working with me. I will honour my commitments and respond to my mentors' communications in a timely manner.

I will initiate weekly meetings with my mentor, Dr. McCann, to discuss my ideas, upcoming events, activities, and any other additional pertinent information.

　　o   I will maintain ongoing and timely communication and collaboration with my mentor throughout my entire DCE.

I will initiate seeking out guidance from my mentor as needed when completing my needs assessment, literature reviews, and additional activities/assignments relative to my doctoral capstone experience.

I will be an active participant during all my meetings (group and individual) and opportunities throughout the upcoming year as evidenced by active listening and full participation.

I will be willing to learn new things, be responsive to both positive and constructive criticism, and be open to others perspectives.

I will initiate feedback requests and implement changes in my ideas/ project based on feedback provided from my mentor in a timely fashion.

Figure 3-2. The mentee portion of a mentee–mentor compact.

Finally, placing an emphasis on developing intrapersonal, interpersonal, and advocacy skills can assist in moving doctoral students from a self-centric model of understanding of the profession to "other-centered," where leading and serving others is at the core of their practice. This movement is critical, particularly when there are consistent findings that the US health-care system does not offer dependable, high-quality care to all people, due in part to the poor organization of the health-care delivery system and limited opportunities within interprofessional education for students to appreciate the dynamic of collaboration outside of their primary discipline (Institute of Medicine, 2011; Zechariah et al., 2019). These changes in thoughts and behaviors can help you be a transformational and servant leader as you graduate and enter the profession (King et al., 2015; Mattila & Dolhi, 2016). Fostering the practice-ready skills to graduate emerging health-care leaders from entry-level occupational therapy doctorate programs will be essential in addressing these systematic issues.

STUDENT SECTION CHAPTER SUMMARY

The doctoral capstone enhances occupational therapy students' abilities to interact, advocate, and collaborate with other health-care professionals in more diverse settings. This process, in combination with a carefully aligned mentorship relationship, will allow programs to graduate into the health-care system not only generalist, practice-ready practitioners but also transformational leaders. There needs to be a clear emphasis on practice-ready skills development that will allow capstone students to positively and confidently work through the human-centered design phases of inspire/ideate and promote more autonomous decision-making. Through the precursory learning activities that have been designed in your coursework and purposeful selection of capstone settings and mentor that facilitate growth in self-regulated learning, leadership, and self-efficacy, you will boldly enter the health-care field as practice-ready professionals!

STUDENT LEARNING ACTIVITIES

1. *Imagery activity.* Picture yourself going through the capstone process. What do you know now that you did not before you embarked on this advanced practitioner phase of your curriculum?
   a. Take a moment to reflect and write down some skills you have developed before, during, and after fieldwork to take inventory of what you need for the capstone.
   b. What are your strengths? What are your areas that need to be developed? How can you create SMART goals around these skills to help you be successful?

2. Think of a task related to your capstone. It could be developing evidence-based questions, embarking on a literature review, or pragmatically preparing for the capstone experience itself. Use Table 3-3 and think through the phases of self-regulated learning.
   a. What questions and answers might you have in each phase of your learning?
   b. Reflect on your motivation and beliefs. How will these characteristics influence each of these phases?

3. Create a capstone experience planning journal. The intent of this journal is to help you set goals for each step of the capstone process. Successful students are known to set goals, monitor their progress, and make plans for how they are going to achieve those goals. In your initial post, think about the following questions:
   a. What are the specific, measurable learning objectives you hope to accomplish during your capstone experience?
   b. What are you going to do to meet these objectives? What do you expect of your faculty and/or capstone supervisor(s) to help facilitate learning?
   c. How are you going to monitor your progress?

Section 2: Educator Focus

Transformational Learning Phases and Framework for the Educator

As mentioned directly within the student section of this chapter, the human-centered design mindsets of learning from failure and promoting reflection through learning are impactful strategies to employ to help students adapt to the transition between the role of doctoral student to emerging practice who is able and willing to navigate the complex health-care landscape. Integrating Mezirow's transformational learning theory, as you are preparing students to be prepared for mentoring relationships and to be practice-ready ahead of their doctoral capstone, here is where a focus on self-examination needs to occur (Mezirow, 1997).

As you design your doctoral capstone preparatory courses, consider how you will incorporate learning activities and assessment methods that challenge students to reflect on their abilities and potential. Your students, and maybe even you as a faculty member or doctoral capstone coordinator, may experience self-doubt or guilt about their readiness or capacity to successfully initiate and/or complete their doctoral capstone. The realization that they must apply theory to real-life situations may raise feelings of inadequacy or fear

(continued)

of failure. In this phase, as educators, we need to ensure that students have meaningful opportunities to examine their own beliefs and feelings in order to develop a meaningful doctoral capstone.

As educators, supporting doctoral students down the learner path throughout the doctoral capstone and experience is one key facet; however, each student much own responsibility for adjusting to the transformation from student to emerging practitioner.

Just as optimism is a key trait that makes a student's experience more productive and enjoyable, as an educator, it is important that you set the tone of optimism in regard to experiential learning, as students will experience a myriad of new exposures. With this come degrees of negative or positive experiences and new relationships. As you navigate the capstone together, keep in mind that optimism can aide your students in how they develop practice readiness and their resiliency when unexpected challenges come their way.

INTRODUCTION FOR EDUCATOR

With increasing complexity in the United States (US) health-care system at all levels and more involved health issues facing society, it is imperative that occupational therapy practitioners be able to meet the needs of their clients, effectively and efficiently, by being prepared to provide advanced-level care immediately upon graduation. Health-care administrators are increasingly challenged to reduce health-care expenditures, leading to diminished opportunities to develop advanced skill competencies after entering the field. The educator will need to ensure that students obtain the additional training in career-ready/practice-ready skills, leadership, and advocacy during their academic preparation before entering the field.

The preparation for occupational therapy students to understand themselves in terms of sociocultural diversity is also of great importance in the current health-care system. Across the world, services are being provided to individuals and populations who historically have not been recipients of occupational therapy interventions (Talero et al., 2015). This shift in care requires a shift in occupational therapy curriculum, as well as opportunities for more diverse interactions while students are still in the educational setting. Taff and Blash (2017) suggested that a more systematized, comprehensive approach must be considered to address the need for a diversely trained and culturally competent workforce in our current health system. Currently, this is an issue because the workforce of practicing clinicians remains at 85% Caucasian and is practicing

in mostly traditional settings (American Occupational Therapy Association [AOTA], 2023). To meet the needs of the focus areas and diversity in populations, capstone experiences may be frequently occurring in emerging areas of practice, such as health and wellness programs, veterans' health, or aging in place, to name only a few of the available unique opportunities.

EDUCATOR REFLECTIVE QUESTIONS

1. What challenges or barriers do you anticipate facing preparing students for their capstone experience?
2. What type of skills or abilities do you think would be essential to address in order for students to overcome these challenges or barriers?
3. What action steps can you commit to taking to supporting practice readiness and the ability to be mentored throughout the capstone?

EDUCATOR OBJECTIVES

By the end of reading this chapter and completing the learning activities, the educator will be able to design teaching methods to meet the stated student learning objectives:

1. Evaluate strategies to address common pitfalls and challenges of the capstone experience.
2. Compare and contrast qualities of a successful fieldwork student vs. the expectations of the capstone student.
3. Compare and contrast mentorship vs. supervision models, and apply best practices to support students throughout the capstone experience.
4. Identify practice-ready and mentorship skills that are instrumental to the successful completion of the capstone experience.
5. Apply concepts of professional identity and professionalism to enhance career readiness through engagement in the capstone experience.

PROMOTING SELF-EFFICACY TO ADDRESS COMMON PITFALLS AND CHALLENGES OF THE CAPSTONE EXPERIENCE

In addition to the resources in the preceding student section, another source to create self-efficacy is through vicarious learning, or having observational experiences provided by a "model" (Bandura, 1997). The work of Bandura (1997) is valuable for occupational therapy educators to prepare capstone students from these younger generations. Effective functioning for the capstone requires skills and efficacy beliefs. Because self-efficacy is influenced by mastery experience, vicarious experience, social persuasion, and physiological state, it is essential for occupational therapy educators to develop capstone preparation curricula aimed at increasing self-efficacy through each of these factors. This understanding of the majority makeup of the capstone student body provides a solid connection between perceived self-efficacy and the emotional intelligence (EI) of a student.

For effective self-regulated learning to take place, students must develop the capability of monitoring what they do and then modifying the skill or strategy appropriately (Boud, 2013). Students also need to have a realistic assessment of their own performance, of what they know, what they still need to know, and the path they will take to bridge theory into practice. In the capstone experience, students are required to be increasingly reliant on their own thinking. The ability to self-assess will allow the capstone student to be a more independent, critical thinker in realistic situations (Boud, 2013; Wald et al., 2015). Using this teaching and learning practice, students can explore greater meaning in the content, and through critical reflection and investigation, they may encounter a fundamental change in their beliefs, feelings, attitudes, perspectives, and assumptions (Costa, 2009; Santalucia & Johnson, 2010).

Ideally, capstone students will have had successful modelling in both their faculty and fieldwork educators before the capstone experience. A strategy students can use during the doctoral capstone experience is to perform their own self-assessment and comparison of capabilities based on the observation of others, such as through a role-play experience. Having the opportunity to role-play or observe their content expert, instructors, or peers in situations such as responding to the reactions of others or facing inaccurate assumptions can affect the student's assessment of self-efficacy. (See Text Box 3-6.)

TEXT BOX 3-6

This process of gathering feedback from various perspectives is often referred to as a 360 review and is discussed in more detail in Chapter 10, which covers evaluation of the capstone.

Following this up with a structured journal prompt or written reflection can help capstone students explore how he or she responded, the differences or similarities with the role-play actors, and how the capstone student would change his or her response in the future if faced with that similar event or situation. Examples of these types of journaling prompts are in Text Box 3-4. Thomas and colleagues (2018) found that through various "soft skills curriculum" role-playing vignettes in which occupational therapy students had the opportunity to watch and reflect, students reported increased awareness of the importance of soft skills and confidence in strategies to navigate difficult clinical situations. Although this source does not provide as strong a

sense of self-efficacy, it can be helpful for students who are struggling with self-awareness (van Dinther et al., 2011). (See Text Box 3-7.)

TEXT BOX 3-7

Navigating Difficulty Situations

Simulating situations in which difficult conversations or disagreements may arise in the clinical setting can provide an opportunity for students to practice soft skills. Here is one way to role-play challenging conversations, in which students can increase their confidence when faced with these situations in the capstone experience:

- Ask students to reflect on a time when they either had a difficult conversation or avoided a topic altogether. Prompt them that it was likely with someone important to them, such as a friend, family member, or classmate. Ask them to think about the perception they had on how the conversation would go (poorly, contentious, etc.).

- Once they have the situation in mind, teach them the SPIKES method and have them replay the conversation with a classmate. The SPIKES method trains them in the following communication techniques:

  - *Setup.* Ensure surroundings are appropriate for this conversation.
  - *Perception.* Ask open-minded questions to ascertain how the individual perceives the situation.
  - *Invitation.* Find out how much information the individual is comfortable receiving or discussing at this time.
  - *Knowledge.* Stick to the facts when possible. Check for understanding as needed.
  - *Empathy.* Respond to individual in a way that acknowledges his or her emotions and reassures that these responses are normal and expected.
  - *Summary.* Determine whether the conversation should continue, or find appropriate closure.

Source: Adapted from Baile, W. F., Lenzi, R., Glober, G., Beale, E. A., and Kudelka, A. P. (2010). SPIKES—A six-step protocol for delivering bad news: Application to the patient with cancer. *The Oncologist, 5*, 302–311.

MOVING STUDENTS FROM ACADEMIC READINESS TOWARD CAREER READINESS

Career readiness has been a continual focal point of professional degree programs both within occupational therapy and in other fields. Although fieldwork education has historically prepared students for generalist, entry-level practice, there is still a gap between what students' vs. employers' feel are career-ready skills and qualities (National Association of Colleges and Employers [NACE], 2024). NACE (2024) defines *career readiness* as "the foundation for demonstrating core competencies that prepare college graduates for success in the workplace and career management." In the NACE 2024 surveys, there were large disparities in key areas of employment between importance versus actual proficiency in eight career readiness competencies. Table 3-2 demonstrates there is now a greater demand than ever for occupational therapy educational programs to develop communication skills, critical thinking, collaboration, and professionalism in all students, which aims to improve long-term employee productivity.

One way to begin to bridge these gaps is through advancing the requirements and challenges of the experiential learning component within all programs. Experiential learning, as described by Kolb (1984), is commonly cited in professional programs in higher education and has relevance for designing successful capstone placements. Kolb (1984) defined *learning* as a four-stage cycle in which students first encounter a "concrete experience," then take the time to reflect on the experience from new viewpoints through "reflective observation." Students then frame their ideas in a different light and assimilate these reflections and ideas into theories during "abstract conceptualization." In the final stage, they test their concepts and beliefs through "active experimentation" (Kolb, 1984). This cycle of learning is important during a capstone experience, due to the increasing demands on the student and the more diverse practice settings and clients they will encounter upon entering this type of placement. The student is challenged through this process at a greater level through the exploration of their learning (Jarvis, 2010; Kolb, 1984, 2014).

Jarvis (2010) suggested that when students begin the fieldwork phase of their occupational therapy education, they encounter a "primary experience of practice that presents them with an array of opportunities for new learning and development" (p. 78). This is equally true for the next phase of experiential learning through the doctoral capstone experience. Jarvis expands on Kolb's theory and defines the complexity of the adult learning process, adding the importance of drawing from past experiences and reflections. This is the area of knowledge that lies between an individual's awareness of an experience (based on the past encounter) and the authenticity of the current situation. When the two reflections begin to separate, questioning or dilemma occurs and learning begins. This is a critical moment for capstone students, as they begin to formulate their clinical questions and create a plan for a capstone experience. Figure 3-3 demonstrates the ongoing cycle that Kolb and Jarvis describe for successful experiential learning.

In addition to the social interaction that occurs in experiential learning, cultural and intergenerational interaction is an invaluable process to their learning experience. Similar to a health-care context, where clients come from diverse backgrounds, experiential learning provides "a trusting and open learning atmosphere, where diverse ideas are shared, considered, tested, and modified" (Biedenweg & Monroe, 2013, p. 931). Of further importance to this interaction, researchers in the field find that the collaboration in these social and cultural contexts resulted in the acquisition of moral values through learning, something that often cannot be taught in the classroom setting (Talero et al., 2015).

Table 3-2. Greatest Reported Gaps in Employer Perception of Importance Versus Proficiency in Career Readiness Skills

COMPETENCY	% OF EMPLOYERS RATING OF IMPORTANCE OF SKILL	% OF EMPLOYERS RATING OF PROFICIENCY OF SKILL
Communication	99.5	55.2
Teamwork	96.5	78.1
Critical thinking	94.9	66.1
Professionalism	91.0	50.0
Equity and inclusion	83.5	70.8
Technology	74.9	81.7
Career and self-development	68.0	47.1
Leadership	55.8	36.8

Source: Adapted from National Association of Colleges and Employers (2024). *Job outlook 2024*. 2024-nace-job-outlook.pdf (naceweb.org).

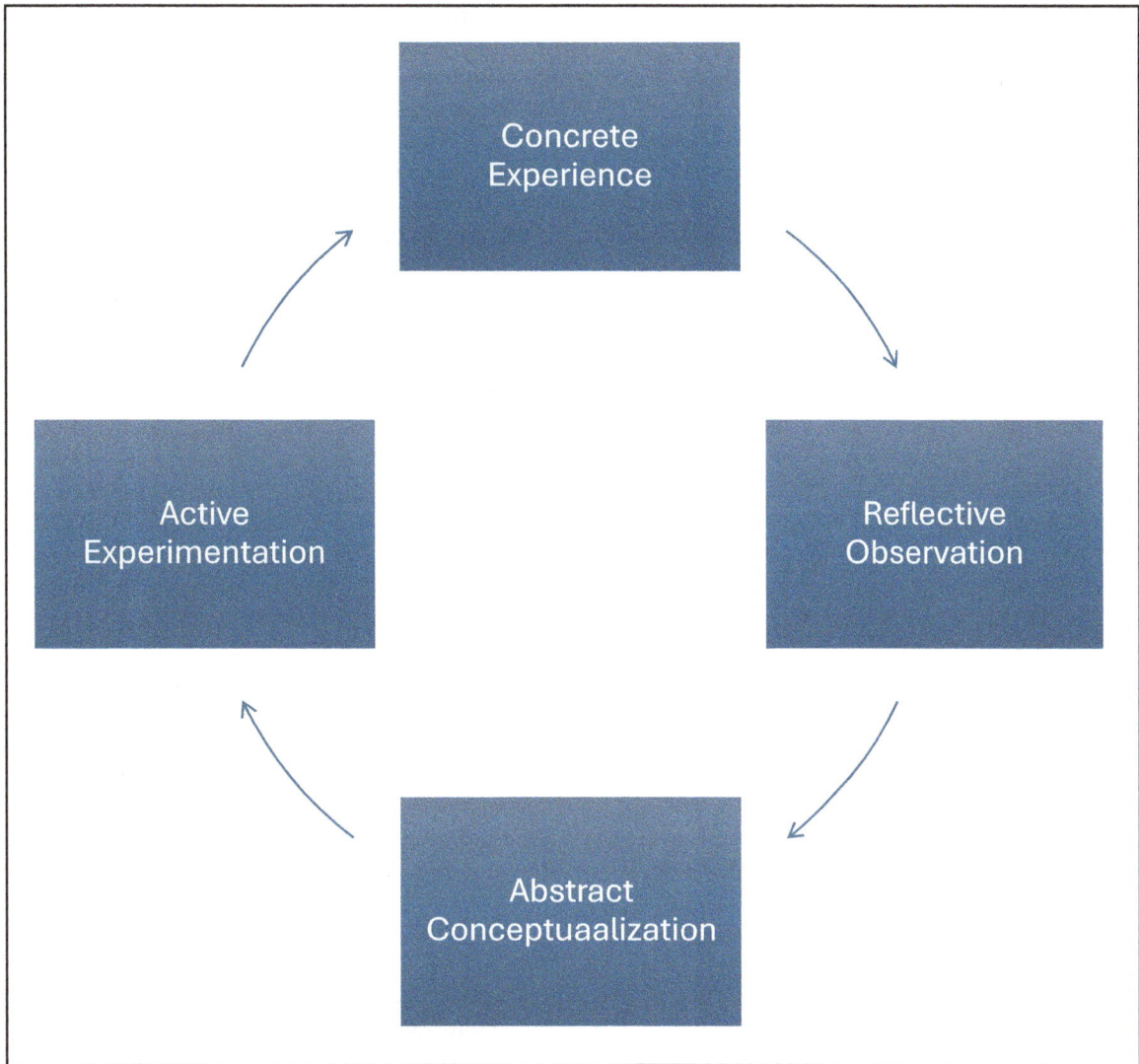

Figure 3-3. Kolb's experiential learning cycle graphic.

Intergenerational perspectives are also important to recognize as you support your students' transition into their capstone experience and project. Generational differences may be challenging, as views and attitudes may create a diverse landscape of experiences and perspectives in the workplace. Generation Z (born between 1995 and 2012) are perhaps one of the most technologically advanced and educated generations in the present day. While having this technological savvy and knowledge of current advancements can be a positive attribute, Generation Z lack exposure to life before the advent of smartphone technology. This gap in personal experience may limit their understanding of how potential clients may continue to use systems and processes before advanced technology, which may further define the gap in understanding with mentors and clients within previous generations (Parker & Igielnik, 2020).

As a result of these learning considerations, the student becomes transformed by their experience on many levels (Jarvis, 2010; Merriam et al., 2007). Examples of these transformations from the literature include increased critical reflection, changed meaning of worldviews and beliefs, increased confidence, and increased connection to themselves and their community, all of which will help bridge the gaps in employment, as shared earlier (Bagatell et al., 2013; Santalucia & Johnson, 2010).

PRACTICE-READY AND MENTORSHIP SKILLS ESSENTIAL FOR CAPSTONE SUCCESS

Occupational therapy educators need to prepare not only what to teach but also how to navigate students through the complexities of self-directed learning throughout their capstone. The role of the educator throughout the capstone is also multifaceted, that of both the instructor and also as mentor. As an instructor, the educator helps the student better understand how to find information and employ problem-based learning solutions that will be essential in idea formation, development, implementation, and evaluation of the capstone. Educators provide structure to capstone through curricular objectives which scaffold and guide the student along the learning path. However, as learners develop both capacity and competency, they must also learn the effective ability to apply learning taken from familiar settings and put this learning into action across new or novel situations during the capstone. Students must also do this in the context of working across new settings within new teams and across, often with professionals from a diverse range of professions.

Although various strategies have been discussed throughout this chapter, there are other, more concrete ways that occupational therapy educators may be able to develop practice-ready skills in capstone students. Through exposure to more diverse learning environments and settings, critical reflection, and an emphasis on interpersonal and advocacy skills, educators and students can facilitate environments or tasks that foster growth, which will transcend beyond the capstone.

First, educators and doctoral capstone coordinators can create unique learning experiences that encourage students *to select non-traditional, community-based, or role-emerging settings.* These types of settings that often provide services to communities or underserved populations where there is no current occupational therapy in practice can provide students with unique opportunities to refine the practice-ready skills discussed in this chapter. Role-emerging experiences offer an experiential learning approach that can better prepare students to be qualified practitioners and enhance a distinctive set of skills that differ from those learned in more traditional placements (Atler & Gavin, 2010; Scaffa & Reitz, 2013). There is also indication that students who participated in role-emerging or community-based fieldwork have positive gains in reflection, knowledge, and overall confidence in areas such as problem-solving, initiative, and creativity in practice (Hoppes et al., 2005). In addition, a different set of skills is often gained in these settings compared with a traditional fieldwork setting, including cultural awareness, therapeutic use of self, and self-efficacy (Atler & Gavin, 2010; Haro et al., 2014).

Another way to develop practice-ready skills and readiness for the mentored experience is *through the use of critical reflection* during the capstone process. Critical reflection is an evidence-based teaching method that can foster personal growth and professional transformation in capstone students. According to Henderson (2010), critical reflection, communication, and support are the key components in fostering students' movement toward transformative learning. When students begin the doctoral capstone process, they are often challenged to question and rethink previously held thoughts and beliefs. Educators can facilitate the student to consider options through exploratory prompts and critical reflection (Matthew-Maich et al., 2010; Mezirow, 1997, 2000). Examples of prompts in the following Table 3-3 can be facilitated through a discussion board or even in a seminar-based in-class discussion. Promoting learning and achievement through critical reflection and self-assessment is an integral component of developing self-efficacy and EI.

As you prepare students to enter the capstone experience and project, it is essential to discuss key differences in relationships they will encounter in the doctoral capstone experience and project. First and foremost is the transition from having a "supervisor" in their fieldwork experiences to a mentor or "content expert" who will serve as a guide, role-model, and key stakeholder during their capstone experience. It is important to provide guidance on establishing and selecting mentorship within the capstone experience and how mentorship differs from aspects of traditional supervision or preceptorship often utilized in health-care settings. It is beneficial to discuss how mentorship relationships foster professional development through planned and deliberate activities with a mentor. While definitions of mentoring vary and there is not a universal standard for these capstone mentorships to evolve, it is generally accepted that mentorship relationships are personal and reciprocal. Unlike fieldwork, where instructors in the field, or "fieldwork educators," have training guidance and formalized programs to help support student interactions in daily experiences, as evidenced by the certification offered within AOTA (AOTA, 2022), for individuals working within fieldwork education, there is no standard equivalent for the site mentor or content expert guidance in the doctoral education program.

It is important to establish the learning foundations for how mentorship functions are complex and multidimensional. Every mentorship relationship is different and may vary due to project goals, population need, organizational context, and experiences of both the mentor and the student. While the ACOTE standards for the entry-level occupational therapy doctoral degree designation include the key component of experiential learning and the inclusion of a mentored capstone experience, quality training or structured guidance on capstone mentorship is largely subjective (Harris et al., 2023). While variation exists in mentorship, it is essential to highlight core behaviors which are most likely to yield a positive mentorship experience and a greater self-efficacy experienced by the student. (See Text Box 3-7.)

Table 3-3. Phases of Self-Regulated Learning During the Doctorate Capstone Experience and Project

SELF-REGULATION PHASE	CAPSTONE PROCESS PHASE	DESCRIPTION	QUESTIONS STUDENTS MIGHT POSE WHILE ENACTING THIS PHASE OF THE CAPSTONE EXPERIENCE
Forethought	Developing and planning phase	Process and beliefs that occur before efforts to learn	• What is the task? What does the capstone assignment tell me to do? • Is it similar to something I have done before? • What information do I need to gather to accomplish this step of my capstone? • How, when, and where should I proceed? • What do I want to gain by completing this capstone project? Why? • Which factors of the project can I control? How will I cope? • Where will I go when I need help?
Performance/action	Implementation phase	Processes that occur during learning and/or activity	• What can I do to stay on track throughout the project? • Am I accomplishing what I set out to accomplish? • Am I being distracted? • Do I actually understand what I am implementing and why? Should I continue working, or is the task complete? • Is it time to seek help? • Do I need/deserve a break or incentive?
Self-reflection	Evaluation phase	Processes that occur after each learning effort	• What is my reaction to the completed project? • What are others' reactions? • Have I taken all the important stakeholders' opinions into consideration? • What are the consequences of these reactions and the outcomes of my work? • Why did I perform well? What did I do poorly? • Did I choose the right steps? What can I do to improve?
Contributing factor throughout all phases	Motivation/beliefs		• Am I capable of completing this capstone experience and project? • Why am I interested, curious, or frustrated? • Can I control my level of success? • Do I care more about the grade or the growth in my learning?

Source: Adapted from Zimmerman, B. J. (2002). Becoming a self-regulated learner: An overview. *Theory Into Practice, 4*(2), 64–70.

TEXT BOX 3-7

Measuring Self-Efficacy

An evidence-based tool you can incorporate into your work with capstone students to help them self-assess areas of self-efficacy is the Student Confidence Questionnaire (SCQ).

The SCQ, originally developed by Derdall and colleagues in 2002, allows students to evaluate their overall confidence in a variety of practice-ready areas. The SCQ is a 40-item Likert scale that assesses the student in the domains of professional competence, communication, adaptability, innovation, risk-taking, supervision, and clinical practice.

Source: Adapted from Derdall, M., Olson, P., Janzen, W., and Warren, S. (2002). Development of a questionnaire to examine confidence of occupational therapy students during fieldwork experiences. *Canadian Journal of Occupational Therapy, 69,* 49–56.

FACILITATING SUCCESSFUL MENTORING RELATIONSHIPS

While the focus of this portion of the chapter has been on preparing the doctoral student for the importance of practice readiness and transitioning them from supervision under the fieldwork experience to a mentor-based program, support for the mentor is essential in order for the student to mutually align and build a positive relationship in the capstone experience to support the student's learning. Being a good mentor requires intentionality. There is no single formula for establishing a mentorship relationship. Expectations of "mentorship" can vary based on the personal experiences of the mentor, their personality and style of leadership, and their primary roles and responsibilities (Pfund et al., 2014). Since doctoral students may elect to complete their capstone experience in a non-traditional setting or even with a non–occupational therapy mentor, content experts who are mentoring a student may not be familiar with the services or roles occupational therapists have in the focused capstone program, leading to gaps or misunderstanding of the process. To alleviate this barrier, preparing the mentor with resources to navigate the capstone experience is essential. These resources can help clear expectations, promote open communication practices, and help the mentor model positive attributes which can bolster their students' confidence in the doctoral capstone experience. The following example provides an overview of an evidence-based approach or tips to developing mentor support and resources which can enhance their confidence and competence in the role too. Text Box 3-8 explores six key behaviors which are essential components of the mentorship experience.

TEXT BOX 3-8

1. *Effective communication.* In a study by Cook (2023), the positive interaction students

TEXT BOX 3-8 (continued)

reported with their content expert may have a direct impact on the student's self-directedness during the DCE. Furthermore, Andonian (2017) noted that a positive correlation existed between a supportive relationship with open and warm communication and student self-efficacy during fieldwork experiences. In addition, content experts were provided with example resources in "dosing" frequency and clarity of feedback related to a variety of situations incorporating constructive feedback since this is also a key element in successfully mentoring students (Pollard & Kumar, 2021).

2. *Aligning expectations.* While the foundational "agreement" of these mutual expectations or the written experiential plan (ACOTE, 2023) is a required element of the entry-level doctoral capstone experience, ensuring that the mentee and mentor take time to outline clear objectives and goals of the doctoral capstone experience can be helpful in avoiding misunderstandings due to prior experiences or expectations changing over time. Evidence supports taking the time in education, particularly graduate student education, in aligning expectations between mentor and mentee in order that both parties are cognizant of the personal and professional expectations which may impact the outcome of the experience for each participant (Huskins et al., 2011; Stephenson et al., 2024).

3. *Assessing understanding.* Developing an understanding of strategies to assess how well a student understands the context of their work can be difficult in any field, but especially when a student is being mentored by a content expert outside of occupational therapy. Assessing understanding within the mentee–mentor relationship is vitally important due to the transfer of often highly complex information. Adams (2015) reported that learning objectives requiring higher levels of cognitive skills can lead to deeper learning and, therefore, greater transfer of knowledge by the student. The importance of assessing understanding is directly linked to the overarching goal of a student attaining an "in-depth" exposure to the area of focus for their capstone experience (ACOTE, 2023).

4. *Addressing equity, diversity, and inclusion.* Diversity in any relationship can offer opportunity or challenge. Learning from individuals different from ourselves can help promote a more vibrant intellectual environment for learning. Recognizing the impact of potential unconscious or conscious bias in our own assumptions takes honest reflection. Byars-Winston and colleagues (2015) identified that cultural diversity awareness can

TEXT BOX 3-8 (continued)

influence how students experience rapport building in a mentoring relationship. The importance of acknowledging factors such as gender, race, ethnicity, as well as many other factors is essential to address as they can influence how mentors and mentees can value diversity, equity, and inclusion in a mentoring relationship.

5. *Fostering independence.* Defining independence and what that looks like is dependent largely upon the setting and the roles within that setting. Providing students with fundamental skills in identifying key strategies to promote their own negotiation of autonomy has been shown to increase a student's sense of ownership and responsibility (Eller et al., 2014). Furthermore, identifying objectives toward goal setting is a key strategy useful in preparing students toward greater independence in a mentored relationship (Lee et al., 2015).

6. *Promoting professional development.* As the mentor–mentee relationship advances, it is essential that students feel comfortable in advancing their goals and reaching for new opportunities during their capstone experience. Mentors must acknowledge their role in promoting the professional development of their students (Byars-Winston & Dahlberg, 2019). By navigating conversations, mentors can help their mentees better balance work demands versus their personal interests and needs (Carmel & Paul, 2015).

MENTORSHIP ALIGNMENT AND WRITTEN AGREEMENT CONSIDERATIONS

Recognizing that mentorships are distinct due to the combinations of skills and experiences each student and content expert bring to the relationship, establishing a written agreement outside of the experiential plan or as part of the experiential plan may be helpful. One such agreement or tool to consider is a mentor compact. A *compact* is a written agreement which can help each member of the mentorship outline their commitment to the mentorship and what needs they envision requiring during the relationship with each other. A mentor compact may provide structure to the goals of the mentoring collaboration and the specific expectations and skills required to work toward those goals. In addition, other items of consideration may include areas mentioned previously in this chapter related to arrangements for meetings and communication frequency, alignment of expectation from each member of the agreement, and support which can be afforded for professional development. Since a mentor compact is a mutual document, each member of the team, both mentor and mentee, has the opportunity to share what works for them and what they can offer to the mentoring relationship in order that each party is clear to

what they are committing to and for how long. Figure 3-4 illustrates what a mentor compact may include and how the agreement may be structured.

FACILITATING A SELF-DIRECTED AND REGULATED LEARNER

Students' ability to be a self-directed and self-regulated learners will lend to their success in the capstone experience and project. In terms of these practice-ready concepts, Gage and Berliner (1991) describe key objectives for self-regulated learning in relationship to educational psychology: (1) to promote positive self-direction and independence, (2) to develop the ability to take responsibility for learning, (3) to develop creativity, and (4) to promote curiosity. One could argue that the inherent nature of the capstone experience addresses each of these objectives by design. These authors also emphasize that knowing how to learn is more important than purely gaining extensive knowledge, and the phases of self-regulated learning in Table 3-3 can help capstone students better reflect and enhance their metacognition on the subject of learning. Students are required to be self-directed in their learning and therefore increase their clinical reasoning, critical thinking, and team-based communication skills (Sadlo, 1994; Scaffa & Wooster, 2004). (See Text Box 3-9.)

TEXT BOX 3-9

Facilitating Self-Regulation and Emotional Intelligence

Keeping in mind that self-regulated learning and EI are explicit, practiced, and implemented over time, how will you help your students get there?

Think of a strategy you can incorporate with capstone students to foster self-regulation of learning and EI. Some evidence-based examples include the following (Zimmerman, 2002):

- Clarifying and modelling what good performance looks like (goals, criteria, expected standards, etc.)
- Facilitating the development of self-assessment and reflection
- Encouraging instructor and peer dialogue about the activity of learning
- Encouraging positive motivational beliefs and self-esteem
- Providing opportunities to close the gap between current and desired performance

EDUCATOR CHAPTER SUMMARY

The occupational therapy doctoral capstone opens up opportunities for students to explore and gain necessary experience in a range of clinical and community settings

---

Commitments of Student Mentor (Dr. Michelle McCann)

I will provide evidence of my qualification and expertise to serve as an OTD Faculty Capstone Chair/Mentor to the mentee's/student's designated focus area.

I will promote open and reciprocal opportunities for role modelling, coaching, professional support, and advocacy through diverse and inclusive experiences.

I will help the mentee reflect and think critically about their program/project and personal goals. I will review and provide feedback to the mentee on progress towards these goals.

I will facilitate the mentee's reflection on and exploration of their interests, abilities, beliefs, and ideas in order to help the mentee realize professional aspirations.

I will provide career guidance by assessing the mentee's academic and professional development and advocate for the mentee where applicable.

I will foster mentee autonomy and be an active participant in redefining the mentorship relationship as the program/project Accomplished in order to respect more peer-like interactions.

I will celebrate accomplishments and provide ongoing support as desired at the culmination of the program/project.

Faculty Capstone Chair/Mentor Signature:

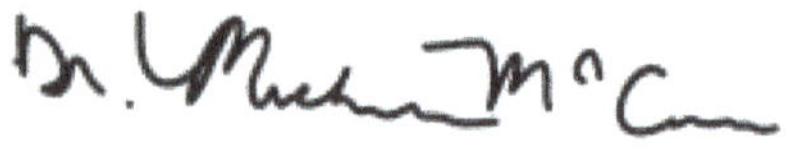

Date: 1/6/2024

OTD Mentee Signature: Alicia Colossi

Date: 1/16/2024

Figure 3-4. Mentorship compact example from the mentor perspective.

above what entry-level fieldwork exposures can prepare a student to envision. Educators must coordinate the blending and application of didactic knowledge and skills with workforce readiness skills, which will enable a capstone student to demonstrate the autonomy and readiness to apply resources and establish mutually beneficial relationships. These relationships can be diverse and complex. Each capstone site has unique needs and expectations based on their prior experiences with present stakeholders. Combined with the partnership of the academic institution and a mentee student, this dynamic can add both exciting and unanticipated demands on each member of the capstone team. Understanding each team member's prior knowledge, sills, and resources at the beginning of each mentoring relationship can help facilitate the practice readiness abilities of each student. In doing so, each member of the team is able to understand the utility of the

capstone and equip themselves with essential readiness to support a successful capstone experience.

ADDITIONAL EDUCATOR RESOURCES
Textbooks

Kolb, D. A. (2014). Experiential learning: *Experience as the source of learning and development*. Pearson Education.

Websites

For a source addressing a variety of topics, see a special issue of *New Directions for Teaching and Learning*, Summer 2011, Issue 126, a Self-Regulated Learning Special Issue on engagement, goal orientation, help-seeking, the role of

Web 2.0, computer-based learning, and more. Available online via Wiley Online Library: http://onlinelibrary.wiley.com/ doi/10.1002/tl.v2011.126/issuetoc.

The Highly Effective Teacher: www.thehighlyeffective-teacher.com

- Developing Self-Regulation
- Use of Mindfulness Exercises in the Classroom
- Incorporating Self-Assessment

Emotional Intelligence Consortium: www.eiconsortium.org

- References for Higher Education

Stanford Teaching Commons: www.teachingcommons.stanford.edu

- Student Self-Assessment

REFERENCES

Accreditation Council for Occupational Therapy Education. (2023). *Standards and interpretive guide.* http://acoteonline.org/accreditation-explained/standards/

Adams, N. (2015). *Bloom's taxonomy of cognitive learning objectives* (pp. 152–153). https://www.ncbi.nlm.nih.gov/pmc/articles/PMC4511057/pdf/mlab-103-03-152.pdf

American Occupational Therapy Association. (2022). Occupational therapy doctoral capstone: Purpose and value. *American Journal of Occupational Therapy, 76*(3), 7613410230. http://doi.org/10.5014/ajot.2022.76S3004

American Occupational Therapy Association. (2023). *AOTA 2023 workforce and compensation survey.* AOTA 2023 Workforce and Compensation Survey Report | AOTA.

Andonian, L. (2013). Emotional intelligence, self-efficacy, and occupational therapy students' fieldwork performance. *Occupational Therapy in Health Care, 27,* 201–215.

Andonian, L. (2017). Occupational therapy students' self-efficacy, experience of supervision, and perception of meaningfulness of level II fieldwork. *The Open Journal of Occupational Therapy, 5*(2). https://doi.org/10.15453/2168-6408.1220

Artino, A. R. (2012). Academic self-efficacy: From educational theory to instructional practice. *Perspectives on Medical Education, 1,* 76–85.

Atler, K., & Gavin, W. J. (2010). Service-learning-based instruction enhances students' perceptions of their abilities to engage in evidence-based practice. *Occupational Therapy in Health Care, 24,* 23–38.

Bagatell, N., Lawrence, J., Schwartz, M., & Vuernick, W. (2013). Occupational therapy student experiences and transformations during fieldwork in mental health settings. *Occupational Therapy in Mental Health, 29,* 181–196.

Baile, W. F., Lenzi, R., Glober, G., Beale, E. A., & Kudelka, A. P. (2010). SPIKES – A six-step protocol for delivering bad news: Application to the patient with cancer. *The Oncologist, 5,* 302–311.

Baird, J. M., Raina, K. D., Rogers, J. C., O'Donnell, J., Terhorst, L., & Holm, M. B. (2015). Simulation strategies to teach patient transfers: Self-efficacy by strategy. *American Journal of Occupational Therapy, 69*(Suppl. 2), 6912185030p1–6912185030p7.

Bandura, A. (1977). Self-efficacy: Toward a unifying theory of behavioral change. *Psychological Review, 84,* 191–215.

Bandura, A. (1997). *Self-efficacy: The exercise of control.* W. H. Freeman.

Biedenweg, K. A., & Monroe, M. (2013). Cognitive methods and a case study for assessing shared perspectives as a result of social learning. *Society & Natural Resources, 26,* 931–944.

Boud, D. (2013). *Enhancing learning through self-assessment.* Routledge.

Byars-Winston, A. M., Branchaw, J., Pfund, C., Leverett, P., & Newton, J. (2015). Culturally diverse undergraduate researchers' academic outcomes and perceptions of their research mentoring relationships. *International Journal of Science Education, 37*(15), 2533 –2554. https://doi.org/10.1080/09500693.2015.1085133

Byars-Winston, A., & Lund Dahlberg, M. (2019). *The science of effective mentorship in STEMM.* The National Academies Press.

Campbell, M. K., Corpus, K., Wussow, T. M., Plummer, T., Gibbs, D., & Hix, S. (2015). Fieldwork educators' perspectives: Professional behavior attributes of level II fieldwork students. *Open Journal of Occupational Therapy, 3*(4), Article 7.

Carmel, R. G., & Paul, M. W. (2015). Mentoring and coaching in academia: Reflections on a mentoring/coaching relationship. *Policy Futures in Education, 13*(4), 479–491. https://doi.org/10.1177/1478210315578562

Carmeli, A., & Josman, Z. E. (2006). The relationship among emotional intelligence, task performance, and organizational citizenship behaviors. *Human Performance, 19,* 403–419. https://doi.org/10.1207/s15327043hup1904_5

Chant, K. J., & Westendorf, D. S. (2019). Nurse residency programs: Key components for sustainability. *Journal for Nurses in Professional Development, 35*(4), 185–192.

Clarke, J., & Foxe, J. (2017). The impact of social anxiety on occupational participation in college life. *Occupational Therapy in Mental Health, 33,* 31–46.

Cook, A. B. (2023). Entry-level occupational therapy doctoral students' self-efficacy for the doctoral capstone experience: A mixed methods analysis. *American Journal of Occupational Therapy, 77*(2). https://doi.org/10.5014/ajot.2023.77S2-PO200

Costa, D. M. (2009). Transformative learning in fieldwork. *OT Practice, 14*(1), 19–20.

Cronin, A., & Graebe, G. (2018). *Clinical reasoning in occupational therapy.* AOTA Press.

Dall'Alba, G. (2009). Learning professional ways of being: Ambiguities of becoming. *Educational Philosophy and Theory, 41,* 34–45.

Deepa, S., & Seth, M. (2013). Do soft skills matter? Implications for educators based on recruiters' perspective. *IUP Journal of Soft Skills, 7*(1), 7–20.

DeIuliis, E., & Hanson, D. (2022). *Fieldwork educator's guide to level II fieldwork* (1st ed.). Routledge.

Derdall, M., Olson, P., Janzen, W., & Warren, S. (2002). Development of a questionnaire to examine confidence of occupational therapy students during fieldwork experiences. *Canadian Journal of Occupational Therapy, 69,* 49–56.

Eller, L. S., Lev, E. L., & Feurer, A. (2014). Key components of an effective mentoring relationship: A qualitative study. *Nurse Education Today, 34*(5), 815–820. https://doi.org/10.1016/j.nedt.2013.07.020

Emmons, R. A., & McCullough, M. E. (2003). Counting blessings versus burdens: An experimental investigation of gratitude and subjective well-being in daily life. *Journal of Personality and Social Psychology, 84,* 377–389.

Everly, J. S., Poff, D. W., Lamport, N., Hamant, C., & Alvey, G. (1994). Perceived stressor and coping strategies of occupational therapy students. *American Journal of Occupational Therapy, 48*(11), 1022–1028. https://doi.org/10.5014/ajot.48.11.1022

Gage, N., & Berliner, D. (1991). *Educational psychology* (5th ed.). Houghton Mifflin Harcourt.

Godwin, K. M., Narayanan, A., Arredondo, K., Miltner, R. S., Bowen, M. E., Gilman, S., Shirks, A., Eng, J. A., Naik, A. D., & Hysong, S. J. (2021). Value of interprofessional education: The VA quality scholars program. *The Journal for Healthcare Quality (JHQ), 43*(5), 304–311.

Goodsett, M. (2021). *"Commitment, respect, and trust: The building blocks of a strong mentoring relationship" from academic library mentoring: Fostering growth and renewal* (Rod-Welch & Weeg, Ed.). ACRL Publications.

Gribble, N., Ladyshewsky, R. K., & Parsons, R. (2017). Fluctuations in the emotional intelligence of therapy students during clinical placements: Implication for educators, supervisors, and students. *Journal of Interprofessional Care*, 31, 8–17.

Gruenberg, K., Hsia, S., O'Brien, B., & O'Sullivan, P. (2021). Exploring multiple perspectives on pharmacy students' readiness for advanced pharmacy practice experiences. *American Journal of Pharmaceutical Education*, 85(5), 8358. https://doi.org/10.5688/ajpe8358

Hardie, P., Darley, A., Langan, L., Lafferty, A., Jarvis, S., & Redmond, C. (2022). Interpersonal and communication skills development in general nursing preceptorship education and training programmes: A scoping review. *Nurse Education in Practice*, 65, 103482. https://doi.org/10.1016/j.nepr.2022.103482

Haro, A. V., Knight, B. P., Cameron, D. L., Nixon, S. A., Ahluwalia, P. A., & Hicks, E. L. (2014). Becoming an occupational therapist: Perceived influence of international fieldwork placements on clinical practice. *Canadian Journal of Occupational Therapy*, 81, 173–182.

Harris, H. L., Kiraly-Alvarez, A. F., Costello, P. J., & Schmeltz, B. (2023). Understanding the doctoral capstone coordinator position: A unique faculty role in occupational therapy education. *The Open Journal of Occupational Therapy*, 11(2), 1–14. https://doi.org/10.15453/2168-6408.2039

Henderson, J. (2010). Transformative learning: Four activities that set the stage. *Online Education*. http://www.uwex.edu/disted/conference/Resource_library/proceedings/28439_10.pdf

Henry-Noel, N., Bishop, M., Gwede, C. K., Petkova, E., & Szumacher, E. (2019). Mentorship in medicine and other health professions. *Journal of Cancer Education*, 34, 629–637. https://doi.org/10.1007/s13187-018-1360-6

Hoppes, S., Bender, D., & DeGrace, B. W. (2005). A service learning is a perfect fit for occupational and physical therapy education. *Journal of Allied Health*, 34, 47.

Huskins, W. C., Silet, K., Weber-Main, A. M., Begg, M. D., Fowler, Jr., V. G., Hamilton, J., & Fleming, M. (2011), Identifying and aligning expectations in a mentoring relationship. *Clinical and Translational Science*, 4, 439–447. https://doi.org/10.1111/j.1752-8062.2011.00356.x

Institute of Medicine. (2011). *Crossing the quality chasm: A new health system for the 21st century*. Report by the Committee on Quality of Health Care in America. National Academies Press.

Jackson, D. (2010). How personal trainers can use self-efficacy theory to enhance exercise behavior in beginning exercisers. *Strength and Conditioning Journal*, 32, 7–71.

Jarvis, P. (2010). *Adult education and lifelong learning, theory and practice* (4th ed.). Routledge.

Keinänen, A. L., Lähdesmäki, R., Juntunen, J., Tuomikoski, A. M., Kääriäinenm, M., & Mikkonen, K. (2023). Effectiveness of mentoring education on health professionals' mentoring competence: A systematic review. *Nurse Education Today*, 121, 105709. https://doi.org/10.1016/j.nedt.2023.105709

Kemp, E., Domina, A., Delbert, T., Rivera, A., & Navarro-Walker, L. (2020). Development, implementation and evaluation of entry-level occupational therapy doctoral capstones: A national survey. *Journal of Occupational Therapy Education*, 4(4). https://doi.org/10.26681/jote.2020.040411

King, J., Barclay, R., Ripat, J., Dubouloz, C. J., & Schwartz, C. (2015). Response shift and transformative learning – do physical therapists and occupational therapists use concepts of change in their clinical practice? *Physiotherapy*, 101, e757–e758.

Kolb, D. A. (1984). *Experiential learning: Experience as the source of learning and development*. Prentice Hall.

Kolb, D. A. (2014). Experiential learning: *Experience as the source of learning and development*. Pearson Education.

Kroll, C., & Delbert, T. (2023). Doctoral capstone: Secrets to student success. *Academic Education Special Interest Section (SIS) Quarterly*. https://www.aota.org/publications/sis-quarterly/academic-education-sis/aesis-8-23?utm_source=SIS%20quarterly%20August%202023

Lave, J., & Wenger, E. (2003). *Situated learning: Legitimate peripheral participation*. Cambridge University Press.

Lee, P. S., McGee, R., Pfund, C., & Branchaw, J. (2015). "Mentoring up": Learning to manage your mentoring relationships. In G. Wright (Ed.), *The mentoring continuum: From graduate school to tenure* (1st ed., pp. 133–151). Syracuse University: The Graduate School Press.

Mahapatra, G. P., Bhullar, N., & Gupta, P. (2022). Gen Z: An emerging phenomenon. *NHRD Network Journal*, 15(2), 246–256. https://doi.org/10.1177/26314541221077137

Matthew-Maich, N., Ploeg, J., Jack, S., & Dobbins, M. (2010). Transformative learning and research utilization in nursing practice: A missing link? *Worldviews on Evidence-Based Nursing*, 1, 25–35.

Mattila, A. (2017). *Perceptions of occupational therapy students participating in role emerging fieldwork at community agencies: An explanatory case study*. Robert Morris University.

Mattila, A. M., & Dolhi, C. (2016). Transformative experience of master of occupational therapy students in a non-traditional fieldwork setting. *Occupational Therapy in Mental Health*, 32, 16–31.

Mayer, J. D., Salovey, P., & Caruso, D. (2008). Emotional intelligence: New ability or eclectic traits? *American Psychologist*, 63, 503–517. https://doi.org/10.1037/0003-066x.63.6.503

McGarity, T., Monahan, L., Acker, K., & Pollock, W. (2023). Nursing graduates' preparedness for practice: Substantiating the call for competency-evaluated nursing education. *Behavioral Sciences*, 13(7), 553. https://doi.org/10.3390/bs13070553

McKenna, J., & Mellson, J. (2013). Emotional intelligence and the occupational therapist. *British Journal of Occupational Therapy*, 76, 427–430.

Merriam, S. B., Caffarella, R. S., & Baumgartner, L. M. (2007). *Learning in adulthood: A comprehensive guide*. Jossey-Bass.

Mezirow, J. (1997). Transformative learning: Theory to practice. *New Directions for Adult and Continuing Education*, (74), 5–12. https://doi.org/10.1002/ace.7401

Mezirow, J. (2000). Learning to think like an adult: Core concepts of transformation theory. In J. Mezirow & Associates (Eds.), *Learning as transformation: Critical perspectives on a theory in progress* (pp. 3–34). Jossey-Bass.

Mitchell, M. M., & Kampfe, C. M. (1990). Coping strategies used by occupational therapy students during fieldwork: An exploratory study. *American Journal of Occupational Therapy*, 44, 543–550.

Mitchell, M. M., & Kampfe, C. M. (1993). Student coping strategies and perceptions of fieldwork. *American Journal of Occupational Therapy*, 47, 535–540.

National Association of Colleges and Employers. (2024). *What is career readiness?* https://www.naceweb.org/career-readiness/competencies/career-readiness-defined/

Noble, C., McKauge, L., & Clavarino, A. (2019). Pharmacy student professional identity formation: A scoping review. *Integrated Pharmacy Research & Practice*, 8, 15–34. https://doi.org/10.2147/IPRP.S162799

Parker, K., & Igielnik, R. (2020). *On the cusp of adulthood and facing an uncertain future: What we know about Gen Z so far*. Pew Research Center.

Pfeifer, T. A., Kranz, P. L., & Scoogin, A. E. (2008). Perceived stress in occupational therapy students. *Occupational Therapy International*, 15, 221–231.

Pfund, C., Branchaw, J., & Handelsman, J. (2014). *Entering mentoring*. W. H. Freeman. ISBN-13 978-1464184901.

Pollard, R., & Kumar, S. (2021). Mentoring graduate students online: Strategies and challenges. *The International Review of Research in Open and Distributed Learning*, 22(2), 267–284. https://doi.org/10.19173/irrodl.v22i2.5093.

Rodger, S., Fitzgerald, C., Davila, W., Millar, F., & Allison, H. (2011). What makes a quality occupational therapy practice placement? Students' and practice educators' perspectives. *Australian Occupational Therapy Journal*, 58, 195–202.

Sadlo, G. (1994). Problem-based learning in the development of an occupational therapy curriculum, Part 2: The BSc at the London School of Occupational Therapy. *British Journal of Occupational Therapy*, 57, 79–84.

Santalucia, S., & Johnson, C. R. (2010). Transformative learning: Facilitating growth and change through fieldwork. *OT Practice, 15,* CE1–CE7.

Scaffa, M. E., & Reitz, S. M. (2013). *Occupational therapy community-based practice settings.* F.A. Davis.

Scaffa, M. E., & Wooster, D. M. (2004). Effects of problem-based learning on clinical reasoning in occupational therapy. *American Journal of Occupational Therapy, 58,* 333–336.

Schunk, D. H. (1989). Self-efficacy and achievement behaviors. *Educational Psychology Review, 1,* 173–208.

Smith, A. L. (2021). Evidence-based practice training in nurse residency programs: Enhancing confidence for practice implementation. *Teaching and Learning in Nursing, 16*(4), 315–320.

Soja, J., Sanders, M., & Haughey, K. (2016). Perceived stressors and coping in junior, senior, and graduate occupational therapy students. *American Journal of Occupational Therapy, 70*(4, Supp. 1), 7011505178p1.

Stephenson, S., Rogers, O., Ivy, C., Barron, R., & Burke, J. (2020). Designing effective capstone experiences and projects for entry-level doctoral students in occupational therapy: One program's approaches and lessons learned. *The Open Journal of Occupational Therapy, 8*(3), 1–12. https://doi.org/10.15453/2168–6408.1727\

Stephenson, S. J., Ivy, C., Vonier, M., & Sweets, D. (2024). Building bridges: A mentor education program for occupational therapy practitioners. *Journal of Occupational Therapy Education, 8*(1). https://encompass.eku.edu/jote/vol8/iss1/19

Stillwell, S. B., Vermeesch, A. L., & Scott, J. G. (2017). Interventions to reduce perceived stress among graduate students: A systematic review with implications for evidence-based practice. *Worldviews Evidence-Based Nursing, 14*(6), 507–513. https://doi.org/10.1111/wvn.12250

Taff, S. D., & Blash, D. (2017). Diversity and inclusion in occupational therapy: Where we are, where we must go. *Occupational Therapy in Health Care, 31*(1), 72–83.

Talero, P., Kern, S. B., & Tupé, D. A. (2015). Culturally responsive care in occupational therapy: An entry-level educational model embedded in service-learning. *Scandinavian Journal of Occupational Therapy, 22,* 95–102.

Thomas, J., Beyer, J., & Sealy, L. (2018). Emotional intelligence: Developing soft skills to Increase student success during fieldwork experience as practicing clinicians. *SIS Quarterly Practice Connections, 3*(2), 8–10.

Torres, K. M., Giddies, L., & Statti, A. (2021). Examining student mentorship experiences in an online program. *Journal of Educational Research & Practice, 11*(1), 320–334. https://doi.org/10.5590/JERAP.2021.11.1.23

van Dinther, M., Dochy, F., & Segers, M. (2011). Factors affecting students' self-efficacy in higher education. *Educational Research Review, 6,* 95–108.

Wake Forest University. (2024). *Defining personal and relationship expectations worksheet.* https://mentoring.opcd.wfu.edu/tools-and-resources/

Wald, H. S., Anthony, D., Hutchinson, T. A., Liben, S., Smilovitch, M., & Donato, A. A. (2015). Professional identity formation in medical education for humanistic, resilient physicians: Pedagogic strategies for bridging theory to practice. *Academic Medicine, 90,* 753–760.

Zechariah, S., Ansa, B. E., Johnson, S. W., Gates, A. M., & Leo, G. (2019). Interprofessional education and collaboration in healthcare: An exploratory study of the perspectives of medical students in the United States. *Healthcare, 7*(4), 117. https://doi.org/10.3390/healthcare7040117

Zimmerman, B. J. (2002). Becoming a self-regulated learner: An overview. *Theory Into Practice, 41*(2), 64–70.

CHAPTER 4

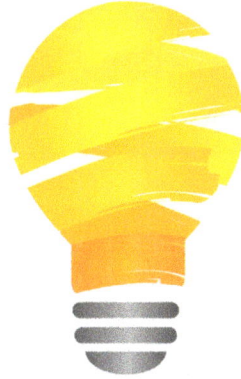

Exploring the Self and Site

Annie L. DeRolf

Section 1: Student Focus

Human-Centered Design Mindsets for Doctoral Students

The development phase of the doctoral capstone involves both self-exploration and the investigation of potential capstone sites. This phase aligns with the inspiration phase within the human-centered design framework. Being inspired and knowing oneself are dynamically interwoven, and self-knowledge will be one of your guiding lights as you explore doctoral capstone sites. The human-centered design mindsets of creative confidence, optimism, and embracing ambiguity will be important for you to hold in mind as you enter this phase of capstone development.

Creative confidence. Creative confidence will empower you to trust your unique skills and perspectives as you navigate the development phase of your doctoral capstone. We are all made to be occupational beings, and creativity involves doing. With creative confidence, you can approach this phase with boldness and innovation.

Embrace ambiguity. Embracing ambiguity will give you "permission to be fantastically creative" (Martin, n.d., par. 1). It will encourage you to be comfortable with the uncertainties and complexities of this phase. By accepting that not all answers will be clear from the start, you can remain open to new insights and opportunities, allowing for a more flexible and adaptive approach to this process.

Optimism. "Optimism is the embrace of possibility, the idea that even if we don't know the answer, that it's out there and that we can find it" (Bielenberg, n.d., Optimism section). This mindset will encourage you to approach the development phase with a positive outlook. By believing that you will find a capstone site that aligns with your values and goals, you will remain motivated and resilient, viewing challenges as opportunities for growth and innovation. This optimistic perspective may help you stay focused on achieving meaningful and impactful outcomes.

DOI: 10.4324/9781003541813-5

INTRODUCTION FOR STUDENTS

The development phase is the first step in the doctoral capstone planning process. Naturally, one of the primary questions you may ask is: "*Where* will I complete my doctoral capstone experience and project?" While this is certainly a critical question, it is not necessarily the best starting point. A more generative inquiry might be: "What do I have to offer, and what do I want to gain from the opportunity to complete a doctoral capstone?" This chapter aims to guide you in exploring yourself and your community by engaging in several reflective action steps, such as creating an identity map, constructing a mission statement, and aligning these with your occupational therapy doctoral (OTD) program philosophy and potential capstone site.

STUDENT REFLECTIVE QUESTIONS

During the development phase of the doctoral capstone, you may find it helpful to reflect on the following questions:

1. What unique skills, experiences, and perspectives do I bring to my doctoral capstone experience and project, and how can they benefit a potential site and/or community?
2. What personal and professional goals do I hope to achieve through my doctoral capstone, and how can these goals shape my mission statement?
3. How can I align my identity, values, and mission with the objectives of my program and the needs of my potential capstone site?

STUDENT OBJECTIVES

After reading this chapter and completing the learning activities, you should be able to:

1. Create an identity map and align with potential capstone sites.
2. Develop a personal mission statement and align with potential capstone site mission statements.
3. Align the personal mission and site mission to the mission and philosophy of the occupational therapy program.
4. Articulate the flow of capstone site communication and site procurement.
5. Create a plan to match with site and site population.

STUDENT IDENTITY MAPPING (SIM)

Acknowledgement. The specific content and guided activities in both student- and educator-focused sections of this chapter related to identity mapping and ethical community engagement are rooted in the work of Dr. Mary F. Price and colleagues. When I began my role as a doctoral capstone coordinator (DCC) at Indiana University Indianapolis (IUI), Dr. Price was the director of faculty development in the Center for Service and Learning, as well as the technical consultant for academic affairs. Dr. Price is a co-developer of the SOFAR partnership model (Bringle et al., 2009), as well as a co-developer of a related tool known as Collaborative Relationship Mapping (ColRM), both of which will be cited and undergird the scope and activities within this chapter. Dr. Price spent considerable time with me and my doctoral capstone students, inspiring the discovery of self and purpose through this framework and these activities, which as we will see, can transform the doctoral capstone development phase.

What Is Student Identity Mapping?

Student identity mapping (SIM) is "a sense-making activity" that invites you to describe, examine, and graphically represent who you are, what you value, and the ultimate purposes of your current and future work (Price, 2019, p. 2). As a doctoral student completing this activity, you are invited to examine yourself as both a professional and an occupational being. In so doing, you will complete this activity in two parts. In Part 1, you will examine your values across your roles as a learner and as an emerging practitioner (EP). In Part 2, you will consider the values you hold alongside your "public purposes" (i.e., professional goals) and how you situate yourself as an EP within the dimensions of justice and social responsibility in collaborative partnerships (M. Price, personal communication, August 17, 2020). (See Text Box 4-1.)

TEXT BOX 4-1

Learning Tips

1. Invest in yourself by making reflective work a priority.
2. Manage and even reclaim time to work on you.
3. Do not rush the process. Break up the work to allow for adequate time to reflect and process your ideas.
4. Allow this to be a guilt-free endeavor. Treat this time like you would if you were working on a project or preparing for an exam.

Source: Price (2019). M. Price, personal communication, August 17, 2020.

Part 1, Steps 1 and 2 of SIM: Guided Reading and Reflection

The sources for step 1's guided reading may be selected by you or your doctoral capstone coordinator (DCC). In the case of my doctoral students, Dr. Price and I assigned Suzanne M. Peloquin's (2005) Eleanor Clarke Slagle Lecture *Embracing Our Ethos, Reclaiming Our Heart* (see Section II for reasoning). After a close reading of Peloquin's article,

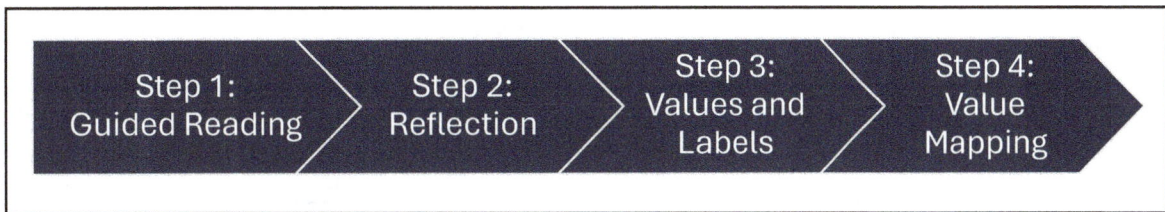

Figure 4-1. Part 1 of the SIM process. *Source:* Figure adapted from Price (2019), p. 3.

Table 4-1 Example Values

ACCURACY	COMPETITION	COMMUNITY	INDEPENDENCE	COLLABORATION	RIGOR
Trustworthiness	Expertise	Discipline	Dialogue	Justice	Inclusiveness
Equity	Reciprocity	Generativity	Entrepreneurialism	Innovation	Democracy
Objectivity	Participation	Fairness	Safety	Practicability	Humility

Note: This table provides examples of values that may inform your work as a doctoral student and EP. This table does not represent an exhaustive list.

reflect on what you read. (See Text Box 4-2 for four tips to enhance your close reading skills and the reflective questions that were assigned to my previous students. These will guide you in assessing your values.)

TEXT BOX 4-2

Learning Tips for Close Reading

1. *Annotate the text.* Making notes in the margins, underlining key phrases, and highlighting important passages will help you engage actively with the text and remember significant or standout details.
2. *Ask questions.* Generate questions about the text as you read. What themes are present? How do different elements of the text interact? What are the author's main points? How do they support their claims and/or ideas? How is the text organized? Do you notice any patterns?
3. *Re-read for deeper understanding.* Close reading often requires multiple readings. Focus on general comprehension on your first read. Re-read to focus on deeper analysis; you can use the previous example questions to facilitate your critical thinking.
4. *Summarize your thoughts.* Summarize your notes in your own words, and try to identify the most relevant details. Using SIM as an example, you can summarize themes in the text and relate them to the reflection questions and values identified.
Source: Proofed (2021). We Are Teachers Staff (2023). Webb (2023).

Reflection Questions

1. List the personal values that you identified within this article. Why did you identify with the values you selected?
2. What professional concepts did you find that resonated with you? Explain.

TEXT BOX 4-2 (continued)

3. The article listed some challenges to an integrative ethos. Did these surprise you? Explain why the challenges did or did not surprise you.
4. Which challenge resonated with you?
5. There are several reflections at the end of the article. Which one fits most with your view of occupational therapy?
Source: M. Price, personal communication (August 17, 2020).

Part 1, Step 3 of SIM: Values and Labels

It is during this step that you will identify the values that inform your work as a doctoral student and EP. Drawing on a non-comprehensive list provided by Dr. M. Price (personal communication, August 17, 2020), identify three to four values from Table 4-1 that are essential to your roles as doctoral student/learner, EP, leader, and advocate. If a value you hold is not listed, please add it.

Next, use the table that follows to spur your thinking, and select two to three that describe *who you are* professionally. As before, if a description you have in mind is not listed, please add it. (See Table 4-2.)

Part 1, Step 4 of SIM: Value Mapping

In this step of the activity, you will draft your identity map. First, consider the relationship among your roles: Is there a connection/intersection among your roles as a doctoral student, EP, leader, and advocate? What is the nature of this connection (e.g., close, siloed, etc.)? The relationships can be represented as a Venn diagram (see Figure 4-2), but you can graphically represent this however this makes most sense to you. Other examples can be noted in Figures 4-3 and 4-4. You can also change the size of the circles to better represent how strongly you identify with each role. This is your map and a product of your own creation!

Table 4-2 Example Role Descriptors

ENTREPRENEUR	RESEARCHER	SCHOLAR	INTELLECTUAL	PUBLIC	EDUCATOR
Organizer	Community-based	Community-engaged	Servant	Translational	Practitioner
Activist	Administrator	Leader	Justice-oriented	Scientist	Academic

Note: This table provides examples of descriptors that may represent or describe the roles you associate with your identity as an EP. This table does not represent an exhaustive list.

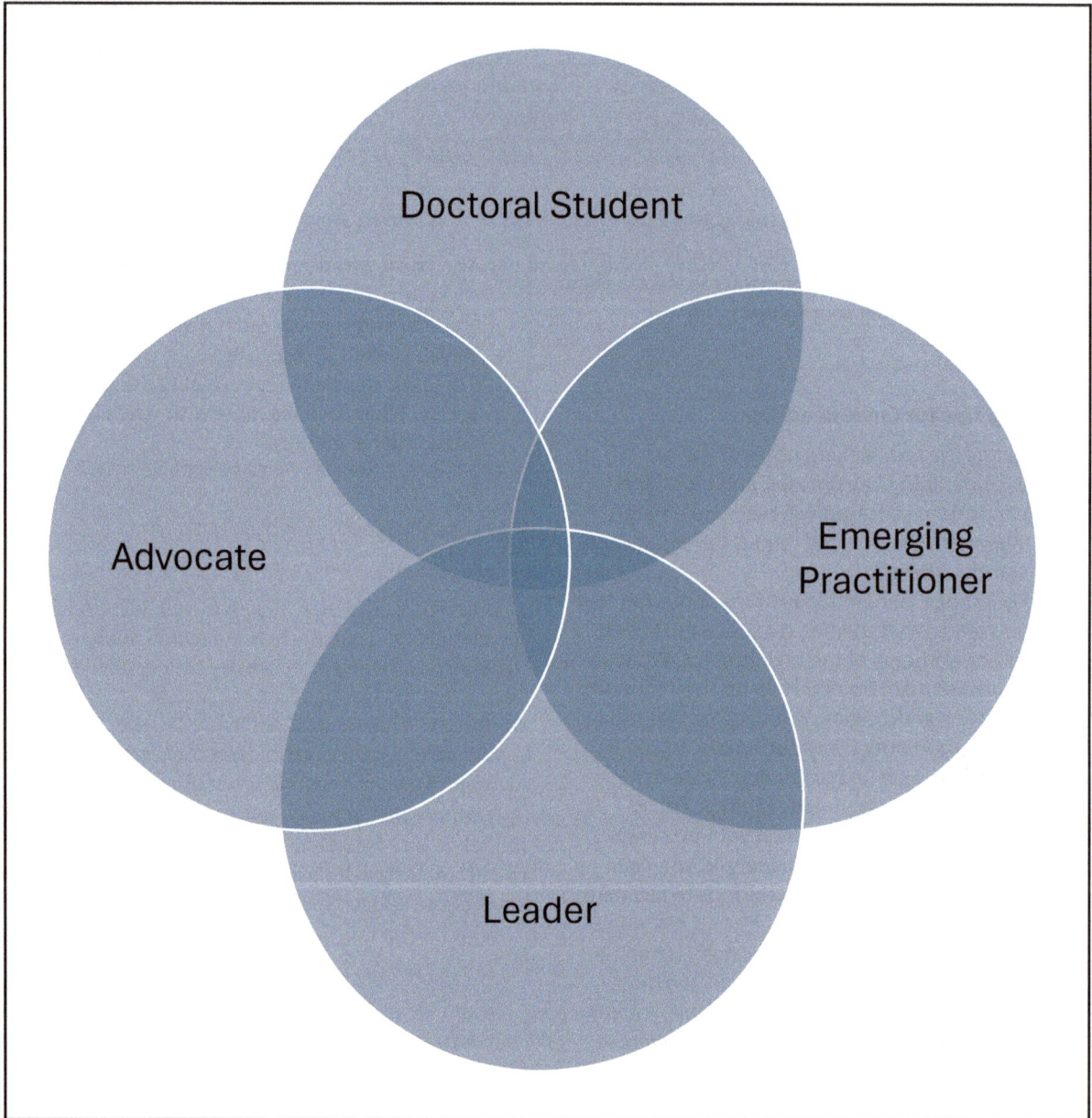

Figure 4-2. Example depictions of relationships among roles. *Source:* Figure adapted from Price (2019).

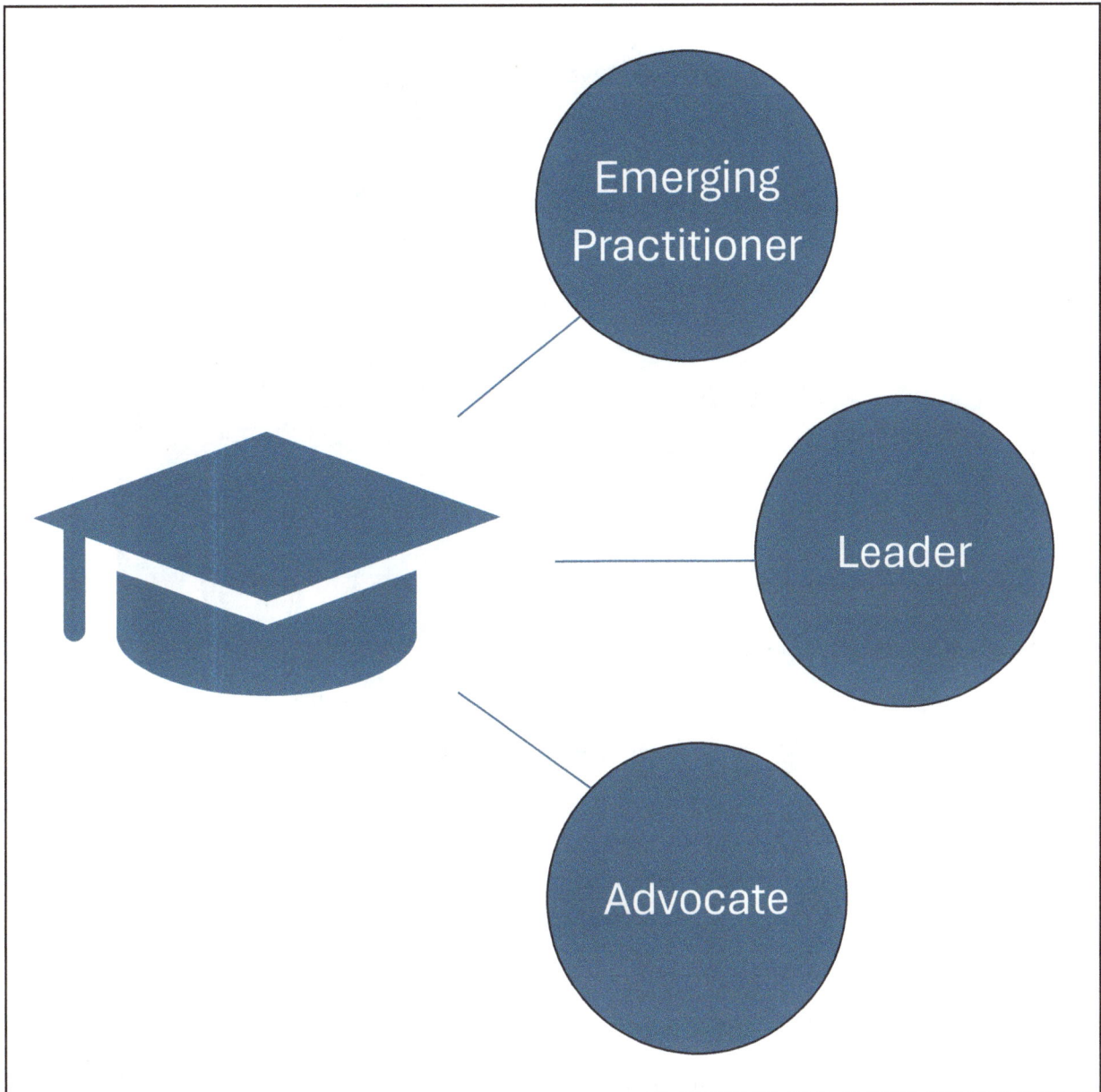

Figure 4-3. Example depiction of relationships among roles. *Source:* Figure adapted from Price (2019).

Once you have a graphic representation of your roles and the relationships among them, add the two to three *descriptors* that you identified in step 3 of who you are professionally. If you used a Venn diagram, these can be added in the center. Next, add to your map the *values* you identified in step 3, and draw circles around the ones that are <u>essential</u> to who you are as an EP.

When finished, you will have completed Part 1, the student values map! (See Figure 4-5 for an example of the map at this stage.) In Part 2 of SIM, you will focus on the "public purposes" of your work and discover how your EP values intersect (2020a). As a result of Part 2, your student values map will be transformed into a completed EP identity map. (See Figure 4-6 for a review of the SIM process.)

Part 2, Steps 1–3 of SIM: Guided Reading, Reflection, and Response

Similarly to steps 1 and 2 in Part 1, you will need to set aside time for guided reading, reflection, and response in Part 2. For these steps, Dr. M. Price (personal communication, August 31, 2020) and I assigned for close reading Aldrich et al. (2017), "Justice and U.S. Occupational Therapy Practice: A Relationship 100 Years in the Making." After reading the article, students reflected upon and answered the following questions:

- "Why is it important for U.S. occupational therapy practitioners to conceptualize their practices more strongly as justice-oriented endeavors?" (Aldrich et al., 2017, pp. 2–3).

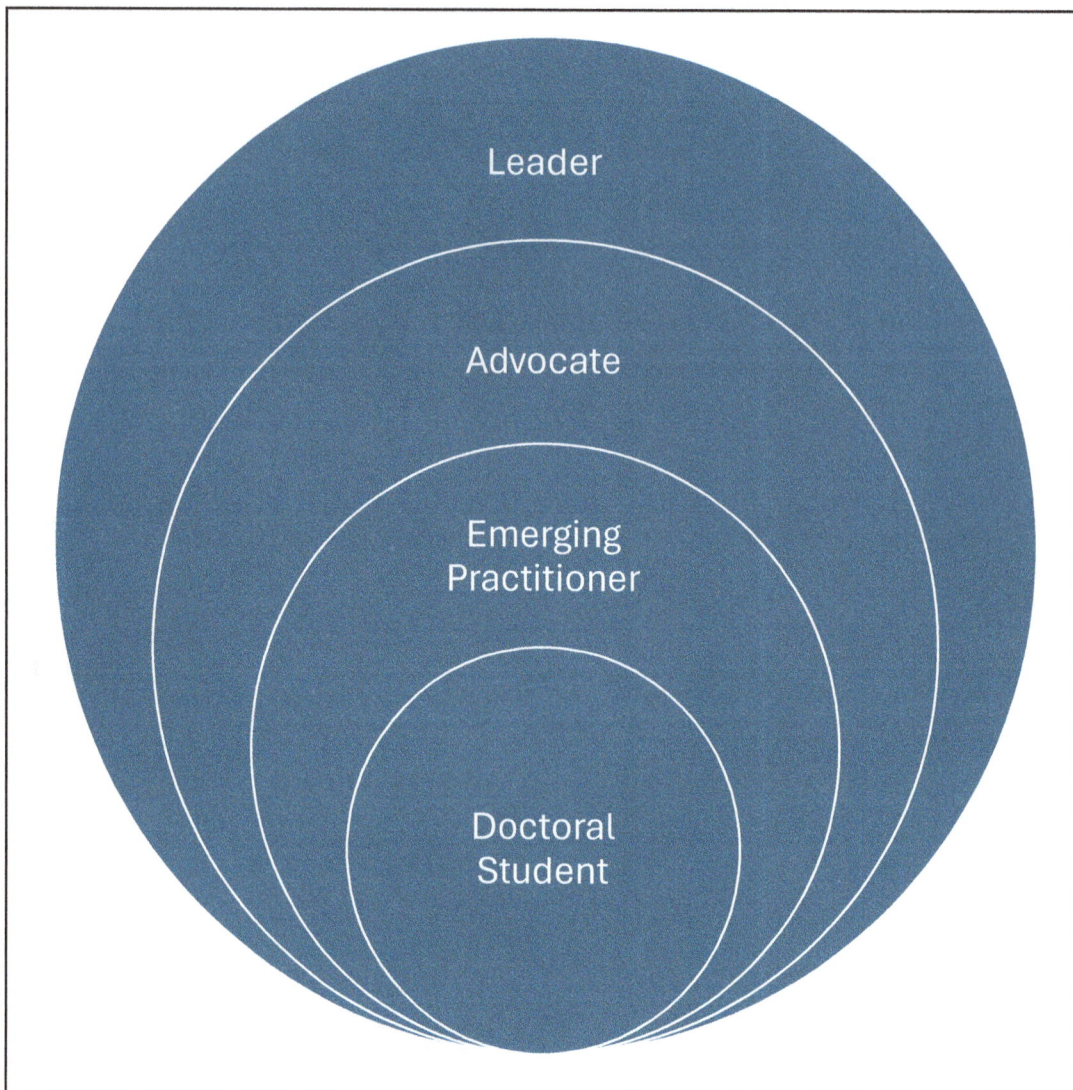

Figure 4-4. Example depiction of relationships among roles. *Source:* Figure adapted from Price (2019).

- How does occupational therapy's ethos match with the idea of occupational justice?
- How does this knowledge affect your view of yourself as an EP? As a student? As a future educator (academic or fieldwork)?
- How does occupational justice fit with your student values map and with your professional descriptions?

Part 2, Step 4 of SIM: Pre-Mapping Questions

Reflecting on the map you created in Part 1, determine the "individual or private" purposes and "public" purposes of your work as EPs and how they relate to your values (Price, 2019, p. 7). Examples of private purposes include getting paid to do the work you love, sharing your love of learning with others, or making discoveries. On the other hand, public purposes work to sustain and enrich a democratic society (Price, 2019). Examples of public purposes include ensuring that all people have equitable access to evidence-based, high-quality health care; improving the quality of life for clients, communities, and populations; promoting adaptation for clients, activities, and/or communities to reduce barriers to full participation in occupation (Price, personal communication, August 31, 2020). You are encouraged to articulate the private and public purposes of the work that is unique to *you* and in your own words.

Consider again the work you do across your roles as a doctoral student, EP, leader, and advocate. Next, illustrate with two to three examples . . .

- How your work may nudge the world closer to achieving the public purposes you cite" (Price, personal communication, August 31, 2020).
- "How you engage your values in support of the public purposes of your work. Make sure to identify relevant values. [NOTE: You may end up revising the values on your map].

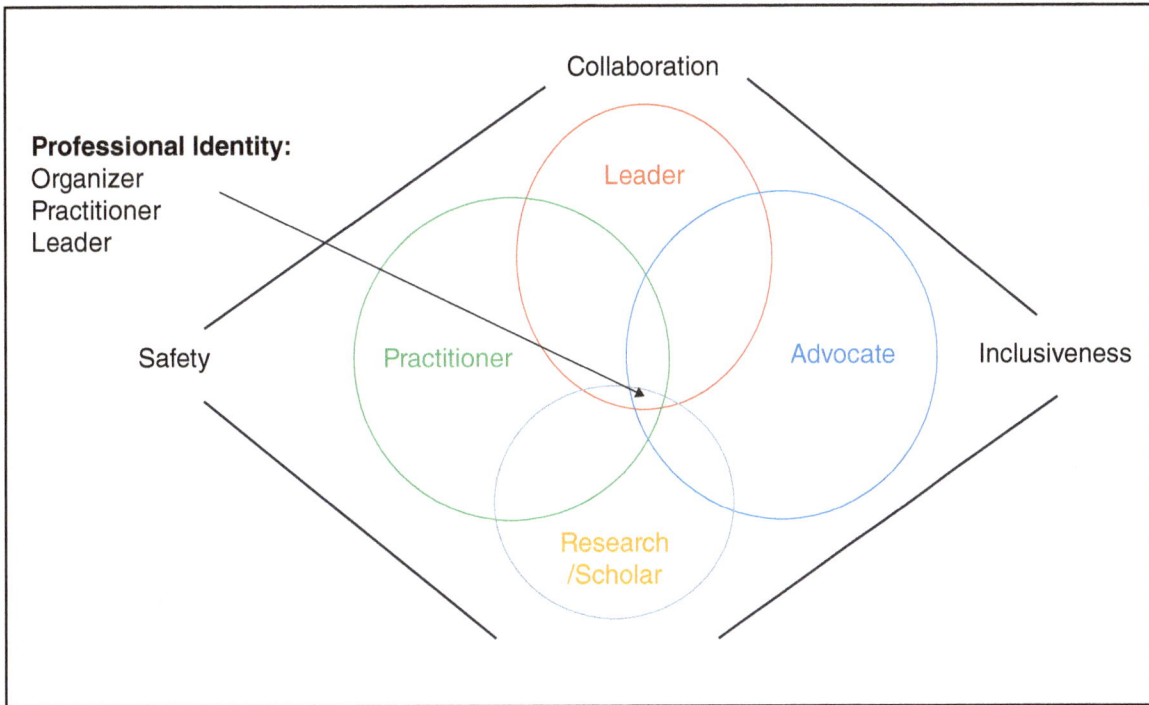

Figure 4-5 Example of a completed "Part 1: Student Identity Map."

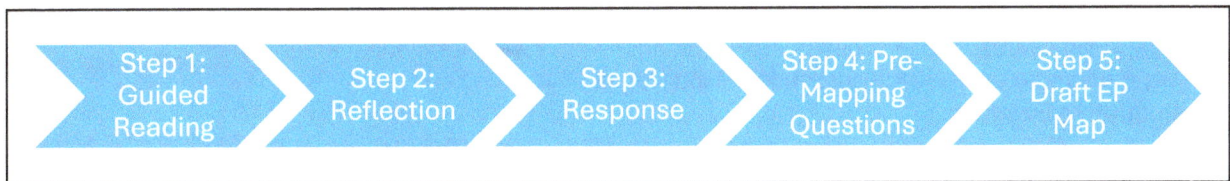

Figure 4-6. Part 2 of the SIM process. *Source:* Figure adapted from M. Price (personal communication, August 31, 2020).

- Place an (*) next to any cited items related to your role as EP.
  (Price, personal communication, August 31, 2020)

For example, perhaps you have . . .
- Completed a rapid systematic review (RSR) on the topic of lifestyle medicine and occupational therapy.
  ○ **Values:** *collaboration, rigor, expertise, holism, quality of life*
- Co-developed a Coalition for Occupational Therapy Advocates for Diversity (COTAD) chapter for your program
  ○ **Values:** *inclusivity, justice, equity, socially responsive health care, education, advocacy*
- Completed a level II fieldwork experience in an inpatient psychiatric setting
  ○ **Values:** *holism, creativity, collaboration, client-centeredness*

After citing your own examples, select one and briefly describe how this particular example (1) engages your values and (2) serves the public purposes of your work.

Part 2, Step 5 of SIM: Draft Your EP Identity Map

Locate the map you created in step 1. Your map should include thus (Price, personal communication, August 31, 2020):

- Your preferred descriptors for yourself as an EP at the center of your map
- The relationships between your roles as an EP, leader, advocate, and doctoral student (i.e., how much you identify with each role and the degree of their overlap)
- Your values (highlight which values are central to you)
- The public purposes of your work (via bullet points or a representation of your choosing)
- The example you chose to illustrate how you engage your values through one of your public purposes

(See following Figure 4-7 for an example of a completed map.)

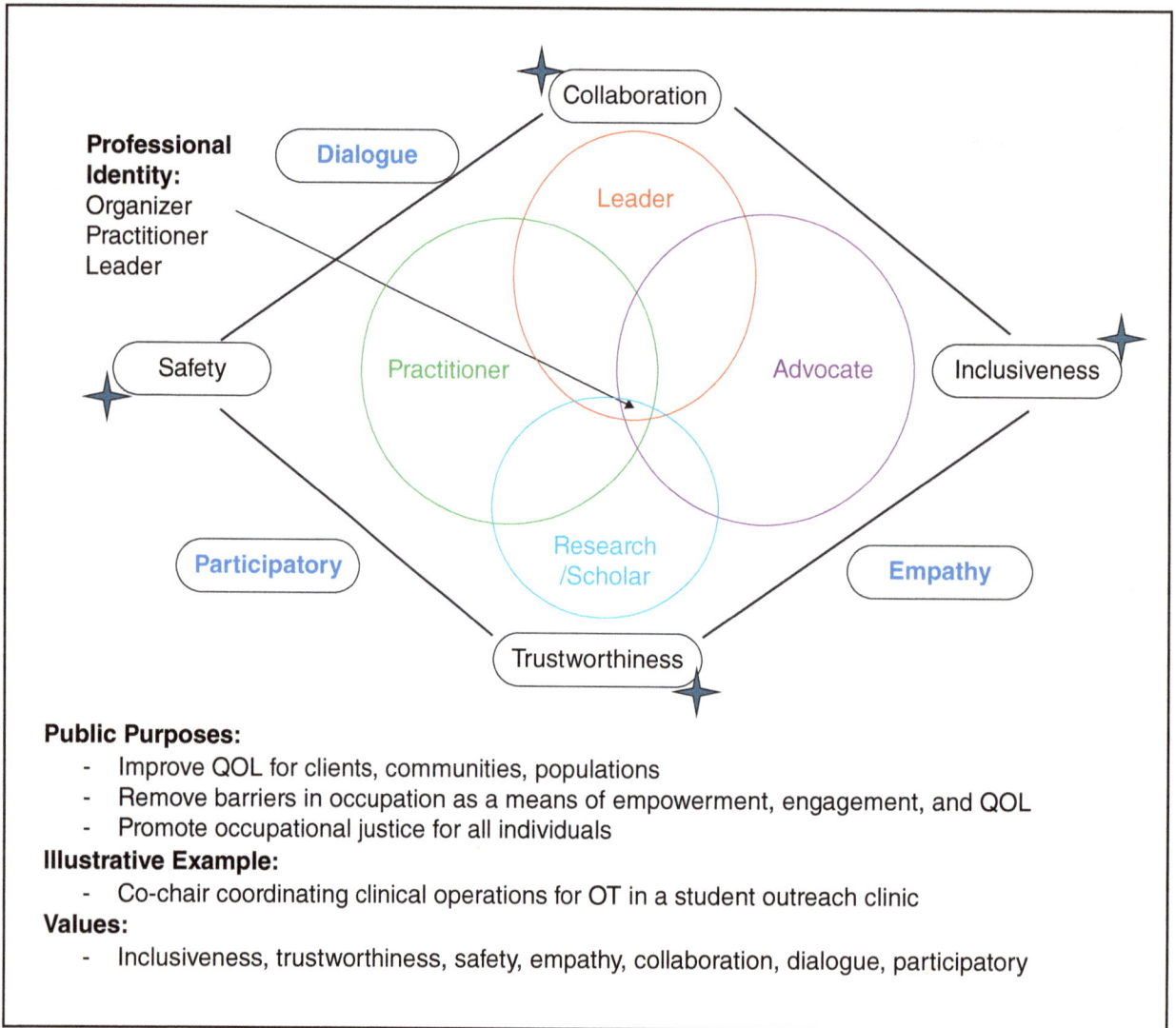

Figure 4-7. Example of a completed Part 2 student identity map.

"Exploring my professional identity was a crucial element in the success of my capstone project. Through reflection on the intersections of my personal values, professional goals, and scholarly pursuits, I gained a clear understanding of my capstone site and purpose. As I navigated the capstone process, I became more aware of how my skills, knowledge, and passion for advocacy and equity needed to be represented with my capstone project. This self-awareness not only guided my project development but also ensured that my capstone was both meaningful and impactful. By intentionally integrating these aspects of my professional identity in this project, I was able to grow my skills as a practitioner through gaining advanced clinical skills in feeding therapy. Through receiving this foundational knowledge, I was able to create a project that reflected my commitment to providing accessible and equitable resources for caregivers on feeding therapy. Ultimately, this exploration contributed to the success of my capstone project, as I was able to grow my skill set in advanced clinical practice. In addition, my site was able to utilize the variety of tools created to support education for providers and caregivers."

– Jocelyne Hernandez, OTD, OTD, Indiana University OTD class of 2023

DEVELOPING A PERSONAL MISSION STATEMENT

After spending considerable time exploring yourself through the SIM activity, it is time to develop your mission statement. Mission statements help identify core values and beliefs, allowing you to prioritize your life. Covey (2004) stated that "a personal mission statement describes what matters most to you, including your vision and values" (pp. 158–159). In addition to the values you have already identified, components of a mission statement include a major life goal, positive language, positive energy, present-tense grammar, and conciseness. An example OTD mission statement could be: "I am dedicated to empowering individuals of all abilities to achieve their fullest potential. I strive to create inclusive and just environments where everyone can thrive. I embrace diversity, advocate for equity, and inspire positive change through compassionate care and innovative solutions." Creating a personal mission statement will guide you as your capstone site is finalized and throughout your capstone experience and project. Now that you have explored who you are as an EP and your core values and constructed your initial mission statement, you can begin to identify sites that align with these aspects. This will assist you and your DCC in determining a final fit.

DETERMINING GOODNESS OF FIT

The purpose of the SIM activity was to guide you through a self-exploration of your identity as an EP, helping you identify your core values and public purposes, the relationships between them, and how they align. With this self-knowledge, you can begin working with your DCC to identify community sites that align with your identity, values, and the mission statement you developed. (See Text Box 4-3 for questions to consider alignment/fit between you, your OT program, and the capstone site.)

TEXT BOX 4-3

Questions to Determine Fit

- What is the mission of the organization? Is there a link to your mission and values? Is there a link to your OT program's mission?
- What clients/populations do they serve?
- What types of professionals and/or which disciplines serve the clients? Are there occupational therapists? Can you identify someone you feel may want to be a content expert?
- What is the organizational structure?
- What types of services are provided?

Empathy Mapping

The American Occupational Therapy Association (AOTA) defines **empathy** as "the emotional exchange between occupational therapy practitioners (OTPs) and clients that allows for more communication, ensuring that practitioners connect with clients at an emotional level to assist them with their current life situation" (American Occupational Therapy Association [AOTA], 2020, p. 20). An **empathy map** is an active exercise used to gain a deeper understanding of a target audience and, typically, customers, users, or stakeholders, by exploring their experiences, feelings, and behaviors. It facilitates the process of connecting with your capstone site and supporting them to meet their needs. Therefore, this can be a great precursor tool before engaging in a full-blown needs assessment process.

To create an empathy map for a potential capstone site or population, identify what the clients or stakeholders

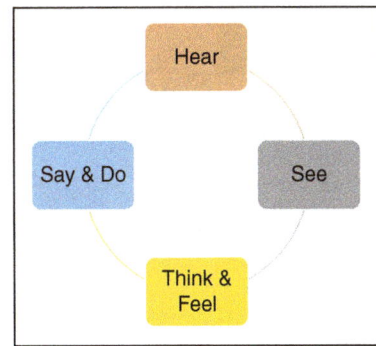

Figure 4-8. Empathy map factors.

at the site might *see, say, think, feel, and do.* Use the results of this to begin to learn more about the practical and emotional aspects of the stakeholders' needs. The use of an empathy map aligns with the holistic and person-centered cornerstones of occupational therapy. (See Figure 4-8.)

Here's an example of an **empathy map** for an **OTD (doctor of occupational therapy) capstone student** planning to work with **adults undergoing cancer treatment**. This map helps understand the emotional, physical, and psychological experiences of these patients to develop a more tailored and empathetic intervention as part of the capstone project.

EMPATHY MAP FOR ADULTS UNDERGOING CANCER TREATMENT

Says (what the patient might say during conversations):
- "I feel exhausted all the time."
- "I'm afraid the treatment will never end."
- "I miss doing things I used to enjoy, like gardening or cooking."
- "I'm worried about how my family will cope when I'm not feeling well."
- "It's hard to keep track of all the appointments and medications."

Thinks (what the patient might be thinking but not necessarily saying out loud):
- "Will I ever feel like myself again after treatment?"
- "Am I going to survive this? What if the cancer comes back?"
- "How will my body handle this treatment in the long term?"
- "Will I still be able to take care of myself and my family?"
- "I wonder how I can stay connected to my loved ones while I'm feeling so sick."

Does (what the patient does in response to their situation):
- Keeps a strict schedule for treatment and appointments.

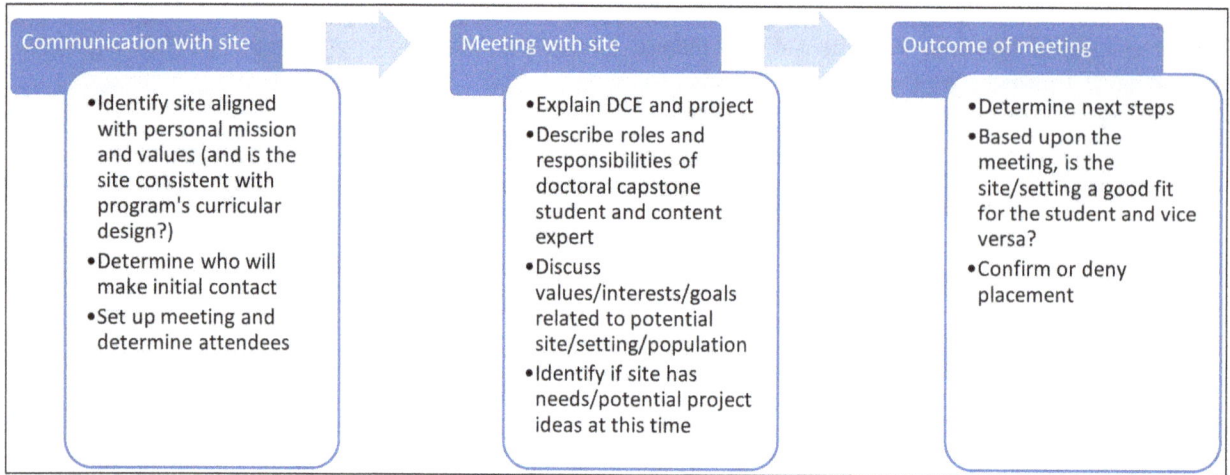

Figure 4-9. Flow of DCE site communication and fit determination.

- Takes breaks during the day due to fatigue.
- Often stays in bed or limits physical activity due to exhaustion or pain.
- May try alternative therapies or seek emotional support from online groups or family.
- Prioritizes rest and recovery, sometimes avoiding social interactions due to feeling unwell.

Feels (what the patient feels emotionally):
- *Frustrated.* Frustrated by the loss of independence and energy levels.
- *Anxious.* About the future, the effectiveness of treatments, and the possibility of recurrence.
- *Isolated.* Especially when they are too tired or sick to participate in normal activities.
- *Hopeful.* Hopeful that treatment will help them heal and regain normal function, though often uncertain about long-term outcomes.
- *Grateful.* For supportive caregivers or medical staff, but sometimes feels a sense of guilt for burdening others.

Empathy mapping is a vital tool in occupational therapy and can support your work as a doctoral student and emerging practitioner (EP). Specifically, this activity supports EPs in their attempts to understand and connect with their clients. By exploring what clients think and feel, say and do, hear and see, capstone students can gain valuable insights into both the practical and emotional aspects of their needs. This process not only enhances communication and emotional connection but also aligns with the human-centered design approach that is fundamental to the development of the doctoral capstone. Ultimately, empathy mapping lays a strong foundation for a comprehensive needs assessment, ensuring the support is effective and site- or population-centered.

DOCTORAL CAPSTONE SITE COMMUNICATION

After engaging in this meaningful reflection of self and potential site, you and your DCC will work together to determine the goodness of fit. First, identify a plan for communicating with the site and setting up an initial meeting. You will want to clarify if the communication should come from your DCC or you. Typically, initial contact communication depends upon the relationship the site has with the school, the relationship the site has with the student, the relationship the site has with the DCC, the type of site, and your program's policy. You will also want to determine who will attend the meeting: you and/or your DCC. (See Figure 4-9 for an example flowchart of site communication and goodness of fit determination.)

STUDENT SECTION CHAPTER SUMMARY

This chapter has provided an activity-based means of entering into the development phase of the doctoral capstone, emphasizing the importance of self-exploration and alignment with potential capstone sites. By adopting human-centered design mindsets such as creative confidence and optimism, you are equipped to navigate this phase with curiosity, innovation, and resilience. Through activities like student identity mapping (SIM), the creation of a personal mission statement, and the building of an empathy map for your future capstone site/population, you will gain valuable insights into your core values and professional goals. These tools will not only assist you in identifying suitable capstone sites but also ensure that your capstone experience is meaningful and aligned with your personal and professional aspirations. As you move forward, remember that this journey is not only about discovering and articulating your unique contributions to the field; it is also about listening to and supporting the strengths and needs of the capstone site for impactful and sustainable outcomes.

Section 2: Educator Focus

Transformational Learning Phases and Framework for the Educator

As students explore their own personal values and beliefs and, simultaneously, attempts are being made to match them with a future capstone site, Mezirow's (1997) transformational learning stage of self-examination is occurring. Your students may experience self-doubt during this stage about their readiness or capacity to both successfully match with a site and also regarding further developing ideas around their capstone experience and project. In this phase, as the educator, you will be guiding the students to examine their own beliefs and feelings as well as "step into the shoes" of the population they hope to be working with to deepen their connection to the future/potential capstone site and population and initiate relationship building. This educator section will explore how you can utilize identity mapping, empathy mapping, and mission statement development to assist your capstone students in exploring their personal belief systems to develop a match with a site and ultimately develop a meaningful and mutually beneficial doctoral capstone.

INTRODUCTION FOR EDUCATOR

In Chapters 3 and 4, the transformational learning stage of *self-examination* was discussed. As you may recall, students can experience self-doubt during this stage about their readiness or capacity to successfully complete their DCE and project. The integration of human-centered design mindsets (e.g., creative confidence and optimism) can significantly enhance the transformational learning experience for students. These mindsets not only foster personal and professional growth but also empower students to undertake innovative and impactful capstone projects. By embedding these mindsets into the capstone coordination process and the development phase of the capstone, DCCs can create a supportive and inspiring environment that promotes transformational learning. This approach not only enhances the quality of the capstone projects but also prepares doctoral students to become confident, optimistic, and innovative practitioners in their field.

EDUCATOR REFLECTIVE QUESTIONS

1. How have you facilitated the exploration of students' values and identities in the selection of capstone sites?
2. What is your current process for communicating with capstone sites?
3. How do you currently match doctoral students with a site or population?

EDUCATOR OBJECTIVES

1. Create an identity map, and align with potential capstone sites.
2. Develop a personal mission statement and align with potential capstone site mission statements.
3. Align the personal mission and site mission to the mission and philosophy of the program.
4. Articulate the flow of capstone site communication and site procurement.
5. Create a plan to match with a site and site population.

STUDENT IDENTITY MAPPING

In Section I of this chapter, doctoral students were guided through a student identity mapping (SIM) activity (Price, 2019). This activity fosters self-reflection through an identification of core values, interests, and identities that shape their personal and professional lives. The beginning of this section will be dedicated to exploring strategies for guiding your students in their "doing" of the activity. This experience fosters collaboration between you and the doctoral student in identifying sites that align with who they are as an emerging practitioner (EP). (See Text Box 4-4.)

TEXT BOX 4-4

Teaching Tip: As DCCs, the benefit of completing our own professional identity maps cannot be understated. Not only will doing so aid you in guiding your students through this activity, but exploring your "integrated identity . . . [is] vital to taking strategic actions that enhance your professional well-being and success" (Price, 2019, p. 2). While you may not consider yourself a community-engaged scholar, our role as DCCs inherently brings public purposes to our work. Reflecting on our public purposes is a process that can elucidate the social responsibility we carry when we consider DC student placements. You can access M. F. Price's (2019) learning resource Scholarly/Professional Identity Mapping (SIM) as an open-access document through the Indiana University

ScholarWorks repository. The assigned readings included in this resource are education-focused, making it ideal for DCCs.

When Dr. Price and I facilitated the SIM activity for my doctoral students, they were given "pre-work," or steps to be completed before the next in-person class. Via Canvas – our institution's learning management system (LMS) – students had access to readings, discussion forums, and pages that outlined each activity step as laid out in Section I. When students commit to completing the SIM activity, the first two steps to be completed are **guided reading** and **reflection** (see Figure 4-1). As previously mentioned, the assigned reading was Suzanne M. Peloquin's (2005) Eleanor Clarke Slagle Lecture *Embracing Our Ethos, Reclaiming Our Heart.*

Ethos is a Greek word that means "character" or "custom" (Merriam-Webster, n.d.). It refers to "the distinguishing character, sentiment, moral nature, or guiding beliefs of a person, group, or institution" (n.d.). In her lecture, Peloquin (2005) adds professional context and elevates the innate poeticism of ethos, stating: "A profession's ethos is an interlacing sentiment, value, and thought that describes its character, conveys its genius, and manifests its spirit" (p. 611).

Ethos, as articulated by Peloquin, encapsulates the core character and guiding beliefs of a profession. By engaging with her lecture, doctoral students are invited to delve into the profound essence of their chosen field. This reflection on ethos serves as a foundational step, enabling students to align their values with the profession's intrinsic principles. Understanding the ethos of occupational therapy helps doctoral students appreciate the moral and ethical dimensions that shape their practice. It fosters a deeper connection to the profession's spirit, encouraging them to embody these values in their own professional journeys – including the DCE. Thus, reading Peloquin's article becomes a pivotal exercise in self-discovery and professional alignment, setting the stage for meaningful and value-driven capstone projects.

Holding this connection in mind, you can construct reflective questions for your students to respond to in step 2. (See Text Box 4-1 in the student section of the chapter for a note on reflective questions.) Via Canvas discussion board forums, students were asked to respond to specific questions, such as:

- List the personal values that you identified within this article. Why did you identify with the values you selected?
- What professional concepts did you find that resonated with you? Explain.
- There are several reflections at the end of the article. Which one fits most with your view of occupational therapy?

Feel free to construct your own reflective questions. If an online discussion forum is not preferred or accessible, your students can prepare individual reflections that can later be discussed in pairs or groups. Students can practice reflective listening and identify points of similarity and difference.

Steps 3 and 4 were also assigned as pre-work for my doctoral students. Outside of class, they identified the values central to their work as EPs and selected identity descriptions that best encapsulated them (M. Price, personal communication, November 11, 2021). They came to class having already drafted their map (step 4), and in-class time was used for discussion. In pairs, each partner can take 3 minutes to share the main elements of their maps, which include their preferred labels (e.g., advocate, practitioner), the focal areas of their work as an EP (e.g., leading, advocacy, research), how strongly they identify with each role and why, and their core values (M. Price, personal communication, November 11, 2021). (See Text Box 4-5 for sample questions that partners can answer for each other during this exercise.)

TEXT BOX 4-5

Teaching Tip: Have both doctoral student partners listen reflectively and intentionally. Consider having them each answer the following:

1. What is one feature that struck you about your partner's story as far as it relates to their EP (e.g., points of consistency and inconsistency, themes you heard that your partner did not note, etc.)?
2. What areas of your partner's work as an EP struck you as a "calling" for them? What about those areas? Get into the details.
3. What are your observations about your partner's expressed values and their relationship to OT as a profession?

Source: M. Price, personal communication (November 11, 2021).

Integrating the SIM activity into this phase provides a comprehensive framework for doctoral students to explore and affirm their professional identities. By engaging in reflective activities and guided readings, such as Peloquin's lecture on our professional ethos, students gain a deeper understanding of the core values and ethical dimensions that define their profession. In so doing, students are better equipped to select capstone sites that resonate with their emerging professional identities. Ultimately, this approach fosters a meaningful and transformative learning experience, preparing students to embark on their doctoral capstone journeys with clarity and purpose.

"Throughout my capstone courses, I engaged in assignments and conversations that helped me explore my passions, values, and interests. Initially, I felt both overwhelmed and exhilarated by the endless possibilities for potential projects I could undertake. With so many areas to explore, narrowing my focus felt like a challenge. My capstone coordinator and I had

numerous discussions about these potential projects and what excited me about each one. When it came time to finalize our projects and sites, I had a solid idea about my project but was unsure how to proceed without selecting a site. Through coursework, assignments, and reflective discussions with my coordinator, we identified a consistent theme in my values and interests: an underlying commitment to occupational justice. This realization led to my placement at a site where occupational justice poses significant barriers to engagement – a gender health clinic. This was a population I had never worked with before, and I felt nervous. However, my prior experiences taught me the importance of approaching the site form a place of cultural humility and amplifying the voices of the community to understand their needs. This site ignited my passion for holistic practice, walking alongside individuals facing systematic barriers that make it difficult to achieve occupational well-being. I couldn't have asked for a better match for my capstone experience.

– Kate Schrader, OTD, OTR,
Indiana University OTD class of 2024

EMPATHY MAPPING

DCCs can guide doctoral students in the empathy mapping activity discussed in Section I of this chapter. Begin by providing a comprehensive introduction to empathy mapping. This should include its definition, purpose, relevance in occupational therapy, and alignment with human-centered design principles. For doctoral students planning their capstone experience and project, mastering empathy mapping is crucial. It equips them with the skills to connect deeply with their target population and/or capstone site, ensuring that their projects are grounded in a thorough understanding of the clients' needs and perspectives. Ultimately, this will lead to more impactful and meaningful outcomes.

Role-Playing

Interactive in-class activities that incorporate role-play can be an effective way to teach empathy mapping to your doctoral students. Role-play can provide an interactive experience, allowing your doctoral students to immerse themselves in the perspectives of clients or stakeholders. What follows is an example of such an activity. (See Appendix 4-C for a rubric that you can adapt as necessary. This rubric can also be used by your doctoral students for peer evaluations.)

- **Objective:** To enable doctoral students to develop a deep understanding of empathy mapping through role-playing exercises, enhancing their ability to connect with clients and stakeholders.
- **Materials Needed**
  - Empathy map templates (printed or digital)
  - Scenario cards with detailed descriptions of different client or stakeholder personas
  - Markers, sticky notes, and large sheets of paper (if using printed templates)
  - Digital tools or software for creating empathy maps (optional)
  - Reflection journals or logs
- **Activity Structure**
  - Introduction (15 minutes)
    - Begin with a brief overview of empathy mapping, its purpose, and its relevance to the DCE and project.
    - Explain the role-playing activity and its objective.
  - Role assignment (10 minutes)
    - Divide doctoral students into small groups (3–5 members).
    - Distribute scenario cards to each group. Each card should describe a different client or stakeholder persona, including background information, challenges, and goals.
  - Role-play exercise (30 minutes)
    - Instruct the doctoral student playing the client or stakeholder to embody their persona as the individual described on the scenario card. (*What do they hear? What do they see? What do they say and do? What do they think and feel?*) (See Figure 4-9 for example.)
    - The other students will interact with the "client," asking questions and observing their responses to fill out the empathy map template.
    - Encourage students to explore what the client sees, says, thinks, feels, and does using open-ended questions and active listening techniques. (See following Figure 4-10.)
  - Group discussion (20 minutes)
    - After the role-play, have each group present their empathy map to the class.
    - Discuss the insights gained from the exercise, focusing on the emotional and practical aspects of the client's needs.
    - Encourage students to reflect on how the empathy map can inform their approach to care.
  - Reflection and feedback (15 minutes)
    - Ask students to write a brief reflection in their journals/logs/etc. about their experience with the role-play and empathy mapping.
    - If time allows, your doctoral students can share their reflections and feedback with the class.
    - Offer constructive feedback and additional insights to help students refine their empathy mapping skills.
  - Integration with capstone projects (10 minutes)
    - Conclude the activity by discussing how the skills learned can be applied to their DCE and project.

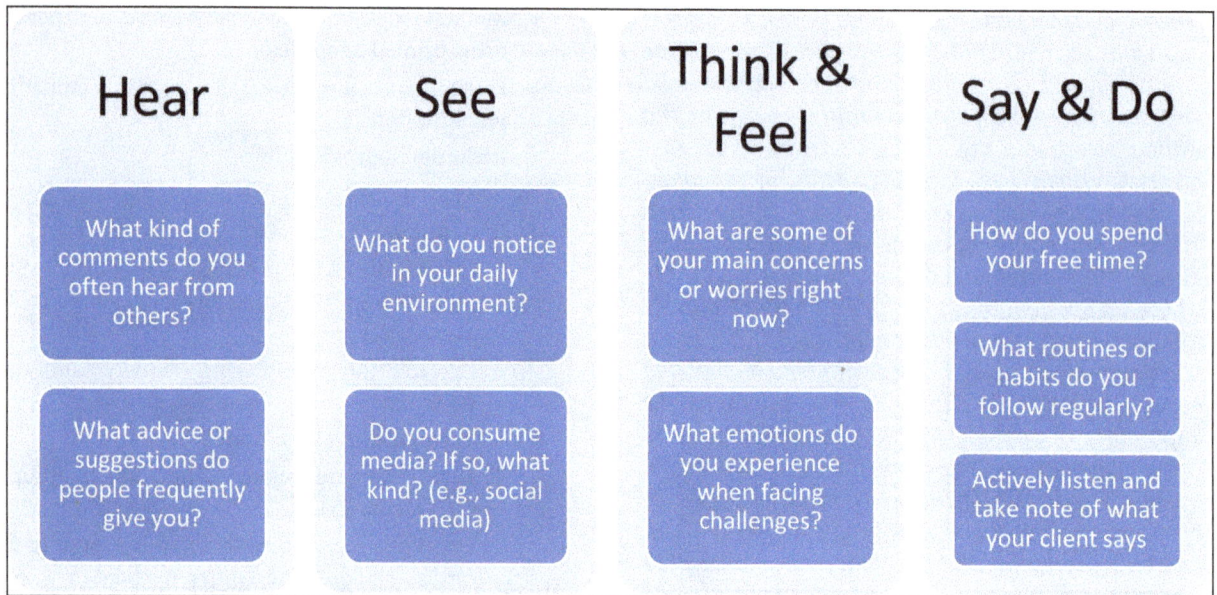

Figure 4-10. Examples of open-ended questions for empathy mapping.

– Emphasize the importance of empathy mapping in understanding the needs of their target population or site and designing effective, sustainable projects.

Completing empathy maps while role-playing aligns well with the principles of transformational learning, which involves a fundamental change in how learners perceive and interpret their experiences. In this activity, your doctoral students can critically reflect on their assumptions and beliefs about the clients or stakeholders they are portraying, helping them question and potentially transform their existing perspectives. Additionally, role-play is an experiential learning opportunity because it requires active engagement and helps solidify new knowledge. Role-playing different personas can facilitate a shift in your doctoral students' worldview. They can gain new insights into their clients' emotional and practical needs, leading to a deeper understanding and empathy. The insights gained from the role-play can be directly applied to doctoral capstone projects, which reinforces the transformational learning process as students implement their new understanding in real-world contexts. Through this empathy mapping activity, DCCs can facilitate doctoral students' critical reflection and perspective transformation.

SITE MATCHING

After completing the empathy mapping and SIM activities, your doctoral students will have a clearer image of their values, who they aspire to be as EPs, and person-centered assessment and communication skills. This is an excellent time for the DC site placement process to begin. (See Figure 4-11 for an example sequence of events for site matching.) At this time, students can begin identifying and exploring traditional, emerging,

and community-based sites. Identifying sites can be done through the following:

- Current sites that have established contracts with the school, including both medical sites (e.g., hospitals, outpatient centers) and community sites
- Sites with which the student has connections that are new to the academic institution (both traditional and role-emerging sites)
- Community sites that have reached out to the academic institution in the past for collaboration

Providing students with a list of available capstone sites can also aid in the site exploration process. In an assignment or classroom activity, doctoral students – with their identity maps and personal mission statements in mind – can explore the mission statements of available sites and refine their preferences based on alignment. This practical exercise not only supports the transformational learning process but also helps students develop critical skills. By integrating the SIM with transformational learning principles, educators can facilitate deeper, more meaningful, and student-centered learning experiences.

You might also consider inviting community members and/or site personnel to your classroom during the development phase. This provides time for sites to discuss their needs and ideas for potential solutions and for the student to get inspired about potential sites that might welcome them as a DCE student. It is an excellent way to exchange ideas and inspire innovative and creative solutions. At the same time, doctoral students need to continue to reflect on the human-centered design mindset of embracing ambiguity. Identifying a site is a process, and there is not a cookie-cutter or perfected method for securing a site that matches the student's interests, values, and goals. Not all sites will be a good match, and not all sites will agree or have the capacity to take a DCE student. This can be frustrating for doctoral students because things may not "fall into place" as they

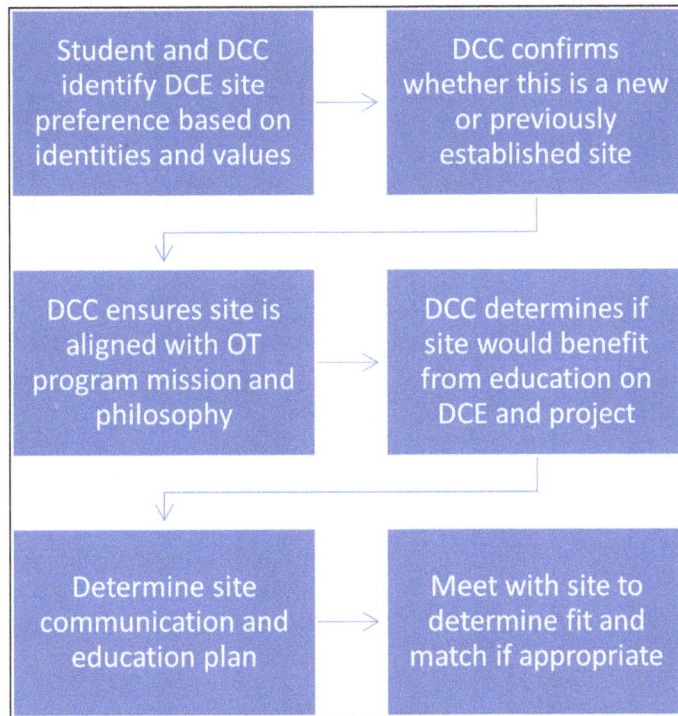

Figure 4-11. Example sequence of site matching and communication process.

would like. They are driving the process and must persevere until a site is mutually agreed on. The process of identifying and securing a DCE site has many ambiguities, and if they can embrace this, it will be a more positive experience.

The Initial Meeting

After collaborating with your student on identifying their initial DC placement preference(s), you and the doctoral student can determine who will initiate the first contact, schedule the initial meeting, and attend the meeting (see Figure 4-7 in the student section of the chapter for a flow of DCE site communication). While communication with FW sites is always mediated by the AFWC, there are instances where doctoral students can initiate communication with DCE sites. This depends on the policy established by the program (see Text Box 4-6 for a tip on developing a policy for site communication), the type of site, the relationship the site has with the DCC, the relationship the site has with the student, and the relationship the site has with the school. As a rule of thumb, DCCs should be the initial contact if a site has been previously used for FW.

TEXT BOX 4-6

Teaching Tip: Developing a policy for the initial communication with a potential content expert is an important first step, and it is recommended that a policy be developed so that all parties understand their responsibilities. One recommendation may be to have this policy in the DCE and project

section of the OTD program's student handbook. A simple statement could be as follows:

Sample Policy: Doctoral capstone students must FIRST identify whether the site they are interested in for their capstone is currently a fieldwork site for the program. If the site IS a current fieldwork site, the DCC will contact the site FIRST to establish the initial interest in taking a capstone student. If the site IS NOT a current fieldwork site, the doctoral capstone student may be the first to reach out to the potential site to describe the DCE and project, but the DCC must be notified that this conversation is taking place.

Once a determination is made as to who will make the initial contact with the site, individual meetings with sites may be an appropriate next step. This can take place over the phone, in person, by video call, or in an introductory email. Communication via email is often one of the first modes of communication to potential sites, so establishing email templates for the capstone student and DCC will help ensure professionalism with the capstone student and reduce time for the DCC. Appendix 4-A at the end of the chapter provides examples of email communications for both the doctoral student and the DCC. If the OTD program is new in the state, or if the program is transitioning from the master of occupational therapy (MOT) degree to an OTD degree, or if the transition has already occurred, meetings with sites are *especially* important. (See Text Box 4-7 for a note on new or transitioning programs.)

TEXT BOX 4-7

Teaching Tip: If the OTD program is new or has transitioned from MOT to OTD, it is recommended that meetings with the DCC and AFWC be set up with fieldwork sites, especially larger hospitals, to discuss how the DCE is different from fieldwork. The goal of these meetings should be to educate the sites on the new ACOTE standards for the DCE and project, discuss your school's process of the DC, and describe the differences between FW and DCE. These meetings can also lead to brainstorming ideas for projects at sites.

The primary purpose of the initial meeting can vary. If the purpose of the meeting is to assess goodness of fit, the goal of the meeting may be to confirm (or deny) the DCE placement. In this case, encourage your doctoral student to research what they can about the site beforehand. They should take the initiative in making note of the site's mission and vision, the clients they serve, the services they provide, and more. It may also be a helpful idea for your doctoral students to prepare an introduction that highlights the values and goals they share with the site. (See Text Box 4-8.)

TEXT BOX 4-8

Teaching Tip: Once students and educators have refined site preferences based upon values, educators can facilitate learning activities for students to explore and align their program's curriculum design and philosophy with the mission statements of the sites they have identified. As an in-class activity . . .

- Ask students to reference their SIM.
- Point students to the OT program's curriculum design and philosophy (e.g., handbook, course syllabi, etc.).
- Ask students to highlight key elements of the curriculum design and philosophy

that resonate with their values and public purposes.
- Distribute mission statements of potential capstone sites.
- In small groups, students analyze these mission statements and identify core values of each site.
- Each student selects one capstone site and uses a Venn diagram to demonstrate alignment between their identity and values, the OT program's mission and philosophy, and the capstone site's mission.
- Have students reflect on how they can apply this to the development phase of their capstone.

During the meeting, the doctoral student should clearly articulate the purpose of the DCE and project so the site can determine whether they can meet the students' educational requirements. It is also important for sites to understand the differences between fieldwork objectives and DCE objectives, which are individualized, specific, and collaborative. Table 4-3 provides potential questions for traditional fieldwork sites.

Overall, the initial meeting should be a time for introductions, education, questions, brainstorming, relating, and perhaps even going on a tour of the site. A "good fit" occurs when all parties (doctoral student, site, content expert, and OT program) are aligned in mission, philosophy, and values and are adequately informed and aware of their roles and responsibilities. If there is a good fit, and if the site and content expert can accommodate the doctoral student through the scheduled dates, then it is a match! (See Text Box 4-9 for a note on initial meeting expectations.)

TEXT BOX 4-9

Teaching Tip: Some sites prefer the prospective capstone student to have an idea for the capstone project at the time of the meeting. This provides DCCs with an opportunity to educate the site on the importance of the needs assessment

Table 4.3 Potential Questions for Traditional Fieldwork Sites

Question 1	Are you familiar with the doctoral capstone experience and project?
Question 2	Have you had any previous OTD capstone students?
Question 3	Where do you see a fit for an OTD capstone student?
Question 4	What types of clients do you serve?
Question 5	What types of services do you offer?
Question 6	What programming do you currently have at the site, and do you have program development needs?
Question 7	Are you doing research, and if so, do you have student involvement?
Question 8	What new initiatives has your organization identified?

Table 4.4 Potential Questions for Role Emerging Fieldwork Site

Question 1	What is the mission of your organization? (This will allow you to determine whether there is a link between the organization and your program's mission.)
Question 2	Who are the clients you serve?
Question 3	What is the organizational structure?
Question 4	What types of professionals serve the clients, and are there any occupational therapists within the organization?
Question 5	Do you have personnel you feel may want to be a content expert, and what are their educational backgrounds? What is their current role within the organization?
Question 6	Do you have students from other disciplines that serve your organization?
Question 7	What are your funding sources?
Question 8	What types of services do you provide?
Question 9	Have you hosted an OTD capstone student in the past?

in doctoral capstone preparation. This prevents a potential misrepresentation of the student's preparedness while simultaneously bringing the doctoral capstone's human-centered design into focus. It may also be helpful to provide the site with a doctoral capstone information sheet to be referenced during the meeting. This sheet can include the dates for the DCE, the purpose of the DCE and project, your program's capstone curriculum, and more. (See Appendix 4-B for an example.)

NEW SITE DEVELOPMENT

The reasons for establishing new DCE sites vary. In some cases, simply exploring your local community and networking with others bring potential partners who align with your program's mission and philosophy into view. In other cases, you may have community-engaged colleagues in your department whose site partner would benefit from a doctoral capstone project. One of your doctoral students may approach you with a new site they have discovered or with which they have a personal connection. DCCs and students can work together to ensure the site is aligned with the student, OT program, and DCE requirements. Table 4-4 includes potential questions for new community and/or role-emerging sites.

EDUCATOR CHAPTER SUMMARY

This chapter focused on strategies for DCCs to guide their doctoral students in their SIM activities and the site matching process. Additionally, this chapter emphasized education and communication as essential steps to capstone site development. Assisting the doctoral student and prospective sites to understand the DCE and project is a critical first step. Once education is initiated, the process of procuring sites will evolve. As relationships build, the

doctoral student will begin to work with the site to develop goals and objectives. Relationship development among the program, doctoral student, and site is essential to build a solid foundation for the DCE and project.

REFERENCES

Aldrich, R. M., Boston, T. L., & Daaleman, C. E. (2017). Justice and U.S. occupational therapy practice: A relationship 100 years in the making. *American Journal of Occupational Therapy, 71*(1), 7101100040p1–7101100040p5. https://doi.org/10.5014/ajot.2017.023085

American Occupational Therapy Association. (2020). Occupational therapy practice framework: Domain and process (4th ed.). *American Journal of Occupational Therapy, 74*(Suppl. 2), 7412410010. https://doi.org/10.5014/ajot.2020.74S2001

Bielenberg, J. (n.d.). *Optimism.* IDEO. https://www.designkit.org/mindsets/6.html

Bringle, R. G., Clayton, P. H., Price, M. F. (2009). Partnerships in service learning and civic engagement. Partnerships: A Journal of Service Learning and Civic Engagement, 1(1), 1–20. https://scholarworks.indianapolis.iu.edu/items/f61a2979-a771-4457-a163-7db39edf873f

Covey, S. R. (2004). *The 7 habits of highly effective people: Powerful lessons in personal change.* Free Press.

Martin, P. (n.d.). *Embrace ambiguity.* IDEO. https://www.designkit.org/mindsets/5.html

Merriam-Webster. (n.d.). Ethos. In *Merriam-Webster.com dictionary.* https://www.merriam-webster.com/dictionary/ethos

Mezirow, J. (1997). Transformative learning: Theory to practice. *New Directions for Adult and Continuing Education,* (74), 5–12. https://doi.org/10.1002/ace.7401

Peloquin, S. M. (2005). The 2005 Eleanor Clarke slagle lecture – embracing our ethos, reclaiming our heart. *American Journal of Occupational Therapy, 59,* 611–625.

Price, M. F. (2019). *Scholarly/professional identity mapping (SIM)* [Learning Resource]. https://scholarworks.indianapolis.iu.edu/items/7486ab96-0c64-4ffd-bbce-a4d39cbcffa8

Proofed. (2021, February 21). *5 tips to enhance your close reading skills.* https://proofed.com/writing-tips/5-tips-to-enhance-your-close-reading-skills/

Webb, T. (2023, April 9). *Close-reading strategies: The ultimate guide to close reading.* Writing with Tyler. https://www.writingwithtyler.com/post/close-reading-strategies

We Are Teachers Staff. (2023, July 31). *Close reading strategies: A step-by-step teaching guide.* We Are Teachers. https://www.weareteachers.com/strategies-for-close-reading/

APPENDICES

Appendix 4-A

EXAMPLES OF EMAIL COMMUNICATIONS

Doctoral Student Contacting a Potential New Site

Dear [Recipient's Name],

My name is [Your Name], and I am a doctoral student in the OTD program at [Institution's Name]. I am writing to inquire about the possibility of completing my doctoral capstone experience and project at [Site's Name]. The dates for this DCE are [Dates].

The purpose of my DCE is to gain advanced skills in a specific area of focus (such as program development or leadership) and to apply those skills through a focused project that meets the needs of [Site Name]. The DCE is required to be 14 weeks in length, and I am required to complete a total of 560 hours (40 hours/week) under the supervision of a content expert. Content experts are not required to be occupational therapists, although they can be. Content experts must have documented expertise in the focus area of the project.

I am particularly interested in [Site Name] because [briefly explain your interest or connection to the site]. I believe that your organization's mission and values align well with my professional values and goals. I would greatly appreciate the opportunity to discuss this further and explore how we might collaborate. Please let me know if we can schedule a meeting at your earliest convenience.

Thank you for considering my request. I look forward to your response.
[Your Name and Email Signature]

Doctoral Capstone Coordinator Contacting a Potential New Site

Dear [Recipient's Name],

I have an occupational therapy doctoral (OTD) student, [Student Name], who is very interested in completing her doctoral capstone experience (DCE) with [Site Name]. Our OTD students are required to complete this 14-week (40 hours/week) placement at a site working with a content expert who does not have to be an OT depending on the site and project. The dates for this DCE are [Dates]. At the start of the DCE, this student will have completed all didactic coursework and both level II fieldwork experiences.

The doctoral capstone is an in-depth experience that allows the OTD student to gain advanced knowledge and synthesize that knowledge into a final project that meets the need of the site. DCE students must be paired with a content expert, or an individual at the site with documented expertise in one of the following focus areas: clinical skills, research skills, administration, program development and evaluation, policy development, advocacy, education, and leadership.

I wanted to contact you to get your thoughts on the possibility of taking an OTD student for their DCE and project. I am attaching a doctoral capstone information sheet for your review. Please let me know if you have any questions or if you would like to talk further.

Kindly,
[Your Name and Email Signature]

Appendix 4-B

EXAMPLE OF A DC INFORMATION SHEET FOR NEW SITES AND CONTENT EXPERTS

This information is based upon the Indiana University OTD curriculum design. Feel free to adapt this to fit your program.

Doctoral Capstone Experience and Project

OTD Class of ****

[Dates of DCE]

Year 2, Summer (May–June ****): T651 Doctoral Capstone Seminar I: Site Development

- Students hear from prior capstone students, content experts and other community partners, and faculty.
- Students submit initial capstone site preferences.
- Begin site placements in July and continue through December ****, with all placements finalized *prior to* the start of year 2, spring term.
- Initiate and finalize or renew affiliation agreements between IU OT and sites.

Year 2, Spring (January–April ****): T780 Doctoral Capstone Seminar II: Needs Assessment

- Students reach out to content experts at the start of the term to schedule the needs assessment interview, typically completed in late February or early March.
- Students begin their literature review.
- Based on needs assessment results, students develop problem statement, purpose statement, and initial goals for the capstone.

Year 3, Fall (6-Week Term, August–September ****): T781 Doctoral Capstone Seminar III: Plan Development

- At the start of the term, students will reach out to content experts to schedule a time prior to the end of 6-week term to review, finalize, and sign student learning plans.
- Students finish their literature review.
- Students collaborate with content expert, capstone coordinator, and faculty to develop their implementation plan, goals and objectives, and their plan for evaluating capstone outcomes.
- Students collaborate with our departmental research coordinator, capstone coordinator, and IRB reviewer to submit their project to the institutional review board (IRB) to receive a determination of exempt, expedited, or non-human subjects research.
- Students receive assigned faculty mentor.

Year 3, Spring (January–April ****): T880 Doctoral Capstone Experience and T830 Leadership Seminar and Capstone Project

- Fourteen-week doctoral capstone experiences begin [Date] and end on [Date].
- Content experts complete in CORE Elms the student's **midterm evaluation** at week 7 and their **final evaluation** at week 14.
- Content experts approve in CORE Elms the students' logged hours; students must complete all 560 hours by the end of the 14th week.
- Doctoral capstone showcase in May ****; content experts are invited to support their students.
- Students submit capstone reports to IUScholarWorks.

Roles and Responsibilities of Content Expert

- Providing résumé to student (who will upload to CORE Elms) in order to verify expertise.
- Providing expertise in their student's area of focus (program development and evaluation, policy development, administration, research, clinical skills, education, and/or advocacy).
- Content experts are *not* required to be an occupational therapist unless* the student will be providing/billing for OT services (per state guidelines, supervision from a certified occupational therapist is required).
- Providing orientation to the site, site personnel, stakeholders.
- Meeting with their student in the spring (February–March ****) for the needs assessment interview.

- Collaborating with the student to develop individual learning objectives in the fall (August–September ****).
- Working collaboratively with the student on their student learning plans and providing signature in the fall (August–September ****).
- Evaluating student performance at week 7 and week 14 in CORE Elms.
- Verifying students' logged hours in CORE Elms.
- Notifying the doctoral capstone coordinator (DCC name) if problems arise, and collaborate with the student, doctoral capstone coordinator, and faculty mentor on plan of correction.

Additional members of the capstone team:

- Here you may list any additional members of your program's clinical education team and their email addresses/ contact information.

Appendix 4-C

EXAMPLE RUBRIC FOR ROLE-PLAY EMPATHY MAPPING ACTIVITY

CRITERIA	EXCELLENT (4)	GOOD (3)	SATISFACTORY (2)	NEEDS IMPROVEMENT (1)
Preparation	Thoroughly prepared; fully understands the persona and scenario.	Well-prepared; understands the persona and scenario, with minor gaps.	Somewhat prepared; basic understanding of the persona and scenario.	Unprepared; lacks understanding of the persona and scenario.
Engagement	Actively engages in role-play, stays in character throughout.	Engages in role-play, mostly stays in character.	Participates in role-play, occasionally breaks character.	Minimal participation, frequently breaks character.
Questioning	Asks insightful, open-ended questions that elicit detailed responses.	Asks relevant questions, mostly open-ended, that elicit useful responses.	Asks some relevant questions, a mix of open-ended and closed questions.	Asks few relevant questions, mostly closed questions.
Listening	Demonstrates active listening; accurately captures client's responses, as demonstrated on empathy map.	Listens attentively; captures most of the client's responses accurately, as demonstrated on empathy map.	Listens but misses some key points; captures basic responses as demonstrated on empathy map.	Poor listening, frequently misses key points, inaccurate responses.
Empathy mapping	Creates a comprehensive and detailed empathy map; covers all aspects.	Creates a detailed empathy map; covers most aspects.	Creates a basic empathy map; covers some aspects.	Incomplete empathy map; covers few aspects.
Collaboration	Works effectively with group members, contributes to discussion.	Collaborates well with group members, contributes to discussions.	Collaborates with group members, contributes occasionally.	Limited collaboration, minimal contribution to group discussions.
Reflection	Provides deep, insightful reflections on the role-play experience.	Provides thoughtful reflections on the role-play experience.	Provides basic reflections on the role-play experience.	Provides minimal or superficial reflections on the role-play experience.
Application	Clearly connects empathy mapping to DCE, demonstrates understanding.	Connects empathy mapping to DCE, shows understanding.	Some connection between empathy mapping and DCE, basic understanding.	Little to no connection between empathy mapping and DCE, lacks understanding.

Scoring
> Excellent: 28–32 points
> Good: 21–27 points
> Satisfactory: 14–20 points
> Needs Improvement: 8–13 points

This rubric can be used by both DCCs and doctoral students. DCCs can decide to have their doctoral students complete peer evaluations, for example. Adapt the rubric as needed.

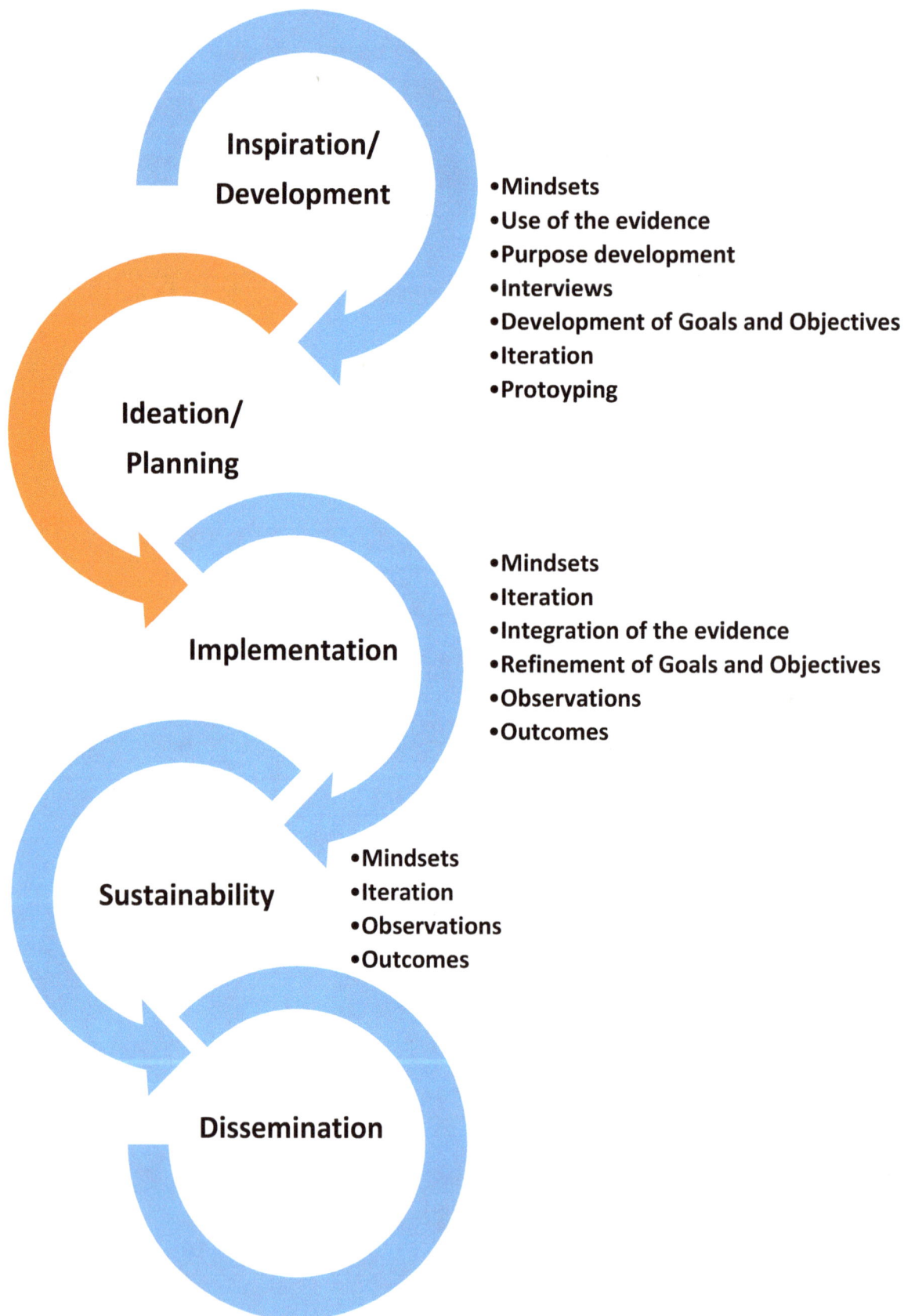

Inspiration/ Development

- Mindsets
- Use of the evidence
- Purpose development
- Interviews
- Development of Goals and Objectives
- Iteration
- Protoyping

Ideation/ Planning

Implementation

- Mindsets
- Iteration
- Integration of the evidence
- Refinement of Goals and Objectives
- Observations
- Outcomes

Sustainability

- Mindsets
- Iteration
- Observations
- Outcomes

Dissemination

Part II. Planning

The second step in the capstone process is **planning** the capstone experience and project, which aligns with the **ideation** process of human-centered design. This phase involves taking the information gathered that allowed the doctoral student to *develop* the problem and purpose to now begin problem-solving and generating ideas to solve a client, group, or population problem. During the ideation phase, the doctoral student is identifying opportunities and locating a site for the capstone. The needs assessment process will begin along with testing and refining possible solutions. Working with people who share the capstone purpose to find real-life solutions is key to this planning phase. Goals and objectives are now finalized to allow for iteration and prototyping to ensure a client-centered approach to the experience.

DOI: 10.4324/9781003541813-6

CHAPTER 5

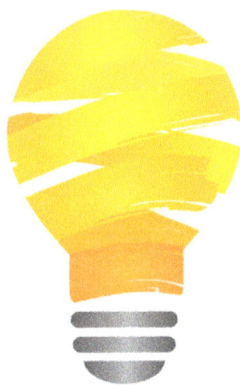

The Literature Review

Allison Bell

Section 1: Student Focus

Human-Centered Design Mindsets for the Doctoral Students

Human-centered design mindset concepts of starting out simple to learn and make your ideas real, giving yourself permission to explore a lot of ideas, and having optimism to drive yourself forward are the vision of this chapter.

Make it. It is important to brainstorm ideas for the capstone experience and project and get those ideas down on paper. What are you most passionate about? What is needed in the community? Think about how what you want to do is within the scope of occupational therapy and what would be the link to occupation.

Embrace ambiguity. You do not know the answer to your problem, and that is okay; be okay with the ambiguity. It will allow you to be more creative as you begin to research your interest area and define your purpose. Be fine with changing direction as you move into the literature. This ambiguity allows you to innovate and create. Looking for a gap or need is important in the development of your problem statement.

Optimism. You do not know the answer yet, and that is fine – staying optimistic that you will find a solution to the problem will lead to the purpose of your capstone. You have a long journey. Stay optimistic – optimism will keep you on track as you move through the process.

INTRODUCTION FOR STUDENTS

Developing a meaningful and robust capstone experience and project requires a demonstration of need coupled with an area of passion for the doctoral student. In keeping with accreditation standards, the occupational therapy doctoral capstone project must be an integral part of the program's curriculum and reflect the ability of the doctoral student to synthesize knowledge in one area of practice, such as clinical practice skills, research skills, administration, leadership, program development and evaluation, policy development, advocacy, education, or leadership (Accreditation Council for Occupational Therapy Education [ACOTE], 2023). Ultimately, the doctoral capstone project must have evidence to support the need and use evidence to develop methods to achieve the desired outcome(s).

The doctoral capstone is an exciting process. It is a systematic yet iterative journey that has the potential to impact *persons*, *communities*, *populations*, and *organizations*. This

DOI: 10.4324/9781003541813-7

- 101 -

chapter examines the process of searching and locating evidence from the literature to develop a problem statement and demonstrate the need for the doctoral capstone project. This process will develop your professional skills and competencies necessary to assume various roles after graduation.

STUDENT REFLECTIVE QUESTIONS

When developing the doctoral capstone, the occupational therapy student may find it helpful to reflect on the following questions:

1. What initial ideas do I have for my capstone project?
2. What are the problems or needs that I have observed?
3. What does the research literature tell you about the problems you observed? How can that knowledge influence your ideas?
4. Why is my idea important? (To me, the profession, individuals, groups/populations).
5. How will the capstone experience influence the project scope and focus?

KEY WORDS

- *Gap problem analysis.* A thoughtful analysis that contrasts what is occurring with what is desired (Davis-Ajami et al., 2014).
- *PICO question.* An interdisciplinary approach to translate a clinical question into searchable terms (Cochrane Linked Data, 2024).
- *Rapid review.* A narrowly focused review to ensure the use of the available evidence in a resource-efficient manner. Resources include time, money, and people (Hamel et al., 2021).

STUDENT OBJECTIVES

By the end of reading this section of the chapter and completing the learning activities, the occupational therapy student should be able to:

1. Determine how to search the literature to provide evidence to support ideas for the capstone project.
2. Develop a synthesis of the relevant literature to answer a clinical question.
3. Use gap analysis to develop a problem statement for the capstone experience and project.
4. Connect the ACOTE areas of focus with Moyers and Quint's (2025) scholarship of knowledge discovery model.

BEFORE SEARCHING THE LITERATURE

All doctoral capstone projects begin with a literature search, as required in the accreditation standards (ACOTE,

2023). This section details the processes of developing targeted clinical and/or doctoral capstone–specific sites, based on questions that result in efficient and effective literature searches. From this search strategy, you will yield research evidence to answer your question. The answer to your question is likely nuanced, requiring your emerging doctoral-level skills where you will synthesize the results to develop a gap analysis statement in which the capstone project can be constructed.

DEVELOPING A FOCUSED QUESTION

The first step in a literature review is developing a focused question to support an efficient search. This essential initial step paves the way for an effective search strategy. Formulating a focused question will assist you in determining whether evidence is relevant to the capstone project.

The pace of publication is daunting, and as an evidence-based practitioner, it can be challenging to keep up with the research evidence that accumulates daily (See Text Box 5-1.) A benefit of a well-developed clinical question is a focused search strategy that yields evidence that directly answers the question, reducing the likelihood of retrieving evidence that is not useful to the proposed question.

TEXT BOX 5-1

A review of publications found that about 80 systematic reviews are published daily (Hoffmann et al., 2021).

The PICO (patient/population/problem, intervention, comparison, and outcome) approach is well described in the interdisciplinary literature (Cochrane Linked Data, 2024). (See Text Box 5-2.) The PICO format transforms the clinical question into a searchable format with narrow search terms. The greater the detail and focus the question has, the better the search terms and, therefore, the greater the likelihood of retrieving evidence that is relevant to the question (Table 5-1).

TEXT BOX 5-2

What is a PICO?

A model that helps break a search into small pieces. The PICO framework is used to create a well-built clinical question into a searchable question to develop literature search strategies for evidence-based practice (Cochrane Library, 2024):

P: Patient, problem, or population
I: Intervention program
C: Comparison, control
O: Outcome

For the capstone project, a PICO can guide the literature search and serve as the foundation for the development of the scholarly project.

Defining a population includes identifying relevant characteristics. This may include not only a diagnosis but

Table 5-1 Building a Better PICO Question

START	BETTER	BEST
In stroke, what treatment is most effective for hemiplegia?	For a woman with chronic hemiplegia, is CIMT or the neurodevelopment treatment/Bobath approach more effective?	For a woman with chronic stroke, is CIMT or neurodevelopmental treatment/Bobath approach more effective for improvement of quality of life?
For people experiencing homelessness, what intervention is best for reducing substance use?	For non-binary teens experiencing homelessness, what interventions are most effective to reduce substance use?	For non-binary teens experiencing homelessness, is harm reduction or cognitive-behavioral therapy approach most effective for reducing substance use?
What assessment is best to measure pain in people with multiple sclerosis?	For relapsing remitting multiple sclerosis, what assessment is best to measure pain?	For relapsing remitting multiple sclerosis, what assessment of pain is most sensitive to change after occupational therapy interventions?
Is group or individual treatment more effective for children with ASD?	For school-aged children with ASD, is group or individual treatment more effective?	For children in high school with ASD, is group or individual training more effective for the development of friendship?
What is the experience of caregivers engaged in a support group?	For informal caregivers, what is their experience when engaged in support groups?	For spouses of people with Alzheimer's disease, what is their experience when engaged in community support groups?
Is anxiety common after concussion?	What is the likelihood of developing anxiety for athletes with post-concussive syndrome?	What is the likelihood of developing anxiety for female high school athletes with post-concussive syndrome?
What are the experiences of people providing care to people with dementia?	What are the experiences of children caring for parents with dementia?	What are the experiences of adult daughters caring for parents with dementia?

Note: ASD = autism spectrum disorder; CIMT = constraint-induced movement therapy.

also variables such as age and chronicity. The PICO format does not simply explore interventions in a traditional sense. Interventions may be a type of treatment (cognitive-behavioral therapy, for example) but can also explore a diagnostic test or prognosis (#3 and #6 in Table 5-1 provide examples). Other examples include education-focused capstone projects exploring the efficacy of high-fidelity simulations.

Not every PICO question requires a comparison. The decision to compare two interventions will be based on the needs of the site and type of project. Finally, a specific outcome is an important last step. Just as occupational therapy treatment goals are client-centered, so should the outcome of a PICO question. It is not enough to ask what is better; instead, identify what is the meaningful outcome of interest and define it.

Questions that are best answered by qualitative/naturalistic inquiry use a different format (Hosseini et al., 2024). The clinical question is framed as population/problem/interest/context (PICo) question. The process of identifying the population or problem is the same as in quantitative research; however, a clearly defined population and context are vital because qualitative research does not aim for results to generalize to a larger population or different context (Howlett et al., 2013). (See example #7 in Table 5-1.) Whether the capstone project focus is qualitative, quantitative, or mixed methods in approach, the ability to construct a robust clinical question will inform the literature search process.

SELECTING A DATABASE

With a solid PICO question, the selection of databases begins. Conducting a literature search involves using web-based search engines and electronic research databases. Electronic bibliographic databases collect and index publications in a focus area. Table 5-2 describes common databases relevant to occupational therapy. To find the right

Table 5-2 Relevant Databases

NAME	AREA OF FOCUS	NOTES
MEDLINE, accessed for free via PubMed	Wide range of literature, including medicine, nursing, rehabilitation therapy, allied health, dentistry, veterinary medicine, health-care system, and preclinical sciences (National Library of Medicine, 2024)	
EMBASE	Wide range of biomedical literature; European database (Elsevier, n.d.)	Similar coverage to MEDLINE, but greater coverage of non-English and European journals
CINAHL	Nursing and allied health literature (including occupational therapy; (EBSCO Information Services, n.d.)	
Cochrane Library	Independent review of clinical effectiveness to inform health-care decision-making (Cochrane Library, n.d.)	
Educational Resource Information Center (ERIC)	Education-related research (Educational Resource Information Center, n.d.)	
PsycINFO	Literature from social and behavioral sciences (PsycINFO, n.d.)	
Google Scholar	Free web-based search engine that indexes citations and full-text articles from a wide range of disciplines (Google Scholar, n.d.)	Results from the searches will typically show the most cited articles, not the most relevant to the search term. The capstone student may find this a resource to discover or browse, *but this is not a systematic approach to a search.*
Occupational Therapy Systematic Evaluation of Evidence (OTseeker)	Critical appraisals of literature relevant to occupational therapy; last updated in 2016 (OTseeker, n.d.).	The critical appraisals may support understanding of a research article; however, they are not a substitution of
Physiotherapy Evidence Database (PEDro)	Critical appraisals of literature relevant to physical therapy. No longer updated (PEDro, 2024).	obtaining and critically evaluating the research considering the clinical question and the context of the DCE site.
Psychological Database for Brain Impairment Treatment Efficacy (PsycBITE)	Critical appraisals of literature relevant to cognitive, behavioral, and other treatments for psychological problems and issues for people with acquired brain injuries (PsycBITE, n.d.)	
REHAB+	Critical appraisals of literature relevant to occupational and physical therapy (Dobbins, 2017)	

database(s), explore what material it covers and develop knowledge of the search features in the database. It is best practice to search multiple databases that are relevant to the content area. A *minimum* of two databases has been recommended for literature reviews to ensure the inclusion of all relevant work (Ewald et al., 2022).

DEVELOPING SEARCH TERMS AND STRATEGY

Search terms are based on the PICO/PICo question; however, each database has different methods to index publications, requiring different search terms for each database selected. The academic librarian can be helpful in tailoring search terms to the selected databases. As seen from the PICO examples in Table 5-1, a well-built clinical question supports more specific search terms. These search terms are words or phrases that describe the key aspects of the PICO question. Individual databases use different search terminologies. For example, MedLine developed medical subject heading (MeSH) terms. The National Library of Medicine developed MeSH to create a controlled and organized lexicon (National Library of Medicine, 2024). MeSH terms are a common vocabulary used to ensure the retrieval of relevant literature. To explain the thinking of a controlled vocabulary, think of searching for a topic or service online. An individual desiring to locate a facility to get a haircut may initially search for the term *haircut*; however, the ultimate term to obtain the exact match for desired services may be best found on a webpage titled "Salon Services."

Each database has different logic for search terms, and not all use MeSH terms. The common vocabulary set in the Cumulative Index to Nursing and Allied Health (CINAHL) is CINAHL subject headings, and EMBASE uses Emtree. This presents another opportunity to collaborate with a librarian to identify relevant databases and tailor search terms to the individual databases.

Finally, consider other terms that may describe a similar concept, to ensure a complete search. For example, spelling differences in the English language, based on region (e.g., orthopedic/orthopadic); outdated terms, such as *Asperger's syndrome* or *pervasive developmental disorder*, when searching for literature on autism spectrum disorder. Table 5-3 provides examples of terms that should be considered based on outdated terms and terminology that is used interchangeably.

After the identification of search terms, Boolean operators, truncation, wildcards, and limits will support the efficient search. Boolean operators connect and define the relationship between search terms. These include the words **AND, OR**, and **NOT**. Using AND to link search terms will yield results that include both terms. OR will yield results that include at least one of the terms. NOT will exclude results based on the search term (EbscoConnect, 2022). Appendix 5-A provides a format to move a PICO question into search terms and strategies. Both CINHAL and EMBASE would be appropriate databases to search for the PICO question, requiring adjustments to the search terms.

Truncation is a strategy to broaden a search, based on variation of word endings. A search with truncation for the root word "child" would search for terms that include child, children, and childhood. Most databases, but not all, denote truncation with an asterisk (e.g., child*). Here is another example of the need for collaboration with the academic librarian.

A wildcard character replaces a single character in a search term. For example, womAn and womEn. This may be denoted with a question mark (e.g., wom?n or orthop?edic); however, there is not a common character across databases, compelling the support and expertise of a librarian.

Most databases also allow the user to limit searches based on characteristics of the article or study, such as language, methodology, age of participants, and publication dates. These filters may help target better the population of interest, such as the age of participants, or may be necessary to ensure rapid utilization of the literature, such as limits to the English language. However, these necessary exclusions, to ensure a rapid review, introduce bias.

The process used to search and select literature should be systematic, although unlikely to be a systematic review. Most doctoral capstone projects will undergo the process of a rapid review of the literature. A rapid review and a systematic review have similarities in that there is a focused question and a systematic search strategy (Smela et al., 2023). Fundamental differences are that rapid reviews have narrow search criteria to answer an urgent policy or practice issue compared to systematic reviews with expansive search criteria to answer a broad question (Smela et al., 2023). Rapid reviews acknowledge the real-world limitations of money, time, and people (Smela et al., 2023). A well-developed PICO question will narrow the search criteria and lead to inclusion and exclusion criteria. In keeping with the stroke example, an example of inclusion criteria would be studies with a population with their first stroke being greater than 6 months before the study.

START THE LITERATURE SEARCH

The work to develop clear search terms and inclusion and exclusion criteria is designed to limit the results to the most relevant. When entering the search query into the selected database, the results are typically presented in

Table 5-3 PICO Search Terms			
P	I	C	O
• Stroke • Cerebrovascular accident (CVA) • Cerebrovascular accident	• Constraint-induced movement therapy (GMT) • Constraint-induced therapy	• Bobath • Neurodevelopmental treatment	• Quality of life

summary format. Like all parts of the doctoral capstone project, the search strategy is iterative and, based on the results obtained, may need to be refined. Even the strongest search strategy will yield irrelevant results. The process of systematically identifying the most pertinent information is the next step in the literature review process.

Table 5-4 is a tool to organize and document the database search strategies, describe the number of articles obtained, and defend the rationale for excluding some. On the basis of the inclusion and exclusion criteria, articles may be excluded based on study design. *Evidence level* refers to a hierarchal categorization of study design, with a higher level of evidence representing designs that have a lower probability of bias (see Table 5-5). The final column in Table 5-4 provides a preliminary assessment of the literature in relation to the proposed project.

SELECTING THE LITERATURE

The next step of the rapid review is to select the relevant articles. As the doctoral student, you should engage in a critical and consistent review of the literature, requiring that they read and analyze a large amount of literature. Screening results for relevance can reduce the volume of literature to only what is relevant.

An initial step in the appraisal process can be a title screen. Many articles may be deemed irrelevant to the clinical question based on the title alone. Articles that are relevant or cannot be excluded based on the title alone move to the next step, an abstract screen, based on the review of the journal abstract (Polanin et al., 2019). If the content is irrelevant to the PICO question, eliminate the article. It is common for a large majority of retrieved articles to be excluded through just the title and abstract screen. Articles that are relevant or cannot be removed based on the abstract alone must undergo a more critical review of the content. This final step is a full-text screen. In this step, obtain the full-text articles and review for relevance (Polanin et al., 2019).

One system to consider using to guide the critical reading of the results derived from the literature search is the preview, question, read, and summarize (PQRS) model described by Cohen (1990). The method has been shown to improve readers' understanding and their ability to recall information (Ulu & Akyol, 2016). In other words, readers are more likely to learn and to learn more of the material they are reading.

Preview. Acquire an overview of the article through a quick scan or skim. Do the main points of the text align with your capstone? Is the article worth a closer read?

Question. Ask questions about what you are reading. Does the article relate to your capstone? What are you learning from the article scan?

Table 5-4 Organizing and Documenting

DATA SOURCE	SEARCH STRATEGY	LIMITS WITH RATIONALE	# RESULTS	COMMENTS ON RESULTS
Database: Date:	List terms and operators used	English only Date Publication type Level of evidence Other		Do the results look like work of interest? Did the results include papers that are known to be relevant?

Source: Adapted from MD Anderson Library: "Excel Workbook to Track Systematic Review Search Results," by Helena VonVille. Licensed under a Creative Commons Attribution-NonCommercial-ShareAlike 3.0 Unported License.

Table 5-5 Levels of Evidence

LEVEL I	Systematic reviews, meta-analyses, randomized controlled trials
LEVEL II	Two groups, nonrandomized studies (e.g., cohort, case control)
LEVEL III	One group, nonrandomized (e.g., before and after, pretest/posttest)
LEVEL IV	Descriptive studies that include analysis of outcomes (single-subject design, case series)
LEVEL V	Case reports and expert opinion that include narrative literature reviews and consensus statements.

Source: Adapted from Sackett, D. L., Rosenberg, W. M., Gray, J. M., Haynes, R. B., and Richardson, W. S. (1996). Evidence based medicine: What it is and what it isn't. BMJ, 312, 71–72. https://doi.org/10.1136/bmj.312.7023.71.

Read. Read the article. Now, read the article again. What information is in the article, and how does it relate to your capstone?

Summarize. Write notes to summarize or paraphrase what you read. Can you summarize how the content of the article helps support your capstone or focus area?

MANAGING THE OUTCOME OF THE LITERATURE REVIEW

In a doctoral project, it is essential to detail the search strategy, as well as the process and results of obtaining the final articles for review. An external reviewer should be able to evaluate the quality of the literature review through an examination of the search strategy.

> Did you know many bibliographic databases allow users to sign up for email alerts for new publications relevant to a search strategy? You can save your search strategy and be alerted of new publications through email.

The Preferred Reporting Items for Systematic Reviews and Meta-Analyses (PRISMA) is an evidence-based minimum set of items for reporting in systematic reviews and meta-analyses. In this minimum set, a recommended diagram depicts how many articles were screened and the process to remove (Page et al., 2021). Although you will most likely not be completing a systematic review, the PRISMA flow diagram is a powerful tool to display the literature review process (Appendix 5-B).

EFFECTIVELY MANAGING THE EVIDENCE

Using reference management program will become a necessity throughout the capstone experience. *Reference managers* are an electronic space to organize, sort, and reference literature when writing. Most systems will organize references by project, save notes on the citation, share with collaborators, develop a reference list in multiple citation formats (e.g., American Psychological Association, 7th ed., Vancouver Style), and accurately develop in-text citations. These programs insert cited sources into a written capstone paper or assist in the manuscript preparation process for a journal (see further discussion in Chapters 11 and 12 of this text). The academic library may offer access to reference managers. There are numerous vendors available, each with different features. Table 5-6 details on key

Table 5-6 Common Reference Management Programs

PRODUCT	MICROSOFT PLUG-IN TO DEVELOP THE BIBLIOGRAPHY AND IN-TEXT CITATION	GOOGLE DOC PLUG-IN TO DEVELOP THE BIBLIOGRAPHY AND IN-TEXT CITATION	PROJECT SHARING WITH COLLABORATORS	OPEN-ACCESS	SAVE PDFS
SciWheel (https://sciwheel.com/)	X	X	X		X
ProQuest RefWorks (https://refworks.proquest.com/)	X		X		X
EndNote (https://endnote.com/)	X	X	X	Basic is free, with limited features.	X
Zotero (https://www.zotero.org/)	X	X	X	Basic is free, with limited storage.	X
Mendeley (https://www.mendeley.com/)	X	X	X		X

features of common programs used by health sciences scholars. However, it is not exhaustive. Developers continually update products, so check with the vendors for the most up-to-date information.

Finally, recognize that search strategies are iterative; when new terms are revealed through article reviews or work is found through citations of reviewed articles, there is a need to return to the databases. Literature searches are time-intensive. You may need references to which the library does not have access. Most academic or professional libraries have a process for an interlibrary loan. Work with the librarian to order what is not available at your institution; however, understand that the time to receive articles may take weeks. Developing rapport with the academic librarian is a must. (See Text Box 5-3.)

EVALUATING THE LITERATURE

The capstone focus is informed by dozens of individual articles, so the capstone student must have a strategy to organize what is read. An evidence table is a good place to start. The structure of the evidence table is not prescriptive and should be adapted based on the question. The evidence table will help you write the justification for the eventual capstone project, so the format should work for the doctoral capstone student (Table 5-7). Recommendations for items to consider include the American Psychological Association citation, the research design, outcome measures used, results, strengths and weaknesses in light of the methodology, and alignment with the specific practice context (external validity). The AOTA's Evidence-Based Review Project provides a coding framework to describe the research design, sample, internal validity, and external validity (Lieberman & Scheer, 2002). Including this coding framework will give a quick snapshot of the relevance of the citation to the population and DCE site.

WRITING THE LITERATURE SYNTHESIS

After the critical appraisal, you will engage in reflection to develop a synthesis of the literature. A *synthesis* is not a list; rather, it is a skilled assessment of the state of the relevant evidence. The goal is to build toward broad statements about what is known (and not known) that are grounded in a deep understanding of the work that has been done. A synthesis will gather all the articles in a narrative form to arrive at a conclusion. The 5Cs (Table 5-8) have been described as a tool to help writers include the

Table 5-7 Evidence Table

CITATION	SUBJECTS	STUDY DESIGN	OUTCOME	COMMENTS ON INTERNAL VALIDITY	APPLICATION TO DCE SITE (EXTERNAL VALIDITY)	COMMENTS	AOTA CODING (I.E., IIA2A; LIEBERMAN & SCHEER, 2002)

Table 5-8 5Cs in Literature Review Writing

Cite	The focus of the paper are the articles you found. Keep the focus on the research and ensure you are appropriately and accurately citing.
Compare	What do you see are common methods, outcome measures, theoretical models, and challenges in the literature?
Contrast	Are there areas where the findings do not align? Offer insight into why that could be, based on deep understanding of the topic.
Critique the literature	Highlight articles with the greatest methodological rigor and those that have the greatest application to the capstone site. Offer analysis based on your deep understanding.
Connect	Connect the work together into a meaningful summary. Link to occupational therapy and to the capstone site.

Table 5-9 Literature Review Structure

Introduction	What is the problem, and why is it important? Consider the clinical question, and give the reader context to understand why asking this question is important. For most doctoral students, the results of your literature search will not give you the background to write this, requiring more investigation. Give data and facts to support your argument. The goal of this section is to convince the reader that asking and answering this question is necessary. *Tip:* The introduction section of the articles you reviewed likely started by explaining the problem. Look at the literature that was cited for justification for this section.
Body	The body of the paper will describe the work that has been done on the problem that was described in the introduction. It is the longest section of the paper and will require thoughtful organization. The similarities that were found during the comparison in the 5Cs (refer to Table 5-7) will provide broad topics that can be addressed in this section. It is important to remember that a literature review is a synthesis. It is not a list of articles and results. The body of the paper gives meaning and context to the research evidence. Conclude the section with a broad statement of what is known about the problem. Aim to answer the clinical question that was posed, recognizing that for many questions, the answer may be there in insufficient evidence.
Limitations	Based on the literature review, there is likely still unanswered questions. Describe what is still unknown. If there is substantial literature on your topic, you may consider what is known specific to the capstone site (unique population or service delivery model). Using the evidence from the literature, conclude with a gap analysis statement. Aligning this statement with the capstone site will better support proposal development.
Conclusion	This is the summary of the paper. It is the last argument of the importance of the problem you are addressing. Restate the main points from the body and limitations sections in a concise and persuasive tone.

necessary elements (Sudheesh et al., 2016) in a way that ensures the writer is not just listing or providing a count of the research evidence. The framework gives you a structure to critically think about each article individually and then connect to each other.

The organization of the synthesis will be influenced by the instructor and the curriculum design. Literature reviews that are developed as a foundation for a research proposal often follow a similar structure that includes defining the problem, synthesizing the evidence, and describing what work remains to be done (Table 5-9).

USING SCHOLARSHIP OF KNOWLEDGE DISCOVERY MODEL TO DESCRIBE THE CAPSTONE PROJECT

Boyer's model of scholarship (1990) has been proposed as a framework to describe the work of occupational therapists (American Occupational Therapy Association, 2009) and to provide a useful framework for the development of

the capstone project. Boyer's (1990) model describes four areas of scholarship. Research and publication are most closely aligned with the scholarship of discovery. This type of scholarship describes the generation of new knowledge (Boyer, 1990). The scholarship of integration refers to the interpretation and synthesis of new knowledge and information (Boyer, 1990). It requires interdisciplinary study and work to coordinate knowledge from multiple arenas (Boyer, 1990). The scholarship of application looks to take new knowledge and develop ways to apply to specific settings or areas (Boyer, 1990). The scholarship of teaching goes beyond providing information. It occurs through carefully planned and evaluated pedagogical procedures delivered by experts in the content area (Boyer, 1990). Table 5-10 provides a snapshot of how to align Boyer's model with the ACOTE focus areas. Table 5-11a provides examples of how to contextualize the development of a capstone project through the lens of Boyer (1990).

Boyer's model is well-established in occupational therapy, but more recently, Moyers and Quint (2025) introduced the *scholarship of knowledge discovery model*. This

Table 5-10 ACOTE Focus Areas Aligned With Boyer's Model

CAPSTONE FOCUS AREA	SCHOLARSHIP TYPE	DESCRIPTION
Research	Scholarship of discovery	Participating in an ongoing study or creating a study. Includes research design and planning, data collection, analyzing data, and summarizing and disseminating results.
Education (academic course development)	Scholarship of teaching	Curricular development and testing of learning outcomes of coursework with occupational therapy or occupational therapy assistant students.
Education (client/family education program)		Curricular development and testing of learning outcomes of coursework with clients and/or their families and caregivers.
Education (staff development program)		Curricular development and testing of learning outcomes of coursework with non-occupational therapy personnel.
Education (textbook or technology development)		Development of publishable teaching materials or teaching technology designed for occupational therapy or other health professional, non-health professional, consumer, or family audiences.
Administration	Scholarship of application	Active participation in the management of occupational therapy departments and/or specialized sites. Examples include working with experienced occupational therapists managing private practices and/or occupational therapy departments in various settings.
Advocacy		Development and testing of a program for consumers' abilities to navigate health systems to improve access to, delivery of, or outcomes of health care.
Program development and evaluation (clinical)		Program development includes implementing or modifying an occupational therapy program in traditional clinical settings (e.g., hand therapy, geriatrics, pediatrics, mental health, rehabilitation, school-based occupational therapy). Program evaluation explores the short- and long-term changes of the program.
Program development and evaluation (community)		Program development includes implementing or modifying an occupational therapy program in role-emerging and community-based settings (e.g., homeless shelters, nonprofit health facilities, criminal justice settings, foster care, adult day care). Program evaluation explores the short- and long-term changes of the program.
Leadership		Collaborating with leaders involved in exercising influence and representing different areas of the occupational therapy profession regionally, nationally, and/or internationally.
Policy development		Drafting strategy plans for the inclusion of school-based occupational therapists in tier 1 (whole school) interventions. These plans would be used for therapists to engage school administration to shift OT resources toward population focuses.
Any of the preceding	Scholarship of integration	Scholarship that creates new relationships between two or more disciplines. Any of the mediums for scholarship listed earlier (discovery, teaching, application) can be used to study the interface between two disciplines.

Table 5-11a Boyer's (1990) Model of Scholarship Aligned With Potential Occupational Therapy Doctoral Capstone Projects

	SCHOLARSHIP OF DISCOVERY	SCHOLARSHIP OF INTEGRATION	SCHOLARSHIP OF APPLICATION	SCHOLARSHIP OF TEACHING AND LEARNING
Types of capstone projects	Projects that may advance the knowledge base of a discipline (testing theories, generating knowledge)	Projects that may cross disciplines to create new ideas and/or perspectives	Projects that strive to connect theory to clinical practice; information is identified and applied.	Projects that examine the teaching-learning process; facilitation of assisting students to understand and apply information
Examples of capstone projects	Exploration of the impact of a novel, occupation-based group intervention to improve health and wellness in people with serious mental illness, guided by cognitive-behavioral therapy.	Interprofessional care planning across disciplines; nursing and occupational therapy collaborating on the impact of medication on falls/patient safety in a nursing home	Development of guidelines to establish a center of excellence in upper extremity rehabilitation	Classroom-based research such as the impact of standardized patient encounters on students' perceived sense of clinical efficacy

model is designed specifically to guide the distinctive scholarly work produced by occupational therapy doctorate students through their capstone projects.

Moyers and Quint (2025) propose ten areas of scholarship of discovery in practice, which include "advocacy/policy development, practice reasoning/decision making, consumer issues, evidence-based practice, implementation science, innovation, leadership/administration, program development and evaluation, quality improvement and teaching/learning" (p. 3).

Review the areas of scholarship of discovery in practice, and begin refining your ideas for your capstone project based on your own career goals and path forward. The following ten areas of scholarship have been adapted from Moyers and Quint (2025):

- *Advocacy/policy development.* Is there a policy you are interested in analyzing, developing, or evaluating through advocacy at your capstone site? In what ways can advocacy impact health and well-being in the context of your capstone population?
- *Practice reasoning/decision-making.* Would you like to explore shared decision-making in a specific practice area? What clinical challenges could you enter at your capstone site where decision-making and clinical reasoning could lead to a solution?
- *Consumer issues.* Are you interested in focusing on client satisfaction and experiences at your capstone site? Are there health literacy issues you could

address to improve the experiences of your clients or the populations you intended to serve?

- *Evidence-based practice.* How can you use evidence to answer a practice question? Would you be interested in developing practice guidelines or policies based on the best available evidence?
- *Implementation science.* Is there a particular intervention strategy you would like to assess for ethical use based on available evidence?
- *Innovation.* Are you interested in technological innovations and generating evidence to support them? For example, could you be exploring smart home technology for older adults, or virtual reality, and seek evidence to back up your interventions?
- *Leadership/administration.* What administrative changes might be beneficial within your capstone site? How could you take the lead in implementing these changes?
- *Program development and evaluation. Many capstone students begin their thought process here.* What program would you like to develop to impact the health and well-being of the population at your capstone site, and how can you evaluate its outcomes? How could it benefit from refinement and evaluation?
- *Quality improvement.* What is the continuous quality improvement (CQI) process at your site? Are there existing programs or processes you feel could be

improved? If so, how could you apply these improvements to enhance the quality of care at your capstone site?

- *Teaching/learning.* What are you already passionate about with regard to teaching and learning theory, and how can you apply this and in-depth knowledge to develop or enhance patient education, fieldwork education programs, or new practitioner mentoring programs?

DETERMINING A PROBLEM STATEMENT AND GAP ANALYSIS FOR THE CAPSTONE

Through a synthesis of the literature, focusing on the doctoral capstone experience (DCE) context, gaps in practice (or knowledge) will become evident. A *gap* is a difference between what is happening and what should be happening. Gaps exist in all areas, including research, clinical practice, and education. The "what should be happening" can be found in peer-reviewed publications, such as research articles, but also includes clinical practice guidelines and standards of practice from accrediting agencies. Stating the gap is the first step in developing a robust capstone proposal. It is not enough to identify what is and what should be; students must be able to articulate what the actual gap is by describing what is happening and contrasting this to the desired action (Davis-Ajami et al., 2014). This is a gap analysis statement.

For example, constraint-induced movement therapy (CIMT) is one of the most well-studied and effective treatments of hemiplegia after stroke. There is a large body of work, with clinical trials and systematic reviews, that supports the intervention; however, CIMT is not widely applied in practice (Morris & Taub, 2014). This is an example of where what should be happening is not the same as what is happening, and the gap is the use of less-supported interventions to address hemiplegia rather than the implementation of a CIMT protocol. Gaps exist for a variety of reasons. A capstone project should use literature to understand both what the gap is and then look for reasons specific to the setting that is addressed. These include gaps in research, education, and practice.

After identifying the gap, it is important to complete another systematic process to understand why the gap is occurring. Gaps exist within a context and involve many stakeholders. A thoughtful examination of why a gap exists, through an examination of the workflow at the DCE site or an interview and observation of the stakeholders, will provide insight into the gap (Davis-Ajami et al., 2014). Chapter 6 discusses the needs assessment process in detail. The literature may also provide insight into the reason for the gap. The clearly articulated reason for why a gap occurs is the problem statement. The problem statement is the foundation on which the capstone proposal is developed. Drawing from the CIMT example earlier in this chapter, the reason for the gap is multifaceted, requiring different problem statements (Table 5-11b).

How might you use the ten areas of scholarship of discovery in practice (Moyers & Quint, 2025) to inspire your problem statement?

Literature must guide how to address the problem, resulting in a new literature search. The problem statement

Table 5-11b Problem Statement Examples

BOYER'S AREA OF SCHOLARSHIP	EVIDENCE	PROBLEM
Discovery	The first multicenter randomized controlled trial of GMT recruited 222 subjects. However, only 6% of screened participants met the inclusion criteria (Wolf et al., 2008).	Subjects in research are not reflective of the population with whom most occupational therapists work. There is a gap in the knowledge on the impact of CIMT on populations that are reflective of typical practice.
Teaching	Only 2.7% of clinicians used all components of CIMT (Pedlow et al., 2014).	Only a small percentage of clinicians (2.7%) are applying CIMT as the protocol described. There appears to be a lack of knowledge of the protocol.
Application	About 75% of occupational therapy/physical therapy participants thought the implementation would be very difficult (Daniel et al., 2012).	Practical barriers toward implementation of best practice exist.
Integration	Use of interdisciplinary framework on knowledge to address any of these problems is an example of the scholarship of integration.	

and the area of focus may lead to another clinical question. For example, if looking to address the problem in education, searches should explore evidence about how to provide education to experienced clinicians, rather than just a general search on education. For example, "Are journal clubs (I) or didactic education sessions (C) more effective to increase therapist (P) competency with novel interventions (O)?"

Real-world problems are often multifaceted. A capstone project is unlikely to address all aspects during the DCE and may only focus on one problem area. The design of the DCE is to give you an in-depth experience in one or more of the focus areas: clinical practice skills, research skills, administration, leadership, program development and evaluation, policy development, advocacy, education, and leadership (discussed in detail in Chapter 2). Appendix 5-C provides inspiration of example PICO questions aligned with the focus areas. Table 5-11c provides examples of how gaps and problem statements aligned with the ACOTE focus areas.

Table 5-11c Example Capstone Focuses

FOCUS AREA	METHOD	GAP	PROBLEM STATEMENT
Clinical practice	Develop advanced skills in the use of CIMT in multiple populations.	A large body of work, with clinical trials and systematic reviews, supports the intervention; however, CIMT is not widely applied in practice (Morris & Taub, 2014).	Only a small percentage of clinicians (2.7%) are applying CIMT as the protocol describes.
Research skills	Develop and deploy feasibility study of CIMT to include subjects that are representative of the context of DCE.	Subjects in research are not reflective of the population with which most occupational therapists work. There is a gap in the knowledge on the impact of CIMT on populations that are reflective of typical practice.	
Administration	Develop workflow procedures to ensure clients who meet inclusion criteria for CIMT are offered service.	Practical barriers toward implementation of best practice exist.	
Program and policy development	Develop a knowledge translation program to improve fidelity to the CIMT protocol in DCE environment.		
Policy development	Develop policies that incentivize therapists to use evidence-based strategies.		
Advocacy	Engage with third-party payers to support reimbursement for hours of CIMT needed to provide protocol with fidelity.		
Education	Develop and implement training for staff at DCE on CIMT protocols.	Only a small percentage of clinicians (2.7%) are applying CIMT as the protocol describes. There appears to be a lack of knowledge of the protocol.	

ROOTING SCHOLARLY INQUIRY AND CAPSTONE IN THEORY

Finally, capstone projects are grounded in theory. A *theory* is a proposed explanation or a generalized statement aimed at explaining a certain phenomenon. *Frameworks* are overall structures that help us organize the elements of the reality we are observing (Cole & Tufano, 2020). The theory and framework chosen will provide the scaffolding to address the stated problem. For example, learning theories, such as adult learning theory (Knowles, 1978) or situated learning (Lave et al., 1991), provide a way to understand how adults (professionals) will access learning and benefit from education.

The theory used to guide the capstone project does not need to be an occupational therapy theory. The integration of interdisciplinary knowledge will strengthen the project. The author of this chapter uses, and has mentored students who have used, theories from psychology, leadership, motor learning, education, and nursing. For example, Frye and Bell (2023) used self-efficacy theory (Bandura, 1977) to guide the development of a self-management program for people with heart failure. In another project, the knowledge to action framework (Sudsawad, 2007) was used to implement a program with nurses to position the hemiplegic arm (Cole & Bell, 2024). These are just a few examples of non–occupational therapy theoretical perspectives that can guide the development of a capstone project. Chapter 8 builds on this notion of using theory and describes how concept maps can be a useful strategy to organize information and depict relationships between concepts, particularly in regard to measuring outcomes and impact of the capstone project.

CHAPTER SECTION SUMMARY

The student portion of this chapter presented recommendations to guide the process of scholarly inquiry for the capstone. Specific steps were presented to help you develop a course of action to build your capstone project. Your capstone project is built out of a gap, defined by the problem identified by you, the capstone student, and guided in the application by theory (Figure 5-1).

Equally important to the capstone being rooted in evidence, the capstone should relate to an area of strong interest and passion of the student. The ideal project should reflect capstone students' interests and help develop skills that will support a professional trajectory. After completion of the capstone experience and project, graduates may be employed in a different practice area or be working with a different population; however, the skill progression that is developed throughout the doctoral capstone process can enhance professional practice and support individual career trajectories throughout your career.

LEARNING ACTIVITIES

1. Reflect on previous work experience or fieldwork experiences.

    a. Identify what was happening and what ideally should be happening.

    b. State the gap.

    c. Describe the influence of knowledge, practice, and research on the gap.

    d. Develop a problem statement.

2. Select from the journal articles you retrieved during a recent literature search. Use the PQRS model to complete the review. Reflect on how you completed each of the four steps:

    P

    Q

    R

    S

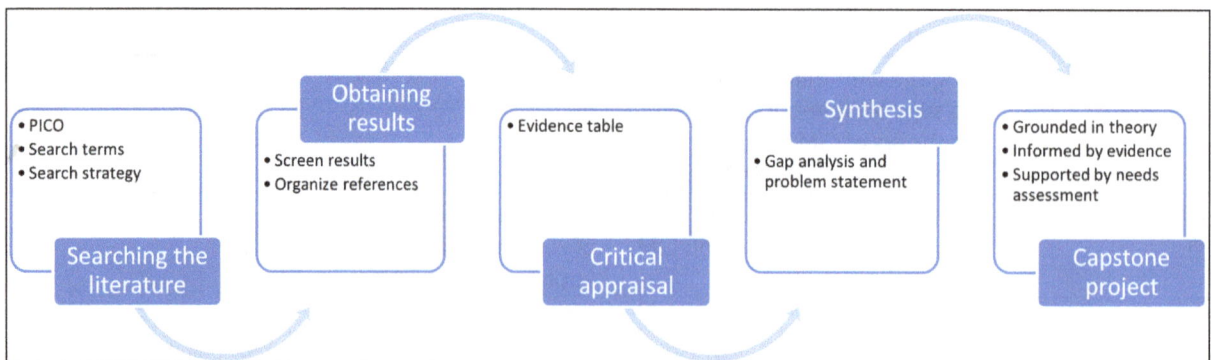

Figure 5-1. Building your capstone project.

Section 2: Educator Focus

Transformational Learning Phases and Framework for the Educator

Engaging in the literature review for a doctoral capstone project closely aligns with Mezirow's critical assessment phase of transformative learning theory (Mezirow, 1997). Mezirow's theory emphasizes the process of critically assessing and reflecting on one's assumptions, beliefs, and knowledge to foster transformative learning. In this context, the literature review acts as a key process for engaging with existing scholarship, critically evaluating and challenging established ideas, and integrating new perspectives. As our students engage with a wide variety of academic and scientific sources, they are naturally prompted to critically assess, and sometimes challenge, their own pre-existing assumptions or understanding about their topic, capstone focus area, or population. This mirrors Mezirow's idea of critically reflecting on assumptions that might have been taken for granted.

As our students initiate and proceed through the literature review, they evaluate the validity, credibility, and relevance of different studies and findings. This process encourages the development of their critical thinking skills, similar to the critical assessment phase, where learners evaluate the strengths, weaknesses, and biases of different perspectives. The process of synthesizing various viewpoints and findings from the literature helps doctoral students develop a deeper, more nuanced understanding of the topic. This synthesis is part of the critical assessment process, where learners consider how different perspectives contribute to or challenge their existing knowledge. Identifying gaps in the literature or inconsistencies in research findings requires a critical mindset. This process helps build the foundation for transformative learning and intellectual growth (Mezirow, 1997).

INTRODUCTION FOR THE EDUCATOR

The design of an entry-level occupational therapy doctoral capstone project must include a literature review (ACOTE, 2023). In many curriculums, students are introduced to completing a literature search and critically appraise research relatively early, perhaps in alignment with other evidence-based practice and research curricular standards. However, in this chapter, the literature review is presented to go beyond critically appraising the methodological rigor to include a synthesis of what is known and what is not relative to students' capstone projects. Developing an adequate synthesis is a complex process with discreet steps. Instructors can support students in this process with instructional materials and assignments that build to the ultimate end product of a doctoral-level synthesis of an important clinical question.

Throughout this section for the OTD educator, generative artificial intelligence (GenAI) tools and strategies will also be introduced and offered. When ChatGPT, the first widely available text-generating AI, became available, the academic discourse surrounded strategies to prevent and detect its use. In this section of the chapter that is geared for the occupational therapy doctoral faculty member, GenAI is offered as a resource that both students and educators should learn to use in a practical and ethical way.

REFLECTIVE QUESTIONS

1. What are the contextual factors of your curriculum and the capstone site? How will the capstone experience influence the project scope and focus?

2. What resources does your institution offer? Consider your department, college/school, the library, and the eventual capstone site. How can those resources support the literature review process?

3. Consider access to databases, librarians, work–study students, and reference management tools.

4. What is your comfort in using emerging technology to support students in completing a literature review?

EDUCATOR OBJECTIVES

By the end of reading this chapter, the educator will be able to apply principles of transformational learning theory to structure learning activities, assignments, and/or assessments in order to promote the capstone student's ability to:

1. Develop strategies for integrating librarian expertise and library resources into course activities.

2. Understand the value of reference management tools and literature review software for organizing and screening search results.

3. Develop rubrics and assessment criteria for evaluating students' work during the literature review process.

4. Construct assignments that help students identify gaps in the literature and formulate problem statements for their capstone projects.

5. Articulate strategies incorporating the ethical use of generative AI tools to support the literature review process.

Objectives modified based on a generative AI response from Anthropic. (2024). Claude [Large language model]. https://www.anthropic.com.

HOW TO SUPPORT STUDENTS IN DEVELOPING A SEARCH STRATEGY

When developing coursework related to literature reviews, engaging a librarian is desirable. High-quality systematic reviews will engage librarians, acknowledging that their expertise is invaluable (Lefebvre et al., 2023). While the doctoral student is unlikely to complete a systematic review, the librarian's role is still essential. Engaging the librarian early in coursework can ensure higher-quality education materials and increase students' comfort with working with these professional colleagues.

Many academic libraries will develop library guides (LibGuides), which are librarian-developed online guides for specific information. These resources are available on various topics relevant to the literature review process. If your library does not have a LibGuide on the topic of interest, you can find one from other institutions. For example, here is a LibGuide made available publicly from Thomas Jefferson University: https://jefflibraries.libguides.com/PICO/BeginningASearch.

How to Support Students in Developing a Focused Question

The first step in the search strategy is the PICO question. While not every clinical question can or should be answered using the PICO format, it is well-known and often familiar to students from previous coursework. Developing the question requires the doctoral student to have some preliminary information about the eventual capstone site, including the population and types of intervention or service delivery models that are feasible in the setting. (See Text Box 5-4.) For example, if a capstone site is a drop-in center for people experiencing homelessness, a literature search on a residential treatment program would not align with the site context. It may be helpful to engage members of the capstone site in developing the PICO question. Consider asking the content mentor to develop a list of questions that students can then develop into the PICO format.

Questions from the content expert may include:

1. Why do consumers choose to come to the drop-in center?
2. For people who are experiencing homelessness, what are their priorities for care?
3. What are common conditions that OTs could address?
4. How can we measure outcomes of a drop-in program?

TEXT BOX 5-4

There are many online platforms for developing PICO questions, including LibGuides and online PICO generators (Research Question Generator – Use The PICOT Framework (picotquestion.com).

How to Support Students in Developing Search Terms and Strategies

Developing a search strategy involves identifying the relevant terms. These terms may be general keywords or specific to the vocabulary of the identified database (MeSH, for example). To assist students in learning the keywords, it is helpful to have them find several relevant articles. The articles do not need to answer the PICO question but rather give information related to the PICO. Most published articles will contain keywords that may be used as they are or used to find the appropriate term in the specified database. For example, when students enter the keyword "autism" into the MeSH thesaurus, they will find the keyword "Autism" is found on the MeSH heading of "Autism Spectrum Disorder," as well as older MeSH terminology that should be included in their search strategy.

After identifying relevant terms, students develop their search strategy. Appendix 5-A is a template developed by academic librarians at Thomas Jefferson University. It is helpful to help students visualize how to construct the eventual search they will execute in the identified database. Learning activities, teaching tips, and assessment strategies for the literature search process are offered in Table 5-12 and Table 5-13.

Support the Student Process to Select and Manage the Literature

After the search strategy is approved and executed, students will have their results. Depending on the topic, it may be a few dozen to several hundred. While it is desirable to limit searches to reduce the number of articles, it is essential to recognize that this is the final stage of doctoral work. Be careful when enacting too many limits for ease and without a strong justification. The accreditation standards require the capstone project to demonstrate in-depth knowledge of the field of study, and so students should have a strong understanding of the literature. While the high numbers can feel overwhelming, faculty and students should reference any systematic reviews they have reviewed in their previous coursework for comfort. For example, a systematic review explored the impact of the CO-OP model on occupational performance after stroke. The search yielded 722 articles, reduced to 8 by removing duplicates and completing a title and abstract screen. The final number was reduced to 7 after a full-text review (Kiriakou & Psychouli, 2024).

To manage a volume of results, students will benefit from tools and procedures to help manage the volume of articles they retrieve. Reference management tools have been described to assist with manuscript development, but they can be useful in the study selection process. For all the tools presented (Table 5-6), students can upload the results of their searches from the different databases into the reference management system and remove duplicates. For most of the tools, students can see the study title and abstract and then complete the first stages of the review process.

Table 5-12 Learning Activities

ACTIVITY	TEACHING TIP	ASSESSMENT
Develop a PICO question	• Engage the capstone site to reflect the needs and priorities. • Use LibGuides. • Use PICO generators.	Students must generate the most appropriate question to ensure they can execute a high-quality search. This assignment should be iterative, with grading reflecting the ability to integrate feedback.
Develop a search strategy	• Use LibGuides. • Find relevant articles to support the identification of keywords. • Engage librarians. • Provide templates to support the organization of search strategy. • Set up email alerts on the search strategy to be notified of the new relevant publications. • PubMed tutorial: https://www.nihlibrary.nih.gov/resources/subject-guides/keeping-current/creating-alerts-pubmed • Check with your library for a LibGuide for other databases.	Students need to generate the most appropriate search strategy. The grading for this assignment should reflect the integration of the LibGuides or librarian instruction. Table 5-13 provides a rubric that includes integration of a librarian in the course.

A higher-level skill for students would be to use tools designed explicitly for literature review. Many university libraries offer access to tools built to facilitate a high-quality systematic review, such as Covidence (Covidence, n.d.) or Rayaan (Ouzzani et al., 2016). Some of these products have introduced machine learning tools (a form of artificial intelligence) to aid the researcher in the screening process, significantly reducing time. Machine learning cannot replace the researcher's review; however, it can speed up the process. There is a learning curve to using these tools, but developing comfort may aid students' future scholarship endeavors.

GUIDING STUDENTS IN EVALUATING THE LITERATURE

An evidence table is necessary to manage the volume of literature that will be reviewed. Evidence tables provide a snapshot of articles in a way that allows the doctoral student to visualize their results, which is a necessary step to synthesize. The format of the evidence table should be influenced by the clinical question and course learning objectives. Table 5-7 is offered as a sample for consideration.

An important prompt in any evidence table should be to consider the application to their specific site. As the doctoral student preparing for the doctoral project, they will need to bring their skills in critical appraisal for methodological rigor and develop a nuanced understanding of how literature is applied in their capstone site. Given the nature of capstone sites, it is very common not to have high-quality evidence that directly answers the question. For example, a student may be exploring trauma-informed care models for people experiencing homelessness and find that most of the available literature is with children. The impact of both the age of the participant and the model of care should be considered when describing the results of the literature for the desired population of people experiencing homelessness. Another example is when the capstone service delivery model does not align with the researched intervention. An intervention might have a dosing of three times a week for six weeks, which far exceeds most service delivery models' scheduling. Students should consider the impact of the site's ability to apply that intervention with fidelity.

GenAI is powerful and can support students' understanding of the often complex and dense literature they read. Understanding the data analysis methods and interpreting the results can challenge students with limited experience in statistical analysis. SciSpace (https://typeset.io/) is a GenAI that is designed to interpret research papers. Students can upload the PDFs of the retrieved articles and ask specific questions or highlight text to

Table 5-13 Search Strategy Grading Rubric

CRITERIA	MEETS EXPECTATIONS	BELOW EXPECTATIONS	DOES NOT SHOW APPLICATION OF COURSE MATERIALS
Follows assignment guidelines	• Three articles are submitted and are relevant to the PICO question. • Appendix 5-A worksheet is submitted as a Word doc. • PICO question is listed on worksheet. • Search "sentence" is written and executed with the number of results.	• Three articles are submitted and are relevant to the PICO question. • Appendix 5-A worksheet is submitted as a Word doc. • PICO question is listed on worksheet. • Search "sentence" is written and executed with the number of results.	Any of the following is true: • Three articles are NOT submitted and/or are relevant to the PICO question. • PICO question is NOT listed on the worksheet. • Search "sentence" is NOT written and/or executed with the number of results.
Search terminology	• Each column of Appendix 5-A has at least five terms per relevant column. • The keywords identified are informed by research articles submitted. • MeSH terms are identified and relevant.	• Each column has five terms per relevant column. • The keywords identified are NOT informed by research articles submitted. • MeSH terms are identified but are not relevant to the PICO question.	• Each column does NOT have five terms per relevant column. • The keywords identified are NOT informed by research articles submitted. • MeSH terms are NOT identified.
Librarian meeting	• Librarians receive articles and worksheet submissions by the due date. Students are on time for the meeting. Students are prepared and engage easily with the librarian. Feedback is accepted.	• Librarians receive articles and worksheet submissions by the due date. Students are on time for the meeting. Students are prepared but require prompting by the librarian to engage in discussion. Feedback is accepted.	• Any of the following is true: Librarians DO NOT receive articles and worksheet submissions by the due date. Students are late or do not show up to the meeting. Students DO NOT engage in discussion, even with prompting. Feedback is NOT accepted.

ask for a plain-language summary. SciSpace can manage multiple articles and generate a table format like what is recommended in Table 5-7. However, like all GenAIs, there are limitations. The output from SciSpace may be inaccurate and should always be reviewed. Instructors can develop learning activities that allow students to see the great value of such tools, along with demonstrating the errors to highlight the need for their critical thinking and expertise. To develop these activities, load articles and ask questions. Note where the GenAI is incorrect to demonstrate this to students. SciSpace was built for research evidence but is not the only GenAI tool. Many of the large language model's AIs (ChatGPT, Claude, Gemini) allow users to upload PDFs and ask questions. Just like SciSpace, the accuracy of the information should be verified.

SUPPORTING THE STUDENTS TO SYNTHESIZE THE LITERATURE

The literature review is done as a foundation for the capstone project and, in many programs, can be considered the first part of a doctoral capstone proposal. The outline recommended to students in Table 5-9 guides them to use the literature to build a problem statement that can become their eventual project.

This chapter guides students through the process of a rapid review. Rapid reviews are an accepted form of evidence synthesis that can be published in peer-reviewed journals. To achieve this, the rigorous process must be documented so a reader can replicate the student's work. The *Rapid Review Guidebook* (Dobbins, 2017), published by McMaster University, provides excellent resources on how to implement and document a rapid review that meets the criteria for peer-reviewed publication.

A narrative synthesis is not the only outcome of a literature review. Critically appraised topics (CATs) are another form of a rapid review suitable for peer-review publication. CATs differ from the narrative review in that they will typically include three to five of the "best available" evidence rather than aiming to understand the full scope of what is known (White et al., 2017). The AOTA evidence exchange contains several CATs on diverse practice areas that follow a consistent structure that includes a clinical question with a scenario explaining the importance of the problem, a summary of the key findings, and then a bottom line for occupational therapy practice.

USING GENERATIVE AI TO SUPPORT STUDENT WRITING

The early discourse around generative AI was focused on concerns for academic integrity, with educators concerned GenAI will now do all student writing. While GenAI is powerful, it is not a replacement for the critical thinking necessary for the doctoral level of scholarship described in this chapter. Students can be guided to use GenAI to support their ability to write a scholarly literature view.

In GenAI, a *prompt* is an input, like a question or a PDF, that communicates with the AI model, from which the response is generated. The quality of the response received is, in part, dependent on the quality of the prompt. Chat GPT-4 was prompted to give examples of prompts that would be helpful to a doctoral student writing a literature review. A sample of the responses follows (OpenAI, 2024):

- "Can you help me create an outline for my literature review on [specific topic]?"
- "What are the essential sections I should include in my literature review?"
- "How can I logically organize the sections and subsections of my literature review?"
- "Can you help me write an engaging introduction that sets up the context and importance of my literature review on [specific topic]?"
- "How can I clearly state the objectives and scope of my literature review in the introduction?"
- "What is an effective way to structure the body sections of my literature review?"
- "How can I write a strong conclusion that summarizes the key findings of my literature review?"
- "What are some effective ways to highlight the implications and future directions of the research?"
- "How can I identify and discuss gaps and limitations in the current literature on [specific topic]?"
- "What are the implications of these gaps for future research?"

- "How can I revise my literature review to improve its clarity and coherence?"
- "Can you help me check my paper for grammar and punctuation errors?"
- "What are the formatting guidelines for a doctoral-level literature review in [specific style guide, for example, APA, MLA]?"
- "Can you help me format my citations and references correctly according to [specific style guide]?"

As you can see, generative AI could support writers as they develop their skills as doctoral-level scholars.

It is not just students who can benefit from GenAI; instructors can too! Try out this prompt in Text Box 5-5 to generate a rubric for a literature review using the outline in Table 5-9.

> ### TEXT BOX 5-5
>
> Please generate a grading rubric for a doctoral-level occupational therapy student that includes criteria for the introduction, literature synthesis, and problem statement. Generate in a table format.

The results will differ for each product the prompt is trialed in and even vary within the same product. The response will likely be a solid starting point for developing a rubric. (See Text Box 5-6.) Just like GenAI does not replace the critical thinking of doctoral students, it cannot replace the instructor with deep knowledge of the content, specific course, and curriculum. Providing more information on course objectives and instructor priorities, like scholarly writing, will further refine the resulting product. Still, with course- and curriculum-specific knowledge, instructors must refine it to meet their needs.

Educators should consider both syllabus-level and assignment-level policies relative to the use of GenAI. Students should also be well informed about the expectation and practice of performing disclosure when AI is used. (See Text Box 5-7.)

> ### TEXT BOX 5-6
>
> Rubrics are not the only place instructors can use GenAI. As noted earlier, the learning objectives for this section of the chapter were developed with the help of Claude 3.5 Sonnet. An early draft of this section was submitted with a prompt for developing objectives. Appendix 5-D shows the output. Note how the final product was influenced by GenAI.

> ### TEXT BOX 5-7
>
> If peer-reviewed publication is the goal, carefully review the desired journal submission guidelines,

as GenAI is explicitly prohibited in some. For reference, the guidelines for AJOT during the publication of this book allow the use of GenAI, with authors disclosing and describing the use (American Occupational Therapy Association, 2023).

EDUCATOR SECTION SUMMARY

The literature review process is a crucial component of doctoral capstone projects in occupational therapy. It serves as the foundation for identifying gaps in current knowledge and practice and justifying the need for the project. Integrating modern tools, including reference management software and GenAI, can enhance this process. The role of the educator is to guide students to responsibly use all available resources, ensuring they understand the tools are resources that can be used to support their own critical thinking and analytical skills necessary to develop into doctoral-level scholars. By fostering these competencies, we prepare our students not only for their capstone projects but also for careers as evidence-based practitioners and potential future scholars in occupational therapy. (See Text Box 5-8.)

TEXT BOX 5-8

The use of GenAI is novel and not without controversy. Students and instructors must understand that GenAI is not always correct. The models make errors and are prone to hallucinations (fabricating data, like a fake literature citation). All AI models are only as strong as their training set, which means the output will be biased based on the data that is available. GenAI is not human and is not responsible for the output (International Committee of Medical Journal Editors, n.d.). The user of GenAI is ultimately responsible for the content, and students should learn how to manage this responsibility.

Other considerations in the use of AI include issues of access. At this time, many tools are available through a freemium model – meaning basic features are available at no cost, while premium features are available with a paid subscription. This may lead to disparities between students with premium access and those without.

For instructors, there are additional ethical concerns. All information that is uploaded into GenAI may become part of the training data. For example, the early draft of this chapter was uploaded and may now be part of the training set. Instructors who use generative AI to assist with grading are taking student work products and distributing them without permission.

Please default to your program or institution's guidelines or policies regarding the use of AI.

ADDITIONAL RESOURCES

Occupational therapy educators and students can refer to other prominent resources for evidence-based practice and research by referring to the following texts that are rated as most frequently used according to the National Board for Certification in Occupational Therapy's (NBCOT) *OTR Curriculum Textbook and Peer-Reviewed Journal Report* (most recent version retrieved from https://www.nbcot.org/-/media/PDFs/2020_Textbook_Report_OTR.pdf)

- Brown, C. (2017). *The evidence-based practitioner: Applying research to meet client needs.* F.A. Davis Company.
- Portney, L. G. (2020). *Foundations of clinical research: Applications to evidence-based practice* (4th ed.). F.A. Davis Company.
- Law, M., & MacDermid, J. (2013). *Evidence-based rehabilitation: A guide to practice* (3rd ed.). Slack, Inc.
- Creswell, J. W., & Creswell, J. D. (2017). *Research design: Qualitative, quantitative, and mixed methods approaches* (5th ed.). SAGE Publications.

REFERENCES

Accreditation Council for Occupational Therapy Education. (2023). *2023 Accreditation Council for Occupational Therapy Education (ACOTE®) standards and interpretive guide.* https://acoteonline.org/accreditation-explained/standards/

American Occupational Therapy Association. (2009). Scholarship in occupational therapy. *American Journal of Occupational Therapy, 63*(6), 790–796. https://doi.org/10.5014/ajot.63.6.790

American Occupational Therapy Association. (2023). Guidelines for contributors to AJOT. *American Journal of Occupational Therapy, 77*(Suppl. 3), 7713430010. https://doi.org/10.5014/ajot.2023.77S3005

Bandura, A. (1977). Self-efficacy: Toward a unifying theory of behavioral change. *Psychological Review, 84*(2), 191–215. https://doi.org/10.1037//0033-295x.84.2.191

Boyer, E. L. (1990). *Scholarship revisited: Priorities of the professoriate.* The Carnegie Foundation for the Advancement of Teaching.

Cochrane Library. (n.d.). *About the cochrane library.* http://www.cochranelibrary.com/about/about-the-cochrane-library.html

Cochrane Library. (2024). *What is PICO.* https://www.cochranelibrary.com/about-pico

Cochrane Linked Data. (2024). *PICO ontology.* http://linkeddata.cochrane.org/pico-ontology

Cohen, G. (1990). Memory. In I. Roth (Ed.), *The Open University's introduction to psychology* (Vol. 2, pp. 570–620). Erlbaum. https://doi.org/10.4324/9781315785127

Cole, E., & Bell, A. (2024). Hemiplegic shoulder pain prevention: A collaborative approach with nursing and occupational therapy in acute care. *Archives of Physical Medicine and Rehabilitation, 105*(4), e84. https://doi.org/10.1016/j.apmr.2024.02.236

Cole, M. B., & Tufano, R. (2020). *Applied theories in occupational therapy: A practical approach* (2nd ed.). Routledge. https://doi.org/10.4324/9781003522591

Covidence. (n.d.). *Better systematic review management.* Covidence. http://www.covidence.org/

Daniel, L., Howard, W., Braun, D., & Page, S. J. (2012). Opinions of constraint-induced movement therapy among therapists in southwestern Ohio. *Topics in Stroke Rehabilitation, 19*(3), 268–275. https://doi.org/10.1310/tsr1903-268

Davis-Ajami, M. L., Costa, L., & Kulik, S. (2014). Gap analysis: Synergies and opportunities for effective nursing leadership. *Nursing Economics, 32*(1), 17–25. https://www.proquest.com/scholarly-journals/gap-analysis-synergies-opportunities-effective/docview/1508688450/se-2

Dobbins, M. (2017). *Rapid Review Guidebook*. National Collaborating Centre for Methods and Tools.

EBSCO Information Services. (n.d.). *CINHAL database*. EBSCO. https://www.ebsco.com/products/research-databases/cinahl-database

EbscoConnect. (2022). *Searching with Boolean operators*. https://connect.ebsco.com/s/article/Searching-with-Boolean-Operators?language=en_US

Educational Resource Information Center. (n.d.). *Frequently asked questions*. https://eric.ed.gov/?faq

Elsevier. (n.d.). *Embase: The comprehensive medical research database*. https://www.elsevier.com/solutions/embase-biomedical-research/embase-coverage-and-content

Ewald, H., Klerings, I., Wagner, G., Heise, T. L., Stratil, J. M., Lhachimi, S. K., Hemkens, L. G., Gartlehner, G., Armijo-Olivo, S., & Nussbaumer-Streit, B. (2022). Searching two or more databases decreased the risk of missing relevant studies: A metaresearch study. *Journal of Clinical Epidemiology, 149*, 154–164. https://doi.org/10.1016/j.jclinepi.2022.05.022

Frye, S. K., & Bell, A. (2023). Heart smart: A virtual self-management intervention for homebound people with heart failure: A pilot study. *Home Health Care Management & Practice, 35*(1), 13–20. https://doi.org/10.1177/10848223221101194

Google Scholar. (n.d.). *About Google Scholar*. https://scholar.google.com/intl/us/scholar/about.html

Hamel, C., Michaud, A., Thuku, M., Skidmore, B., Stevens, A., Nussbaumer-Streit, B., & Garritty, C. (2021). Defining rapid reviews: A systematic scoping review and thematic analysis of definitions and defining characteristics of rapid reviews. *Journal of Clinical Epidemiology, 129*, 74–85. https://doi.org/10.1016/j.jclinepi.2020.09.041

Hoffmann, F., Allers, K., Rombey, T., Helbach, J., Hoffmann, A., Mathes, T., & Pieper, D. (2021). Nearly 80 systematic reviews were published each day: Observational study on trends in epidemiology and reporting over the years 2000–2019. *Journal of Clinical Epidemiology, 138*, 1–11. https://doi.org/10.1016/j.jclinepi.2021.05.022

Hosseini, M. S., Jahanshahlou, F., Akbarzadeh, M. A., Zarei, M., & Vaez-Gharamaleki, Y. (2024). Formulating research questions for evidence-based studies. *Journal of Medicine, Surgery, and Public Health, 2*, 1–5. https://doi.org/10.1016/j.glmedi.2023.100046

Howlett, B., Rogo, E., & Shelton, T. G. (2013). *Evidence-based practice for health professionals. An interprofessional approach*. Jones and Bartlett Learning.

International Committee of Medical Journal Editors. (n.d.). *Defining the role of authors and contributors*. ICMJE. https://www.icmje.org/recommendations/browse/roles-and-responsibilities/defining-the-role-of-authors-and-contributors.html

Kiriakou, A., & Psychouli, P. (2024). Effects of the CO-OP approach in addressing the occupational performance of adults with stroke: A systematic review. *The American Journal of Occupational Therapy, 78*(2), 1–7. https://doi.org/10.5014/ajot.2024.050131

Knowles, M. S. (1978). Andragogy: Adult learning theory in perspective. *Community College Review, 5*(3), 9–20. https://doi.org/10.1177/009155217800500302

Lave, J., Wenger, E., & Wenger, E. (1991). *Situated learning: Legitimate peripheral participation*. Cambridge University Press.

Lefebvre, C., Glanville, J., Briscoe, S., Featherstone, R., Littlewood, A., Metzendorf, M.-I., Noel-Storr, A., Paynter, R., Rader, T., Thomas, J., & Wieland, L. S. (2023). Chapter 4: Searching for and selecting studies Version (6.5). In *Cochrane handbook for systematic reviews of interventions*. https://training.cochrane.org/handbook/current/chapter-04

Lieberman, D., & Scheer, J. (2002). AOTA's evidence-based literature review project: An overview. *The American Journal of Occupational Therapy, 56*(3), 344–349. https://doi.org/10.5014/ajot.56.3.344

Mezirow, J. (1997). Transformative learning: Theory to practice. *New Directions for Adult and Continuing Education, (74)*, 5–12. https://doi.org/10.1002/ace.7401

Morris, D. M., & Taub, E. (2014). Training model for promoting translation from research to clinical settings: University of Alabama at Birmingham training for constraint-induced movement therapy. *Journal of Rehabilitation Research and Development, 51*(2), 9–17. https://doi.org/10.1682/JRRD.2014.01.0008

Moyers, P., & Quint, N. (2025). The issue is-discovery of knowledge in practice. *American Journal of Occupational Therapy, 79*, 7901347010. https://doi.org/10.5014/ajot.2025.050880

National Library of Medicine. (n.d.). *PubMed*. https://pubmed.ncbi.nlm.nih.gov/

National Library of Medicine. (2024). *Welcome to medical subject headings*. https://www.nlm.nih.gov/mesh/meshhome.html

OpenAI. (2024). *ChatGPT [Large language model]*. https://chat.openai.com/chat

OTseeker. (n.d.). *Welcome to OTseeker*. http://www.otseeker.com

Ouzzani, M., Hammady, H., Fedorowicz, Z., & Elmagarmid, A. (2016). Rayyan – a web and mobile app for systematic reviews. *Systematic Reviews, 5*(1), 1–10. https://doi.org/10.1186/s13643-016-0384-4

Page, M. J., McKenzie, J. E., Bossuyt, P. M., Boutron, I., Hoffmann, T. C., Mulrow, C. D., Shamseer, L., Tetzlaff, J. M., Akl, E. A., Brennan, S. E., Chou, R., Glanville, J., Grimshaw, J. M., Hróbjartsson, A., Lalu, M. M., Li, T., Loder, E. W., Mayo-Wilson, E., McDonald, S., . . . Moher, D. (2021). The PRISMA 2020 statement: An updated guideline for reporting systematic reviews. *BMJ, 372*, 1–9. https://doi.org/10.1136/bmj.n71

Pedlow, K., Lennon, S., & Wilson, C. (2014). Application of constraint-induced movement therapy in clinical practice: An online survey. *Archives of Physical Medicine and Rehabilitation, 95*(2), 276–282. https://doi.org/10.1016/j.apmr.2013.08.240

PEDro. (2024, April 2). *Welcome to PEDro*. https://www.pedro.org.au/

Polanin, J. R., Pigott, T. D., Espelage, D. L., & Grotpeter, J. K. (2019). Best practice guidelines for abstract screening large-evidence systematic reviews and meta-analyses. *Research Synthesis Methods, 10*(3), 330–342. https://doi.org/10.1002/jrsm.1354

PsycBITE. (n.d.). *NeuroRehab evidence resource*. http://psycbite.com/web/cms/content/home

Sackett, D. L., Rosenberg, W. M., Gray, J. M., Haynes, R. B., & Richardson, W. S. (1996). Evidence based medicine: What it is and what it isn't. *BMJ, 312*, 71–72. https://doi.org/10.1136/bmj.312.7023.71

Smela, B., Toumi, M., Świerk, K., Francois, C., Biernikiewicz, M., Clay, E., & Boyer, L. (2023). Rapid literature review: Definition and methodology. *Journal of Market Access & Health Policy, 11*(1), 1–7. https://doi.org/10.1080/20016689.2023.2241234

Sudheesh, K., Duggappa, D. R., & Nethra, S. S. (2016). How to write a research proposal?. *Indian Journal of Anaesthesia, 60*(9), 631–634. https://doi.org/10.4103/0019-5049.190617

Sudsawad, P. (2007). *Knowledge translation: Introduction to models, strategies, and measures*. National Center for the Dissemination of Disability Research. https://ktdrr.org/ktlibrary/articles_pubs/ktmodels/ktintro.pdf

Ulu, H., & Akyol, H. (2016). The effects of repetitive reading and PQRS strategy in the development of reading skill. *Eurasian Journal of Educational Research, 63*, 225–242. https://doi.org/10.14689/ejer.2016.63-13

White, S., Raghavendra, P., & McAllister, S. (2017). Letting the CAT out of the bag: Contribution of critically appraised topics to evidence-based practice. *Evidence-Based Communication Assessment and Intervention*, *11*(1–2), 27–37. https://doi.org/10.1080/17489539.2017.1333683

Wolf, S. L., Winstein, C. J., Miller, J. P., Thompson, P. A., Taub, E., Uswatte, G., Morris, D., Blanton, S., Nichols-Larsen, D., & Clark, P. C. (2008). Retention of upper limb function in stroke survivors who have received constraint-induced movement therapy: The EXCITE randomised trial. *The Lancet Neurology*, *7*(1), 33–40. https://doi.org/10.1016/S1474–4422(07)70294–6

APPENDICES

Appendix 5-A

PICO Terms List Worksheet

PICO Question:

Databases Searched:

Inclusion and Exclusion Criteria:

- Patient characteristics:
- Study types: systematic reviews__ meta-analyses__ randomized controlled trials__

Cohort __ case controlled__ other__

- Date of publication (years):
- Languages:

Search Terms:

P				I				C				O
OR				OR				OR				OR
OR		AND		OR		AND		OR		AND		OR
OR				OR				OR				OR
OR				OR				OR				OR
OR				OR				OR				OR

Appendix 5-B.B
PRIMSA Diagram

This work is licensed under CC BY 4.0. To view a copy of this license, visit https://creativecommons.org/licenses/by/4.0/

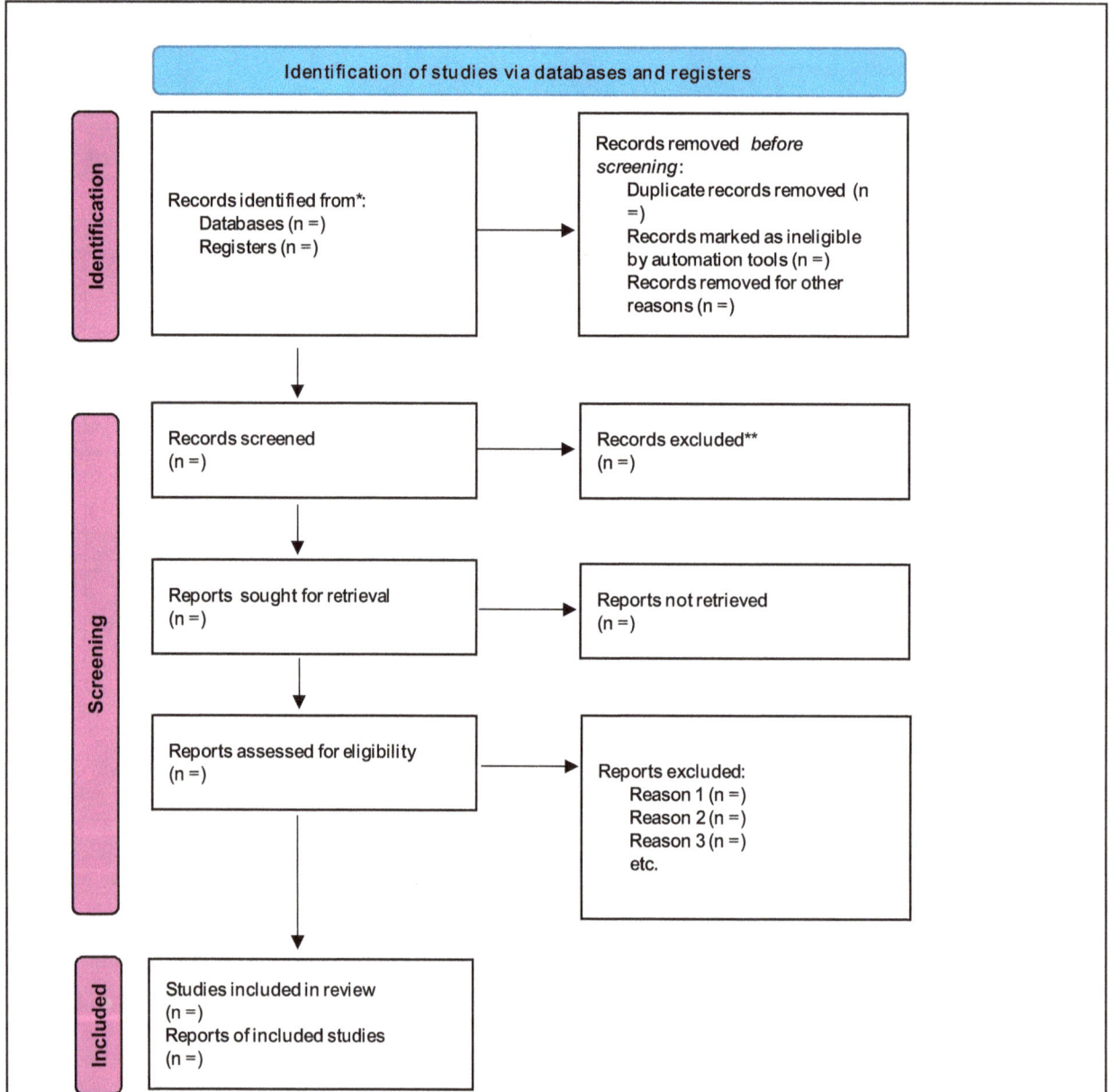

*Consider, if feasible to do so, reporting the number of records identified from each database or register searched (rather than the total number across all databases/registers).

**If automation tools were used, indicate how many records were excluded by a human and how many were excluded by automation tools.

Source: Page, M. J., McKenzie, J. E., Bossuyt, P. M., Boutron, I., Hoffmann, T. C., Mulrow, C. D., Shamseer, L., Tetzlaff, J. M., Akl, E. A., Brennan, S. E., Chou, R., Glanville, J., Grimshaw, J. M., Hróbjartsson, A., Lalu, M. M., Li, T., Loder, E. W., Mayo-Wilson, E., McDonald, S., … Moher, D. (2021). The PRISMA 2020 statement: An updated guideline for reporting systematic reviews. BMJ, 372, 1-9. https://doi.org/10.1136/bmj.n71

Appendix 5-C
SAMPLE PICOs USING FOCUS AREAS

FOCUS AREA	SAMPLE PICO(S)
Clinical practice	• What is the effect of equine-facilitated wellness therapy on the quality of life for adults with substance use disorders? • Do classroom-level interventions for elementary students with emotional disturbances reduce maladaptive behaviors and improve academic performance?
Research	• Are sensory-based strategies effective at reducing negative behaviors in long-term care facilities? • For surgeons, what is the likelihood that occupational therapy–ergonomic interventions decrease work-related musculoskeletal disorders (MSDs)? • Are individuals with a history of opioid addiction who are prescribed Suboxone alone more likely to report relapse than those individuals who utilize cognitive behavioral strategies along with Suboxone?
Administration	• What is the impact of participation in occupational, physical, and speech therapy on hospital admission after discharge for skilled nursing facilities? • What is the effect of mechanical lifting equipment on work-related injuries for occupational therapists when compared to traditional manual lifting for patient care?
Leadership	• In occupational therapy leaders, how does participating in an evidence-based leadership curriculum vs. not participating affect staff retention, staff satisfaction, and quality of care? • How does transformational/complexity leadership style, compared to transactional leadership style, affect occupational therapy practitioner retention and satisfaction?
Program development and evaluation	**Clinical** • Does a community transition programming during inpatient rehabilitation improve community mobility and social participation once discharged to home? • What is the effectiveness of mindfulness practice on people with chronic pain for work-related outcomes?
	Community • Does an occupational therapy–led tai chi group reduce falls in community dwelling? • What is the effect of occupational therapy in addressing the transition from school to work with individuals with an intellectual or developmental delay?
	• What is this impact of an education program for occupational therapists on occupational justice on the well-being and quality of life of those residing in long-term care facilities? • How will policy development and education to occupational practitioners on issues of sexuality and the importance of addressing the sexuality needs of rehabilitation patients affect patient quality of life?
Policy advocacy	• For children with disabilities, do peer-mentored programs facilitate participation in 4-H (a nonprofit organization for youth)? • For refugee families from Somalia, how can occupational therapy have a positive effect on their occupational performance as they begin the process of resettlement?
Education	• Among OTD students, does taking the NBCOT certification exam within two months of graduating result in higher pass rates compared to taking the exam later? • Should health professionals' education and training institutions use simulation methods to support successful completion of clinical rotations?
Theory development	• Will a gender-as-occupation model improve occupational therapy practice for transgender and gender-non-conforming individuals?

Appendix 5-D

INITIAL EXAMPLE OF EDUCATOR SECTION OBJECTIVES BEFORE USING GENAI

1. Design a curriculum module that guides students through the process of developing a focused PICO question and comprehensive search strategy.
2. Create instructional materials that demonstrate the effective use of reference management tools and literature review software for organizing and screening search results.
3. Develop rubrics and assessment criteria for evaluating students' evidence tables and literature syntheses.
4. Plan learning activities that incorporate ethical use of generative AI tools to support the literature review process.
5. Construct assignments that help students identify gaps in the literature, and formulate problem statements for their capstone projects.
6. Design instructional approaches to teach different types of literature reviews, including rapid reviews and critically appraised topics (CATs).
7. Create guidelines for students on properly documenting their literature review process to meet academic and publication standards.
8. Develop strategies for integrating librarian expertise and library resources into literature review instruction.
9. Design assessments that evaluate students' ability to critically appraise research for both methodological rigor and real-world applicability.
10. Create a framework for providing constructive feedback on students' literature reviews throughout the iterative process of their capstone projects.

CHAPTER 6

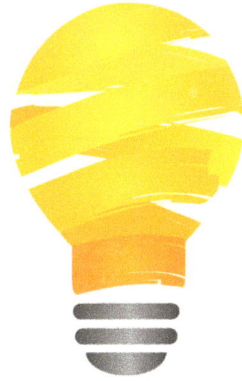

The Needs Assessment

Erika Kemp and Paula J. Costello

Section 1: Student Focus

Human-Centered Design Mindsets for Students

Human-centered design is centered on designing for and with the individuals involved. Therefore, your needs assessment becomes central to the process of creating your capstone project and places value on the co-creation with your site. HCD embraces creativity, and to have **creative confidence**, you must not self-censor or have preconceived notions of what will or will not work for your community partners. As you build trust and empathy with them, your needs assessment becomes a tool for discovering what the people want and need. You will need to lean into ambiguity as you begin to prototype solutions to address these needs.

INTRODUCTION FOR STUDENTS

Similar to the literature review, a *needs assessment* is defined as a required preparatory activity for the doctoral capstone project. This chapter provides information to guide the planning and execution of the capstone needs assessment, which must be completed prior to the commencement of the capstone experience (Accreditation Council for Occupational Therapy Education [ACOTE], 2023; D.1.3). A needs assessment is the first step in any program development or improvement planning and, therefore, may be intertwined with the literature review and may not necessarily feel sequential. This chapter will provide students with a framework to guide their needs assessment planning and implementation and examples of methods for data collection and analysis. Depending on the institution's integration of curriculum in their capstone program, the results of the needs assessment can be used to further develop capstone experience learning objectives within the experiential learning plan or better define the focus of the capstone project and its related goals and objectives. Examples of actual doctoral capstone student needs assessment application to the experience and project will be used to illustrate this process.

STUDENT REFLECTIVE QUESTIONS

During the planning phase of the doctoral capstone, the occupational therapy student may find it helpful to reflect on the following questions:

1. What information do I already have available from the literature review or other conversations with my site that can be a starting point for the needs assessment?

DOI: 10.4324/9781003541813-8

2. How will I maintain an open mindset and creative confidence as I plan, collect data, and prioritize results from the needs assessment?

3. How do I deal with change? As you learn from your capstone state city holders what their wants and needs are, how will you respond to changes in your original goals and objectives for your capstone project?

STUDENT OBJECTIVES

By the end of reading this chapter and completing the learning activities, the students should be able to:

1. Identify the steps involved in the needs assessment process.
2. Create a site-specific plan for the needs assessment.
3. Determine how theory is applied to the needs assessment process.
4. Identify gaps between the evidence and the literature, and the capstone site and/or population.
5. Analyze needs assessment data, and understand how this will be applied to the capstone proposal development.

INTRODUCTION

A needs assessment is a systematic method of identifying and addressing needs for groups of individuals, communities, organizations, or a population. There are many frameworks available to help guide the capstone needs assessment process from planning and data analysis for decision-making to implementation and evaluation of project outcomes. Needs assessments can be as informal as interviewing your site mentor/content expert, or as formal as gaining institutional review board approval to conduct surveys, focus groups, or interviews with the capstone site organization members or program participants. Often, the needs assessment is an iterative process, revisiting each step to refine objectives and plans as the project evolves. This is important to realize ahead of time: things will change, and change reflects that you are meeting the needs of your community partner.

A needs assessment typically involves several key steps to identify and measure needs (sometimes known as "gaps"), as well as the desired outcomes of a group of people (Altschuld & Kumar, 2010; National Institute for Children's Health Quality, 2024). Figure 6.1 illustrates the general steps in the needs assessment process.

The general steps of a needs assessment applied to the capstone planning process are:

1. Define your project goals and objectives.
   a. These will change over time as you begin to collaborate with your site and collect and analyze the needs assessment data.
2. Understand the context and engage with the stakeholders.
   a. You will need to use several data points to understand the layers of context at your community site.
3. Evaluate the scope and complexity.
   a. You only have 14 weeks; consider what is feasible and what is sustainable when you leave.
4. Consider available resources.
   a. The confines of the real world. This is where evidence meets practice.
5. Pilot and adapt through program evaluation.
   a. Always consider sustainability and what is feasible for the site as you exit.
   b. This final phase is usually happening during the actual capstone experience.

Although there are general steps to guide the needs assessment, there are also more specific theoretical frameworks that can guide the process. This next section of this chapter will introduce you to two distinct models: PRECEDE–PROCEED model (Green & Kreuter, 2005) and appreciative inquiry (Cooperrider & Srivastva, 1987).

PRECEDE–PROCEED MODEL

The PRECEDE–PROCEED model was created by Lawrence Green in 1974 and has been widely used in health program planning, implementation, and evaluation for assessing health needs and designing effective interventions. It is an outcomes-oriented approach which begins with the end in mind. It is a comprehensive framework which allows for multifactorial causation of health risks from individual behaviors to social influence and environmental affordances. Its participatory approach encourages the involvement of the community from the ideation and planning process through implementation and evaluation (Green & Kreuter, 2005).

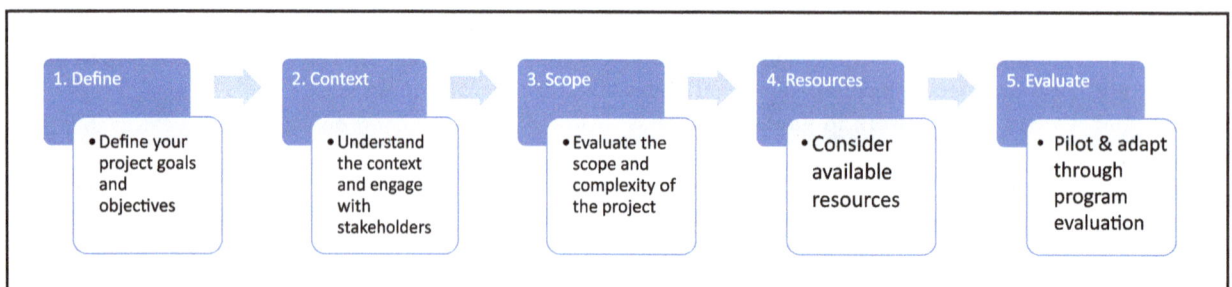

Figure 6.1. General steps of a needs assessment.

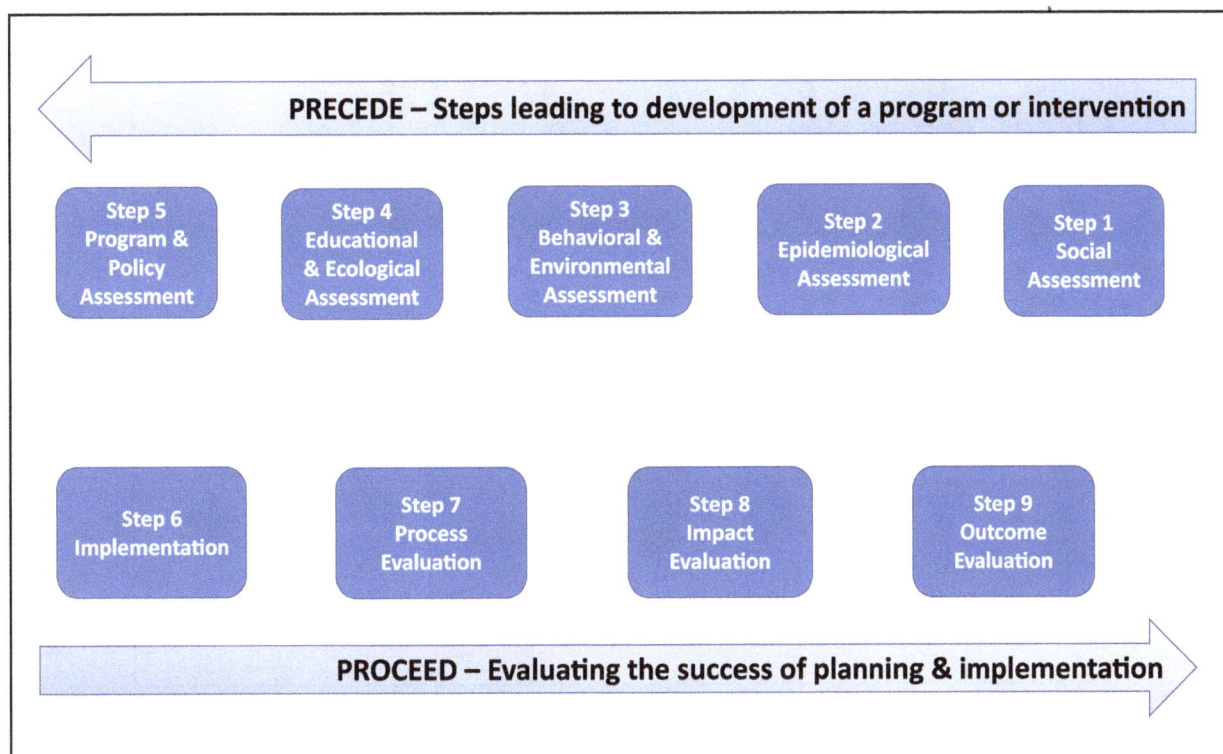

Figure 6.2. PRECEDE–PROCEED model. *Source:* Adapted from Green and Kreuter (2005). *Health promotion planning: An education and ecological approach* (4th ed.).

PRECEDE–PROCEED is an acronym. PRECEDE stands for *predisposing, reinforcing, and enabling constructs in educational/environmental diagnosis and evaluation* (University of Kansas, 2024). The PRECEDE aspect of the model addresses the process of assessing and planning when developing a program or conducting a needs assessment. This includes steps or phases 1–5 of the model. The aspects of each step will be described in more depth as you move through this chapter, and the process is illustrated with case vignettes.

PROCEED stands for *policy, regulatory, and organizational constructs in educational and environmental development*. The PROCEED aspect of the model addresses the implementation and evaluation of a program or project. Use of the PRECEDE–PROCEDE model is an iterative process that focuses on data-driven decision-making, encouraging the group to continually evaluate the progress and adjust at any point in the process. Figure 6.2 depicts the steps of the PRECEDE–PROCEED model.

APPRECIATIVE INQUIRY

Appreciative inquiry (Cooperrider & Srivastva, 1987) is a strengths-based approach to organizational change and development with applications in organizational, community, and leadership development. Instead of focusing on deficiencies or problems, the focus shifts to the "positive core" of strengths, successes and potentials, or opportunities. Appreciative inquiry features a collaborative process focused on finding what works well and envisioning a desired future delivered through use of the 5D cycle of defining, discovery, dream, design, and destiny/delivery. (See Figure 6.3, the 5D cycle of appreciative inquiry.) Used within the process of conducting a needs assessment, this approach will generate appreciative questions to guide whichever method is applied for further exploring the best of past experiences, sharing of critical values, and envisioning a vision for the future.

Five core principles underlie the philosophical base of appreciative inquiry and include constructionist, simultaneity, poetic, anticipatory, and positive principles. These principles provide guidance when applying this model to the capstone needs assessment process and help in formulation of the questions asked within data gathering.

1. *Constructivist.* Reality is subjective and constructed within the social context of words and language. The positivity of words matters when constructing interview questions.

2. *Simultaneity.* Inquiry starts the change process, so the minute we ask a question, we begin to make change.

3. *Poetic.* What we choose to study can make a difference, and teams or organizations are sources for our inquiry through questions.

4. *Anticipatory.* Positive and hopeful images for the future serve to move systems toward these images in positive ways.

5. *Positive.* Positive questions increase the positive core and provide the momentum for large-scale change (Cooperrider & Whitney, 1999).

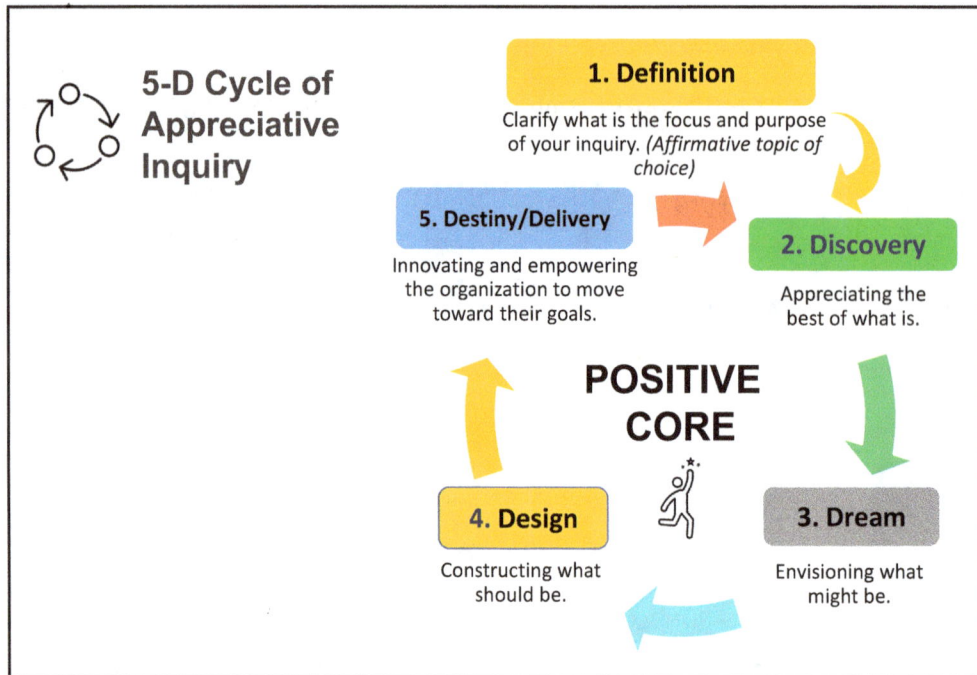

Figure 6.3. The 5D cycle of appreciative inquiry. *Source:* Adapted from Stavros, J., Godwin, L. N., and Cooperrider, D. L. (2015), in W. J. Rothwell, J. M. Stavros, and R. L. Sullivan (eds.). *Practicing organization development: Leading transformation and change* (4th ed.).

This next section of the chapter will demonstrate how each of these frameworks can be applied to the steps of the needs assessment process applied to doctoral capstone planning.

STEP 1: DEFINE PROJECT GOALS AND OBJECTIVES

Where to begin? This step of needs assessment is often the first step in the entire capstone planning process, may be the one you revisit the most, and therefore may be the one that will change the most as you go. Needs assessment processes ensure that projects take multiple perspectives and data points into consideration to give the project the best possible chance of success and longevity. The first perspective to include is your own. What interests you? Why were you drawn to this topic, site, and/or content expert to serve as your mentor? You already began this when you chose your specific topic and began exploration of yourself and site (Chapter 4), and you will revisit this step as you learn more about the context of your population, and again as you determine your individual learning objectives and project implementation. (See Chapter 7 for more discussion on the experiential plan.)

Capstone Student Vignettes

Student A wants to learn more about the role of occupational therapy in the acute care phase of cancer treatment. This was identified as an interest initially during a guest lecture in the acute care course in the OT program. Student A connected with the individual after the class for more information. They learned that this site has a physician interested in involving more therapy at the start of lengthy hospitalizations. This physician wanted to see a preventive therapy program to help clients keep their strength and ability to engage in activities of daily living (ADLS) during the intensive inpatient stay rather than waiting for the deconditioning to occur. The student worked with the doctoral capstone coordinator (DCC) to initiate a formal affiliation with the site, establish the capstone site placement, and define the content expert/site mentor to be the OT at the hospital that worked on that unit. Student A's initial goals were to learn in-depth knowledge about managing fatigue with individuals that have cancer, to learn how to create this preventive program for the unit, and to learn more in-depth clinical skills in the acute care environment.

Student B has an interest in increasing available activities for individuals with low vision in the community. They had personal experience with a family member being unable to enjoy community recreational experiences due to visual impairment. They were connected to the local zoo by the DCC to discover what the zoo was already doing and working on in this area. While the initial project goals were broad, Student B knew they wanted to learn more about universal design and use of tactile maps to engage individuals with low vision.

Student C, Sam, has expressed an interest in specialized clinical skills related to upper extremity performance. Working with their DCC, they have secured a site in a university medical center–affiliated hand clinic. Their initial learning objectives have focused on advancing specialist skills related to hand conditions, leadership in entrepreneurship, and are hoping to address a clinic need through the capstone project. After completion of the literature review, they have identified several gaps in the literature, including limited consensus on use of standardized therapy protocols, a need for better integration of patient occupational preferences in goal development, and a need for determining cost-effectiveness of OT services. These stimulate several areas to focus on for the capstone project as they begin to engage the clinic therapists through the needs assessment interview.

PRECEDE–PROCEED Model

If you are using PRECEDE–PROCEED, you begin to identify the project goals through the first phase: *social assessment*. In this phase, you will determine the social context of a given population and work to figure out the social problems and needs of the community, usually in an area of health, such as quality of life, and key social issues and priorities of the community (Gielen et al., 2008). Data to gather may include population characteristics and trends, housing conditions, education levels, crime rates, employment rates, availability of community services and organizations, and cultural and social norms, such as traditions, beliefs that influence community life, as well as structure of social networks and supports. Data may come from public records and reports, informal conversations with the content expert, members of the community and your faculty advisor/mentor, and even online posts and culture.

Capstone Student Vignettes

Student A already had learned a lot about the social factors through initial conversations with the content expert. They learned that deconditioning is a problem in the bone marrow transplant (BMT)/hematology unit as many patients were discharged with lower levels of independence than when they were admitted. This led to poorer outcomes, including discharge to higher levels of care, such as subacute rehabilitation, and sometimes even rehospitalization. Most patients received an initial evaluation at admission and were immediately discharged due to their current level of occupational performance. During their stay, the combination of lack of mobilization/activity and effects of treatment led to deconditioning, yet there was no mechanism to re-refer these clients and there was no prevention program in place. The implementation of such a program was difficult due to staffing shortages, time restraints, and reimbursement difficulties.

Student B had a lot of knowledge about the social context of navigation in the community for

individuals with low vision due to her personal experiences. The social assessment included discovering that the built environment is geared toward sighted people, given the dominance of sight as a sensation that guides experiences in society. Upon talking with family members, they narrowed in on wayfinding as a barrier that exists to exploring community spaces. Through conversations with the content expert at the capstone site, it was discovered that there were knowledge gaps about accessibility options for this population, but that a priority for the zoo was to increase accessibility to populations with a variety of disabilities.

Appreciative Inquiry

In this approach, the first *D* of the 5D cycle, *define*, aligns with the first step of a needs assessment. You will work to clarify the project purpose and what needs to be achieved for the specific community where you will be implementing the capstone. Again, this may change as you work through your 5D cycle; be open to the possibilities! This step will identify the topic or generative question that will guide the full inquiry by setting the stage for what the organization or community wants to explore and enhance. Methods to gather data at this stage of the assessment may include an electronic, phone, or email survey sent to site clinicians or program participants to better understand their interests to be focused on for the needs assessment. An interview with leadership or the content expert is the recommended methodology for best integrating the 5D cycle within your needs assessment.

Capstone Student Vignettes

Student C, Sam, starts their needs assessment by planning the questions for the needs assessment interview to help the site define the focus of the inquiry. When they meet with their content expert, they begin by asking, "What general topic would you like to focus on?" Sam shares what they have gathered from the literature review and aligns this with several areas of needs or areas of inquiry collected from the clinical staff. Sam helps flip the statements to be positive opportunities to address through the capstone project as a clearer focus for the project develops.

STEP 2: UNDERSTAND CONTEXT AND STAKEHOLDERS

This is the step that is most widely recognized as the needs assessment as it involves the participation with stakeholders to ensure diversity of voices is represented in the assessment (Altschuld & Watkins, 2014). In this step, the needs assessment seeks to better understand the context in which the problems or opportunities exist, and how the stakeholders perceive the context as supporting or creating barriers to meeting the desired outcomes they are seeking. It is important to value the experiences of individuals of every age, national origin, race, ethnicity, gender, sexual orientation, ability status, and other identities as you engage with stakeholders. Students are encouraged to consider their own identities and positionality in relation to the identity of the participants and community stakeholders from which you are collecting data. You may need to explicitly state this positionality with your stakeholders or engage in reflexivity as you work through the needs assessment.

Again, the two frameworks provide structure for approaching this step of the needs assessment.

PRECEDE–PROCEED Model

The second phase of this model is the *epidemiological assessment*. This helps understand the health determinants contributing to the specific health problem, such as prevalence and incidence rates, population characteristics, and access to and utilization of health-care services in the area. Sources of this data may include public health records from local, state, and national health departments; census data; and surveys of the community members. You also want to gather more information on the medical diagnosis if applicable, and its symptoms, in this phase.

The next two phases are best thought of together. The *behavioral and environmental assessment* focuses on identifying specific behaviors and environmental conditions that impact the health issue identified; it looks at what people do and the context in which they do it. The last phase, *educational and ecological assessment*, focuses on the underlying factors that influence these behaviors and environmental conditions; it looks at why people behave the way they do and what supports or hinders those behaviors. You will start by identifying both risk behaviors and protective behaviors the community engages in, such as smoking, diet, exercise, substance abuse, and adherence to medical advice. The environment is also considered as to how it may contribute to health behavior. This may include physical environment like air and water quality, housing conditions, recreational facilities, and transportation availability and social environment, such as social determinants of health, socioeconomic status, education levels, and community safety. Much of this data may be collected through informal conversations with content experts or community members and may be continued at the start of the experience with direct observations of the community to confirm. Some of this information may also come from the literature review and public records. All this helps you determine the predisposing, reinforcing, or enabling factors present in the population and/or environment and may help you refine what your program is going to target for your specific site.

Capstone Student Vignettes

Student A continues with the needs assessment by looking into the literature on cancer and deconditioning. They discovered that 2.8 million adults were hospitalized with cancer in the year 2017 alone, illustrating the high rates of admission for oncology patients (Hargraves et al., 2021). Cancer patients may experience fatigue from the diagnosis itself but also experience adverse effects due to treatment protocols that can exacerbate fatigue and prevent participation in daily life (Dougherty et al., 2017). They learn about hospital-associated deconditioning and its associated effects, including mobility limitations, functional dependency, and falls (Suriyaarachchi et al., 2020). When sharing this information with her site, they discover that this literature lines up with what is happening there, thus identifying a need for this type of preventive programming. They also learn that the staff are aware of both physical activity and mindfulness approaches to help decrease fatigue and increase energy, but that these are being implemented without consistency on a case-by-case basis. The behaviors in which patients currently engage while inpatient is more in line with rest and passive activity, which is commonly thought to help when one is sick. The staff enabled this "restful sick" patient behavior due to their high demands of other job duties, with good intentions. In these informal conversations with the site, they discovered that many staff were open to change and interested in what else could be done for these clients to help maintain their current level of activity.

Student B begins the epidemiological phase by discovering the different types of visual impairments, and how each one has unique challenges. They discover that there is a high population in the area most likely because the state school for the blind is located in the same city. They decided to focus on challenges that arise from low vision or blindness and use of sensory cues in the environment for wayfinding/orientation and mobility. In the next phase, it was discovered that this population was not visiting the zoo due to difficulty with navigation while there, as well as lack of community-based transportation to get there. They discovered that the zoo had many programs, including educational programming and conservation efforts in addition to open visiting hours, but that all these were designed for the public. In the environmental phase, they learned about built environments, and that the zoo had many competing auditory, tactile, and olfactory sensory cues that made use of sensory cues difficult for orientation and mobility. While the zoo had some exhibits with braille text, it was difficult for the individuals to locate and visit those exhibits.

Appreciative Inquiry

The second *D* in the 5D cycle is *discover*. In this step, you will begin to appreciate the best of what currently exists, the best of "what is." Data for this may come from conducting formal or informal interviews with community members and engaging in storytelling to discover stories of success, strengths, and experiences (Stavros et al., 2015). This often will focus on past initiatives and experiences that were successful and had high engagement in the community. This may require you to carefully consider the guiding questions to ask of community members and then dive into the data gathered to determine what factors made those initiatives successful to ensure those factors are present in future projects (Stavros et al., 2015).

Capstone Student Vignettes

Sam continues with their interview of the content expert, asking questions to better understand and appreciate what the best lived experiences have been of the clinicians and clients at the site. "Can you describe a time for me when you felt you were at your best in providing services to a client? What did that look like, and how did you feel? What was it that made this situation so positive for you or your clients?" Sam asks these questions to discover what works at this site when excellence is being demonstrated. They hear stories of clients setting and meeting their personal goals and regaining function to return to their preferred daily activities. Sam asks additional probing questions to better understand the factors that made the difference in these positive stories that were shared.

STEP 3: EVALUATE THE SCOPE AND COMPLEXITY

The next general step in a needs assessment is to evaluate the scope and complexity of the problem. You will need to carefully consider the scope of what you can take on as a capstone student. A 14-week experience is very short in comparison to what is needed to make lasting change within an organization or community. As you begin to create your actual program/project, you need to hold this concept in your mind.

PRECEDE–PROCEED

The last step of PRECEDE before moving to PROCEED is *health program and policy development*, where you will identify and develop the appropriate intervention that encourages desired and expected changes of your community. This is often where skills in evidence-based practice are required and useful. Some occupational therapy programs may now step over to have students complete a comprehensive literature review to discover what

intervention or programming has been shown to be effective for this specific population. Within this step, you will consider which active ingredients of an intervention or program are most effective and carefully consider each one to determine if it will fit your specific site. This usually includes discussions with site staff and content experts to determine how the proposed evidence-based intervention aligns with their site, population, and current practice patterns. This step of *integrating* the known evidence with the community's unique needs is critical to ensure success.

Capstone Student Vignettes

Student A turns to the literature review to determine what the best evidence-based or evidence-informed protocol may be for this type of programming. She already learned that the site was interested in both physical activity and mindfulness/relaxation approaches, and that the main goal of the program would be to decrease the rate of deconditioning. She designed a scholarly question she could answer through a comprehensive systematic literature review: For inpatient cancer patients, does a multimodal program including both exercise and relaxation components decrease the deconditioning rate during the inpatient stay? The active ingredients discovered in the evidence for this program should include physical activity five times a week (stretching/yoga, aerobic exercise, resistance training) and relaxation breathing techniques twice a week. Key outcome measures addressed fatigue symptoms. The next step was to translate these active ingredients and outcomes measures to her specific site. She discovered that her site already used the Brief Fatigue Inventory and the AM-PAC "6 clicks." She translated the physical activity to available activities and ADLs in a "usual" hospital day that would require little staff supervision and created materials for the relaxation breathing activities.

Student B completes a comprehensive scoping review to answer the following question: What sensory cues or supports are most effective at increasing wayfinding abilities in adults with low vision in their environment? She found evidence that supported the creation and use of tactile maps and ground-surface indicators for unsafe terrain or drop-offs. The zoo did not currently have any tactile maps or robust ground surface indicators but was interested in more information.

Appreciative Inquiry

The third *D* in the 5D cycle using an appreciative inquiry approach to the needs assessment is *dream*. You will want to support the stakeholders to envision "what could be." Encourage leveraging past achievements, and combine those with the stakeholders' wishes, hopes, and inspirations for the future. This phase encourages aspirational thinking and creativity, which is often prompted by asking a "provocative question or proposition" which is challenging and promotes creativity without constraint. Provocative propositions help bridge "what is" to "what could be" (Center for Appreciative Inquiry, n.d.). Starting from this "dream" of the site's vision may seem incongruent with the needs assessment phase of considering the scope and complexity of the site's needs and resources; however, it is through this provocative visioning that creativity is fostered and opportunities become more visible. Data in this step may be gathered through workshops or focus groups with community members or structured formal or informal interviews with members and leadership.

Capstone Student Vignettes

Student C, Sam, next asks the content expert to use these successes cataloged in *discover* to project and envision aspirations for the future, posing a "provocative proposition." "If you were to secure a large funded grant or philanthropy gift that enabled you to purchase time, goods, or services to design your dream clinical program, what would that look like?" This question helps the site envision her ideal situation for the clinic and set a goal that they can then work together to identify the steps to reach this vision and encourages her to freely be creative with confidence and without being encumbered by any real or imagined restrictions or boundaries.

STEP 4: CONSIDER AVAILABLE RESOURCES

Like the previous step, you have already gathered much of this information about your capstone site through the phases already completed in either approach. The student and capstone team should again pause to consider available resources of the site and the academic program. Is the proposed program still too big in scope? What equipment and personnel are available between both the site and the school to oversee the implementation? It is prudent to consider the sustainability of the project after the student exits at this point in the needs assessment as well. If this project is discontinued in 14 weeks, will the community members be harmed? Is this project able to be executed by laypersons? Is this project able to be implemented without occupational therapy supervision? Are different professionals available to assist in carrying it out that may have overlapping scopes of practice?

PRECEDE–PROCEED

Before implementing your program fully, you will want to do an administrative and policy assessment. Most often, this is started before you arrive on-site and is completed once you are there. Arrival on-site gives such a plethora

of information that one cannot learn about from afar, no matter how thorough your needs assessment may be before beginning the experience. The administrative and policy assessment allows you to take the program you have created from your literature review and prior steps of the needs assessment and really see if it is possible within the confines of your site. What resources are actually available? Are there legal or other policies that are in conflict with what you propose to do?

Capstone Student Vignettes

Student A discovers that there are policy and administrative barriers to this program, including facility policies for reimbursement and billing code usage, shortage of staff to run the program, and high daily caseload for therapy and nursing staff. This information leads them to think about the sustainability of this program when the capstone experience is done, helping make some alterations to the scale of what they plan to implement. This also leads them to think about the additional learning objectives they might create, including learning about reimbursement mechanisms and administrative policies regarding staff positions at the site. This process of the needs assessment altered the initial project and objectives to better match the site's needs and the students' interests. What began as a unit-wide program run by a skilled therapist daily was modified to a program initiated at evaluation by a skilled therapist, daily activities implemented by the patient with occasional assistance from patient care attendants, and relaxation training by a skilled therapist as part of the therapy plan of care.

Student B takes the findings from the literature search to the zoo and, through conversation, discovers that financial and time barriers will not allow the zoo to add ground surface indicators at this time, but that tactile maps would be something they would like to explore. Student B adds learning more about ground surface indicators to her list of other learning objectives she would like to accomplish during the experience but sets that aside for now. Student B and the content expert determined that the zoo could contribute financial resources to create at least a prototype tactile map for trial use, and that this could be accomplished in the 14-week time frame.

Appreciative Inquiry

The fourth *D* in the 5D cycle is *design*. Students will work to determine "what should be" in collaboration with their site mentor, content expert, and faculty mentor. They will work to develop their project's actionable plans to achieve the envisioned future. While working on the design phase, it is again essential to consider the scope and complexity of the project and the available resources of the site to be dedicated to the project.

Capstone Student Vignettes

Sam's provocative questions have prompted the clinic staff to "dream" of an individualized and tailored program of interventions and minutes devoted to treatment that are optimal for each client. They have a current convenient and efficient scheduling system that allows clients to schedule online, cancel, and reschedule appointments that tie directly to the other record functions. However, they are not clear if the 30- or 40-minute time slots really are optimal, and they do not currently know how satisfied their clients are with their therapy outcomes. They begin to plan a quality improvement (QI) project that will provide client satisfaction information, use of goal attainment scaling for client outcomes, and collect data on optimal length of treatment sessions to reach client goals.

STEP 5: PILOT AND ADAPT THROUGH PROGRAM EVALUATION

While this topic is covered further in Chapter 7, on project implementation, and Chapter 8, project evaluation, it is helpful to know that each of these needs assessment frameworks also provides guidance on how to pilot the program you have comprehensively designed and use that data to suggest quality improvement for future iterations.

PRECEDE–PROCEED

The last phase of this needs assessment model overlaps with the final step of the needs assessment and allows for an iterative process to arrive at the best possible program. PROCEED stands for *policy, regulatory, and organizational constructs in educational and environmental development.* As is seen in Figure 6.2, moving through the phases of PROCEED allows you to evaluate how well you accounted for each of the planning phases, and adjust as you go. PROCEED allows you to create a comprehensive evaluation of the program you have co-created with your site. It can include evaluation of the process of implementation (what changes had to be made for administering the program), the impact of the program on participants and their behaviors, and the evaluation of the outcome (did your program actually affect the health problem you initially had targeted?).

Capstone Student Vignettes

As Student A got ready to begin her 14-week capstone experience, she walked through the phases of PRECEDE once more to confirm each of the decisions she made about the alterations to her initial project and objectives. These decisions were made

as she fit her evidence-informed program to the specific behavioral and environmental needs of her site. Some of these alterations included adjusting her initial program from unit-wide to one that could be completed on an individual basis, and some that would become part of the nursing staff's responsibilities. Part of this adjustment also meant decreasing the frequency and duration of the program that she had found was most effective in the literature review. She also adjusted the physical activity metrics to match occupations rather than just exercise, specifically aligning occupations to metabolic equivalent of task (MET) levels for use by the clients and staff of the unit. She selected processes and outcomes she was going to monitor as she went so she could determine if the program and carryover activities were feasible, acceptable, and sustainable by not only the client(s) she would serve during the experience but also the therapy staff, administrators, and entire unit. She determined the methods to collect the data she identified and set up touch points with her content expert and faculty advisor throughout the experience to help her monitor and make adjustments to the program.

Student B also walked back through the phases of PRECEDE to confirm each of the decisions made and landed on the creation and use of tactile maps for community members to use while at the zoo. To evaluate her project's success, she outlined a set of steps she would take to create the tactile maps with the zoo. She engaged two community members to help trial-use of the tactile maps and make changes based on their feedback.

Appreciative Inquiry

The last *D* of the 5D is destiny/delivery, to "create what will be." You implement and sustain the change, focusing on embedding new practices and ensuring ongoing support and adaptation (Stavros et al., 2015). This step ensures that mechanisms are established for ongoing feedback and improvement. Depending on your institution's policies, this might include developing an application for determining the need for research board approvals. Looking ahead to sustaining your project, this may include finding a student in the next cohort interested in carrying on the next phase of the project, or discussions and consultations from a practicing OT about similar needs in their own practice. Deliver/destiny – creating what will be, that is, identifying how the design is delivered and how it will be embedded in groups, communities, and organizations.

Capstone Student Vignettes

Sam and the content expert decide that there is a need to gather more information from clinicians and patients across the clinical practice locations through a formal process of data collection using an anonymous survey and de-identified patient records. This will require an institutional review board approval for non-human research, and Sam begins designing the quality improvement project survey and the IRB determination application, guided by their faculty mentor and capstone coordinator. They gain additional information from the content expert for the survey content, determine the application to use for the survey, decide which data analysis tools to use and how to best deploy the survey to patients.

CONCLUSIONS AND NEXT STEPS

The needs assessment allows you to gather information that will mutually benefit the capstone site and population and support your own goals and objectives. Because the needs assessment process is iterative, this process can alter your initial capstone project's goals and learning objectives for the experience. When that happens, it means you did an excellent job designing your project to meet the needs of your unique community partner. Every capstone project takes unexpected turns, and everyone is unique. Remember this entire process is iterative. Trust the steps you are taking, gather as many data points as you can from multiple viewpoints, and enjoy the co-creation process! Your next step is to solidify your experiential plan and program evaluation as you inch closer to the implementation phase. Know in advance that even once your DCE begins, you will be revisiting the needs assessment process. Know that your project may even change slightly again once you arrive and begin to be fully immersed in the context of your site. This is okay; just revisit the steps of the needs assessment, make the necessary changes, and begin again. This is not a failure; this is how programs are created, adjusted, and trialed in real life. It is the ultimate learning experience of implementing evidence into practice and is a skill you will use time and again as practicing clinicians.

STUDENT SECTION CHAPTER SUMMARY

This chapter has illustrated how you can use a guiding framework, theory, or model to walk through the process of conducting a needs assessment. The needs assessment is an interactive and iterative process between you and your capstone site and related stakeholders. You may need to revisit each step of the needs assessment several times before you have fully gathered enough information. This process may happen before, alongside, or after your literature review, depending on your own program's capstone curriculum. This needs assessment data provides the foundation upon which to determine the next steps for your capstone.

Section 2: Educator Focus

Transformational Learning Phases and Framework for the Educator

Engaging in the needs assessment for the doctoral capstone aligns with Mezirow's recognition of shared experiences phase, which is a crucial part of his transformative learning theory (Mezirow, 1997). This phase involves learners recognizing that their personal experiences are not isolated but are shared by others. In the context of a doctoral capstone project, a needs assessment often requires the researcher to understand the perspectives, challenges, and needs of a particular community, organization, or group.

During their needs assessment, our doctoral capstone students gather rich information from multiple stakeholders at their capstone site to identify common challenges, issues, and needs. This process encourages the capstone student to recognize that their individual experiences or assumptions about a problem or gap may not be universal. Our students must acknowledge that others have shared, and potentially different, experiences that shape the needs they are assessing.

By analyzing data collected from various sources, the capstone student can identify patterns or trends in the experiences and needs of different individuals or groups. This process mirrors the recognition of shared experiences phase, as it requires learners to move beyond their own perspective and recognize that others' experiences may be similar or different but still part of a larger, shared context.

A key component of the needs assessment is the capstone student's ability to listen to and empathize with those being studied. This is important for accurately identifying and understanding the shared experiences of others. Mezirow's theory emphasizes the importance of perspective-taking and empathy-building, and the needs assessment process provides an opportunity for researchers to develop a more empathetic and holistic understanding of the people or communities they are studying (Mezirow, 1997). As an educator, within this phase of the doctoral capstone, it is important to engage in various strategies that promote reflection, empathy, and recognition of common experiences among diverse groups. By facilitating these mindsets, it not only enhances our students' academic growth but also prepares them for critical engagement with real-world issues as they inch closer to entering practice.

INTRODUCTION FOR EDUCATOR

This chapter uses two different approaches to illustrate how the use of a theory or framework can guide the needs assessment process. Choosing a framework that fits your occupational therapy program's curriculum design and the mission and goals of your institution can help tie up all the threads of learning your students have been engaged in. Is your program focused on complex medical problems, rural or urban health access, leadership, advocacy, community-based programming, service, etc.? What skills beyond practice excellence do you want your students to begin to exhibit to others? The needs assessment provides the opportunity to pivot programs to the needs of those your students are serving and the sites they are partnering with for capstone. It also provides an opportunity to think realistically about what can and cannot be accomplished in 14 weeks. In some ways, as their faculty or doctoral capstone coordinator, your job is also to help them realize they cannot change the world in 14 weeks but can begin to develop the scholarship and leadership skills needed to address the needs of communities and populations.

EDUCATOR REFLECTIVE QUESTIONS

1. Consider which comprehensive planning framework might best fit your curricular design and institute mission/vision.
    a. Are there theories or frameworks that your students are already familiar with and have used in other preparatory courses, such as those teaching program development, population health, or health disparities?
    b. Consider how your curricular threads in student learning outcomes may influence your approach to the needs assessment process through a particular framework.
2. Consider the methods of the needs assessment. Will these need to be formalized through an IRB process at your school?
    a. Will students formally report on survey or interview results, which might require this determination?
    b. Will less formal methods be used, which likely do not require this level of approval?
3. Consider the timing for your full capstone planning and execution and where the needs assessment fits within the sequence.
    a. What is done before level II FW?
    b. Do you see them again before execution of the experience?
    c. What types of coursework are you using to teach them the needs assessment process?
    d. How does your literature review interface with your needs assessment?

EDUCATOR OBJECTIVES

By the end of reading this chapter, the educator will be able to apply principles of transformational learning theory to structure learning activities, assignments, and/or assessments to promote the capstone student's ability to:

1. Choose a needs assessment framework that matches your curricular design best.
2. Create a plan and design learning activities and assessment methods to scaffold students through the needs assessment process.
3. Support students' analysis of needs assessment data to understand how this will be applied to the capstone proposal development.

EDUCATOR CONTENT

This next section of the chapter will focus on strategies and teaching tips for educators supporting capstone students.

Determine How Theory Is Applied to the Needs Assessment Process

As the occupational therapy faculty member or doctoral capstone coordinator, you will need to first choose whether you want to use a theoretical framework to formally root how students will learn about and implement the needs assessment. You may also need to consult with your program director (or curriculum committee) to ensure that the chosen framework aligns with your program's curricular threads and the institution's mission/vision. It is possible that your program has something in another course, like health management planning, that you can scaffold from and leverage within the doctoral capstone process. In addition to the two models presented in this chapter, there are many others, some of which flow directly into program development, and others that can be more malleable to practice, administration, or other areas of focus for the capstone. Some others to consider include the Center for Disease Control and Prevention (CDC) Program Evaluation Framework (Kidder et al., 2024) and the Rand Foundation's Getting to Outcomes Planning Tool (Chinnman et al., 2024).

Identify the Steps Involved in the Needs Assessment Process

Once you have chosen your framework, you will need to consider how students will learn this additional framework before applying it on their own. If this is a theory that was already taught in a prior didactic course, then the capstone courses can merely point back to that content, saving the initial teaching time. It may be helpful to consider creating templates or assignments for each step of the needs assessment to help students walk through the process. Appendices 6.A and 6.B are assignment examples that you could embed or adapt into your doctoral capstone curriculum, specific to the needs assessment, using the PRECEDE–PROCEED and appreciative inquiry models. This includes example assignment guidelines and rubrics to evaluate student performance with the needs assessment. It will also be important to consider timing with the literature review; is this being done before, after, intermittently? Needs assessment is inherently something that is returned to time and again, which is not often made clear to students. The ACOTE standards do not specify that the needs assessment needs to be done after the literature review; it merely lists them in that order and requires completion of both prior to capstone implementation. It may be possible to have parts of the needs assessment due at the same time as part of the literature review, as is illustrated in the PRECEDE–PROCEED examples earlier.

When considering the design of the actual courses, there are several considerations. The first is timing of completion – meaning, determining the time points in which students are completing each of the phases, and how you want to handle the iterative nature of the needs assessment within courses. There may be more than one point in time that students are engaged in these tasks and updating their written needs assessments. In this case, there is not one course focused on needs assessment, but it is an iterative assignment revisited in two or three different capstone-related courses. A second consideration is how you want to see students engaged in the completion of the needs assessment. Do you want them to use publicly available data, do additional literature searches, conduct formal face-to-face or virtual interviews, or make use of email communications or informal conversations to gather the needed information? If capstone sites are near where the student is residing, it may be feasible to spend some time immersed on-site to learn about the site's culture to assist in completing the needs assessment. These on-site hours would be built into the preparatory course and would not count toward the total capstone experience hours.

Determine the Site-Specific Plan for the Needs Assessment

As your students begin to plan their needs assessment, some questions often come up regarding whether what they do for the needs assessment steps is considered human subject research. Use of research methods provides a systematic and rigorous approach to setting up a project but does not always mean it qualifies as research. It will be important to have conversations ahead of time with your institution's IRB for not just the execution of the project but also the planning phases. This will be discussed further in Chapter 7. Needs assessments can include formal methods, such as semi-structured interviews, focus groups, and surveys. They can also be completed through

informal methods of conversations, observations, or email exchange. You'll want to consider the intent of what is being done by the student, as well as whether this data collected is to create generalized knowledge, how it will be shared either internally or externally, or whether it is being gathered for improvement of one specific site's offerings.

Identify Gaps Between Evidence in the Literature and the Capstone Site and/or Population

Once the needs assessment data is gathered, students will need to compare what is happening at their site to what they found in the literature. You can set up activities to help them compare these two using a simple chart, as seen in Appendix 6.C. Students then will begin the decisions about which gaps they want to fill with their project. This may include considering what to add/change to an existing protocol or program to improve client care or decisions on how much of the program they can develop in 14 weeks, including whether or not they will be able to implement the actual program in that time frame. Sometimes, using an established evidence-based program in a different context or with a different population can meet the student's desire to work with clients and the site's needs to serve their clients. Sharing evidence such as this article by Hemmingson et al. (2013) that reports on the use of the YEAH (Young Adults Eating and Active for Health) that used the PRECEDE–PROCEED model can provide an example for students to better understand the process and the possible outcomes. Using such a framework for the needs assessment provides the data to assist in decisions about the scope and complexity of the capstone project. Appendix D provides an example of what the final needs assessment documentation might look like.

Analyze Needs Assessment Data, and Understand How This Will Be Applied to the Capstone Proposal Development

Analysis of the needs assessment data provides a data-based decision about the focus and scope of the capstone project. The need for development of a specific program might be identified, but the time needed to develop the program, plan the evaluation, implement the program, and assess the outcomes may be beyond the scope of the 14 weeks. Many students want to work with clients and implement their project, but sometimes projects need to be scaled back. Consider other ways for students to interact with clients through additional learning objectives if their site is not yet ready to implement the amazing evidence-informed program your student has developed. Scaling back might include translating a previously published program to be implemented at this site with a different population or the same population but a different setting, developing a program evaluation plan for a current site program, or developing the new program with plans for the next student to implement. At this point, you may need to reflect on your curriculum design.

When analyzing the needs assessment data, you should also consider if your capstone program or students are focused on knowledge translation, program development, quality improvement, or other projects that might use a research methods approach. Each of these foci may require a different approach to needs assessment data analysis. Chapter 8 will dive deeper into program evaluation and sustainability concepts.

Assignments/Curricular Structure

At what point does your program have the student begin to work on the learning objectives and activities that need to be done during the capstone experience? Some programs choose to have students start with the project first and then plan the experience around execution of the project. Others might start wider with the students' general learning desire for the experience and identify the site's strengths, then narrow down the actions needed to complete the specific project. Knowing this sequence of approach will help to situate your needs assessment within the overall capstone process as a whole.

EDUCATOR CHAPTER SUMMARY

This chapter provides the student and the educator with guidance to complete the needs assessment, a required element of the doctoral capstone project. It includes application of theory or frameworks to guide the process with examples using two frameworks to illustrate each step of the process.

REFERENCES

Accreditation Council for Occupational Therapy Education. (2023). *Standards and interpretive guide* [PDF]. https://acoteonline.org/accreditation-explained/standards/

Altschuld, J., & Kumar, D. (2010). Needs assessment: An overview (Book 1). In J. Altschuld (Ed.), *The needs assessment kit*. SAGE Publications, Inc.

Altschuld, J. W., & Watkins, R. (2014). A primer on needs assessment: More than 40 years of research and practice. *New Directions for Evaluation*, *144*, 5–18. https://doi.org/10.1002/ev.20099

Center for Appreciative Inquiry. (n.d.). *Generic process of appreciative inquiry*. https://centerforappreciativeinquiry.net/resources/the-generic-processes-of-appreciative-inquiry-5ds/

Chinnman, M., Shearer, A. L., & Acosta, J. D. (2024). *Getting to outcomes™ planning and evaluation tool*. RAND Corporation. https://www.rand.org/pubs/tools/TLA1363-1.html

Cooperrider, D. L., & Srivastva, S. (1987). Appreciative inquiry in organizational life. In R. W. Woodman & W. A. Pasmore (Eds.), *Research in organizational change and development* (pp. 129–169). JAI Press.

Cooperrider, D. L., & Whitney, D. (1999). *A positive revolution in change: Appreciative inquiry*. Corporation for Positive Change.

Dougherty, M., Tolbert, K., Kusumoto, M., Greenberg, N., & Smith-Gabai, H. (2017). *Oncology: Occupational therapy in acute care* (2nd ed., H. Smith-Gabai & S. Holm, Eds.). AOTA Press.

Gielen, A. C., McDonald, E. M., Gary, T. L., & Bone, L. R. (2008). Using the PRECEDE-PROCEED model to apply health behavior theories. In K. Glanz, B. K. Rimer, & K. Viswanath (Eds.), *Health behavior and health education: Theory, research, and practice* (94th ed., pp. 407–434). Josey-Bass.

Green, L. W., & Kreuter, M. W. (2005). *Health promotion planning: An education and ecological approach* (4th ed.). McGraw Hill.

Hargraves, J., Change, J., Kennedy, K., Sen, A., & Bozzi, D. (2021). *Health care cost and utilization report* (p. 10). Health Care Cost Institute.

Hemmingson, K., Lucchesi, R., & Kattelmann, K. (2013). Project YEAH – American Indian: Tailoring a web-delivered weight maintenance intervention for American Indian college students *Journal of Nutrition Education and Behavior*, *45*(Suppl. 4), S36.

Kattelman, K., White, A. A., Greene, G. W., Byrd-Bredbenner, C., Hoerr, S. L., Horacek, T. M., Kidd, T., Colby, S., Philips, B. W., Koenings, M. M., Brown, O. N., Olfert, M., Shelnutt, K. P., & Morrell, J. S. (2014). Development of young adults eating and active for health (YEAH) internet-based intervention via a community-based participatory research model. *Journal of Nutrition and Education Behavior*, *46*(2). https://doi.org/10.1016/j.jneb.2013.11.006

Kidder, D. P., Fierro, L. A., Luna, E., Salvaggio, H., McWhorter, A., Bowen, S.-A., Murphy-Hoefer, R., Thigpen, S., Alexander, D., Armstead, T. L., August, E., Bruce, D., Nu Clarke, S., Davis, C., Downes, A., Gill, S., House, L. D., Kerzner, M., Kun, K., . . . CDC Evaluation Framework Work Group. (2024). CDC Program evaluation framework, 2024. *MMWR Recommendation Report*, *73*(No. RR-6), 1–37. https://doi.org/10.15585/mmwr.rr7306a1

Mezirow, J. (1997). Transformative learning: Theory to practice. *New Directions for Adult and Continuing Education*, (74), 5–12. https://doi.org/10.1002/ace.7401

National Institute for Children's Health Quality. (2024). https://nichq.org/blog/seven-steps-conducting-successful-needs-assessment/

Stavros, J., Godwin, L. N., & Cooperrider, D. L. (2015). Appreciative inquiry. In W. J. Rothwell, J. M. Stavros, & R. L. Sullivan (Eds.). *Practicing organization development: Leading transformation and change* (4th ed.). Wiley.

Suriyaarachchi, P., Chu, L., Bishop, A., Thew, T., Matthews, K., Cowan, R., Gunawardene, P., & Duque, G. (2020). Evaluating effectiveness of an acute rehabilitation program in hospital-associated deconditioning. *Journal of Geriatric Physical Therapy*, *43*(4), 172–178. https://doi.org/10.1519/JPT.0000000000000238 (Original work published 2001)

University of Kansas. (2024). *Precede-proceed*. The Community Tool Box, Chapter 2, Section 2. Center for Community Health and Development. https://ctb.ku.edu/en/table-contents/overview/other-models-promoting-community-health-and-development/preceder-proceder/main

APPENDICES

Appendix 6.A PRECEDE–PROCEED Worksheet

Appendix 6.B Appreciative Inquiry 5D Cycle Needs Assessment Assignment Overview, Template, and Rubric

Appendix 6.C Needs Assessment Decision Chart – Literature Review Focus

Appendix 6.D Needs Assessment Assignment Write-Up Template

Appendix 6.A

PRECEDE–PROCEED Worksheet

PRECEDE–PROCEED Needs Assessment Worksheet

Organization Name

Organization Background

- Website:
- Mission and Vision:
- Setting:
- Population(s) Served:
- Services Offered:
- Programs Offered:

PRECEDE–PROCEED Model

Reminders:

- PRECEDE and PROCEED are acronyms.
- PRECEDE (predisposing, reinforcing, and enabling constructs in educational/environmental diagnosis and evaluation) – describes the process that precedes, or leads up to, the development of a program (or an intervention).
- PROCEED (policy, regulatory, and organizational constructs in educational and environmental development) – describes how to proceed with the program (or the intervention).

PRECEDE Phases	What do you already know from: • Literature? • Theory? • Community partner?	What do you need to find out from: • Literature? • Theory? • Community partner?
Phase 1: Social and Situational Analysis What are the community's needs or problems?	Literature/theory (*include in-text citation*): • Community partner:	Literature/theoretical search: • Community partner questions:
Phase 2: Epidemiological Assessment What are the health and well-being needs within the community? For example, what are some objectives set by Healthy People 2030?	Literature/theory (*include in-text citation*): • Community partner:	Literature/theoretical search: • Community partner questions:
Phase 3: Behavioral and Environmental Assessment What are the behavioral risk factors or supports? What are the environmental risk factors or supports?	Literature/theory (*include in-text citation*): • Community partner:	Literature/theoretical search: • Community partner questions:
Phase 4: Educational and Ecological Assessment What intervention approaches support positive outcomes in this population or setting?	Literature/theory (*include in-text citation*): • Community partner:	Literature/theoretical search: • Community partner questions:

Phase 5: Administrative and Policy Assessment What support and infrastructure are needed to make the program a success (i.e., funding, policies, procedures, and community involvement)? Make sure to consider budget, space, timeline, and personnel.	Literature/theory (*include in-text citation*): • Community partner:	Literature/theoretical search: • Community partner questions:
Phase 6: Implementation *How would you monitor program processes in order to make adjustments as needed?*	Literature/theory (*include in-text citation*): • Community partner:	Literature/theoretical search: • Community partner questions:
Phases 7–9: Evaluation *7 Process evaluation: How will you know that the program is implemented as planned? How will you measure goals attainment? How will you know if the needs of the population were addressed?* *8 Impact Evaluation: How will you evaluate the short-term impact of the program? For example, attitudes and knowledge.* *9 Outcome Evaluation: How will you evaluate the long-term impact of the program? For example, behaviors, quality of life, and community needs.*	Literature/theory (*include in-text citation*): • Community partner:	Literature/theoretical search: • Community partner questions:

Appendix 6.B
APPRECIATIVE INQUIRY 5D CYCLE NEEDS ASSESSMENT ASSIGNMENT OVERVIEW, TEMPLATE, AND RUBRIC

ASSIGNMENT OVERVIEW

Description: Students will schedule a meeting with their capstone site mentor or other site representative to complete the capstone needs assessment. The Appreciative Inquiry 5D Cycle will be used to plan and implement the meeting. The template for this assignment is on the learning management system and provided here.

ASSIGNMENT COMPONENTS

Students will submit the following:
- **Meeting agenda and question outline** – follow the 5D cycle.
- **Meeting notes** – summarize your interview and observation findings.
- **Action plan** – based on your needs assessment findings, identify 1–3 short-term goals using the SMART format to support your capacity to develop a strong capstone project statement of need and project methods to be submitted for approval.
- **Proposed project objective** – based on the outcomes of your needs assessment meeting, what do you anticipate the objective of your capstone project to be?

Grading Rubric: Doctoral Capstone Site Needs Assessment

CRITERIA	POSSIBLE POINTS
Meeting Agenda and Question Outline Follows the 5D cycle, including: • Introduction • Definition • Discovery • Dream • Design • Destiny/delivery • Wrap-up and action planning	2.5
Meeting Notes Summary of your interview and observation findings. Can be written in an outline or narrative format.	2.5
Action Plan • One to three short-term goals for the semester based on the needs assessment findings. • Goals written in SMART format and that support the students' capacity to develop a strong project proposal. • Each goal includes a clear due date and action steps to achieve the goal.	4
Tentative Project Objective	1
TOTAL	10

Doctoral Capstone Project
Appreciative Inquiry Needs Assessment TEMPLATE

Student Name:
Site Name:
Site Mentor Name:
Faculty Mentor Name:
Other Meeting Participants:

Meeting Agenda and Question Outline (_____ min)
1. **Introductions (____ min)**
   a.
2. **Definition (____ min).** Clarify what is the focus and purpose of your inquiry. (Affirmative topic of choice.) Reframe the problem statement into a desired state, and identify key ideas and topics of inquiry.
   a. **Hint:** Include the questions you anticipate using in your interview as bullet points under each step.
2. **Discovery (____ min).** Appreciating the best of what is. Collect stories from stakeholders with a focus on their lived experience rather than opinions.
3. **Dream (____ min).** Envisioning what might be. Pose a "provocative proposition" to help the stakeholders think about a shared vision for the future.
4. **Design (____ min).** Constructing what should be. Collaborate with the stakeholders to develop a plan of action.
5. **Destiny/delivery (____ min).** Innovating and empowering the organization to move toward their goals. Support the organization to move toward its vision for the future.
6. **Wrap-Up and Action Planning (____ min).**

MEETING NOTES

Provide a copy of your meeting notes here. You may format your notes in paragraph or bullet form.

ACTION PLAN

Based on your needs assessment findings, identify one to three short-term goals for the semester (ensure that you are using the SMART format). Your goal(s) should support your capacity to develop a strong project abstract and research methods–based proposal. The aim is to ensure that your proposal will be ready to submit for research approval by the IRB prior to implementation of capstone if needed.

Goal 1 (SMART)
- **Date Due:**
- **Action Steps:**
- **Notes:**

Goal 2 (SMART):
- **Date Due:**
- **Action Steps:**
- **Notes:**

Goal 3 (SMART):
- **Date Due:**
- **Action Steps:**
- **Notes:**

Tentative Project Objective or Guiding Question:

Appendix 6.C
NEEDS ASSESSMENT DECISION CHART – LITERATURE REVIEW FOCUS

A fillable table or chart may help guide students through the process of comparing what they find in the literature for best practice with the needs assessment process to help them create their clinical guideline/program guideline for their actual project. This can be used to help them track the process of moving evidence into practice and identifying real-world barriers that they may be able to help eliminate with their capstone projects. The following is a fictitious example and is not rooted in actual literature.

	THE LITERATURE SAYS	MY SITE CURRENTLY DOES
Who? What type of client?	Left neglect s/p R CVA	Left neglect s/p R CVA
Outcome measure	Section GG ADL	Section GG ADL
Key assessments	Clock drawing	Informal field cut testing
Intervention key ingredients	Tactile cues, visual scanning instruction, dual task training	Verbal cues, tactile prompts during sessions
Frequency/duration	5× a week for 30 minutes	5× a week, but does not focus on this task each day
Discharge criteria	When able to scan to left independently	When d/c to home from rehab

Appendix 6.D
NEEDS ASSESSMENT ASSIGNMENT WRITE-UP TEMPLATE

This is an example of a needs assessment assignment/template that the student would turn in. Appendix 6.B is the planning tool, and this is the written document that is completed.

Resources: Kattelman et al. (Mar 2014). "Development of Young Adults Eating and Active for Health (YEAH) Internet-Based Intervention via a Community-Based Participatory Research Model," *Journal of Nutrition and Education Behavior,* 46(2). DOI:https://doi.org/10.1016/j.jneb.2013.11.006

Each bolded heading in the following should have between 250 and 400 words.

Introduction: Start with your literature review clinical question (PIO/PICO/PCC), then your site's name and general info (XX Regional Medical Center, large acute care hospital with oncology-specific units). 1 paragraph

Process of Needs Assessment: Just the chart here (fill in the boxes in what follows with your information, which phases of PRECEDE–PROCEED did you complete? What was your data source, and what did you do to get that data? This should be the quick version of your planning chart (Appendix 6.B), your methods of the needs assessment process).

PHASE	DATA SOURCE	TASKS/ACTIVITIES
Epidemiological	Franklin Co Auditor CDC website National Autism Society; textbook, additional citations, etc. (just author, year)	Obtained local and national numbers; major symptoms and features of diagnosis
Social	Site mentor Client	Conversation with site mentor, interaction with targeted population during level I or level II or other personal experience
Etc.		

Epidemiology Assessment: Describe the condition, signs, symptoms, prevalence, incidence, severity, available programs, potential role of OT, and your rationale for why this problem is so important.

Social Assessment: Describe the social factors that contribute to this problem, the barriers to addressing it, and the existing supports for addressing it. Identify the social challenges you will address in your program (include readiness to change, such as health belief model, or TTM). (Subjective evaluation of social factors impacting their condition may come from mentor talking about how their clients are impacted.)

Administrative/Policy Plan: Describe the administrative and organization concerns that will be important to consider before you implement your program – consider data you will need, data sources, interview questions, etc. (talk to site, investigate staffing, restrictions, policies, may not know all this right now).

Behavioral Assessment: Describe the behaviors that are linked to the problem you identified in the social and/or epidemiological assessments. These include the individuals' behaviors directly related to the disease/condition (e.g., vaping among teens), the behaviors of others that affect the individual (e.g., peer group that vapes), and the behaviors of "decision-makers" (e.g., school administrators who install detectors in schools to reduce opportunity). These are supports and barriers.

Environmental Assessment: Describe the environmental supports, barriers, risks of the site (staff, patients) or community, as appropriate to the specific capstone.

Educational/Ecological: If applicable, analyze the predisposing, enabling, and reinforcing factors related to the behavioral and environmental factors that, if modified, can change behavior.

Summary of Needs Assessment (250 words): What are the major factors you discovered for this population, intervention, and/or facility? At this point in time, based upon what you know, does this project topic seem acceptable? Will your site be supportive of implementing your program/protocol? As is or with changes?.

CHAPTER 7

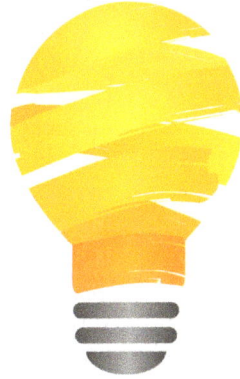

Determining the Experiential Plan for the Capstone Experience and Project

Julie A. Bednarski and Elizabeth D. DeIuliis

Section 1: Student Focus

Human-Centered Design Mindsets for the Doctoral Student

The human-centered design mindsets of optimism and empathy will be important for you to embrace as you enter this final planning phase. Keeping optimistic and practicing empathy will allow you to delve deeper into the needs of the site, ensuring a client-centered approach and providing a meaningful project outcome.

Empathy. This is the time for you, as a capstone student, to "step into the shoes of your site" and begin to understand its needs to problem-solve solutions. This problem-solving will lead to more individualized goals and objectives and will create a meaningful experience for both you and your site. Spend time building the occupational profile with your content expert, who most likely is your mentor on-site. For your project to be successful and have sustainability, you need to listen to your clients and understand their problems and needs.

Optimism. Be optimistic! By having a mindset of optimism, you will continue to try as hard as possible to find solutions to problems and develop goals that will be meaningful. Keep that attitude of optimism as you complete the final planning phase.

INTRODUCTION

This chapter provides recommendations to guide you, the doctoral student, in developing the *experiential plan* for your doctoral capstone. Formerly referred to as the memorandum of understanding (MOU), the experiential plan is a mechanism designed to communicate an understanding of various terms and activities of the doctoral capstone and to help create a partnership among the parties involved. The main rationale for having a formal experiential plan is to set expectations for the doctoral capstone and achieve a mutual understanding between all members of the capstone team. The process of developing the plan ultimately helps build confidence and trust among the capstone team (the student, doctoral capstone coordinator, faculty mentor, and content expert). This experiential plan will serve as a key document during the planning and implementation phases of your doctoral capstone. Proactive and ongoing planning, communication, and collaboration among your capstone

DOI: 10.4324/9781003541813-9

team are important to ensure success. In this planning stage, you will be working collaboratively to (1) finalize the problem statement and purpose to frame the capstone experience and project, (2) develop an experiential plan to include your individualized specific objectives for the capstone experience, a plan for evaluation, supervision, and mentoring, and determine the responsibilities of all parties (Accreditation Council for Occupational Therapy Education [ACOTE], 2023).

STUDENT REFLECTIVE QUESTIONS

When finalizing the planning of the doctoral capstone, capstone students may find it helpful to reflect on the following questions:

1. How do you feel your communication is with your content expert at your doctoral capstone site? What are the barriers to communication? What is going well with communications between you and the site? Do you need any assistance from your program's doctoral capstone coordinator?

2. Spend a moment thinking about and articulating the difference between your capstone experience and your capstone project to a family member. Are you clear on the differences?

3. How have you begun to plan for your project? Are you comfortable articulating your plan and purpose to others? Describe to a friend or family member your plan for your capstone experience. Does it make sense to this person?

4. Reflect on the goals you hope you to achieve both through the capstone experience and the project; visualize the steps you will need to take to achieve your goals.

STUDENT OBJECTIVES

By the end of reading this chapter and completing the learning activities, the student should be able to:

1. Compare and contrast the experience vs. project purpose and plan.

2. Create a finalized problem statement to frame the capstone experience and project.

3. Collaborate with the faculty mentor and content expert to develop individualized specific doctoral capstone experience objectives.

4. Collaborate with the faculty mentor and content expert to create a plan for evaluation, supervision, and mentoring during the capstone experience.

5. Determine responsibilities of the capstone student, faculty mentor, and content expert as identified and agreed upon.

6. Finalize the experiential plan and agreement for the doctoral capstone.

7. Determine the capstone project purpose and set goals.

8. Create plan for the institutional review board process for the capstone project.

When trying to finalize the purpose of your doctoral capstone, it is important to remember that there are two distinct parts of the doctoral capstone, which include the experience and the project. Your doctoral capstone experience is the 14-week period of time that you will be spending and learning at a specific site. The capstone project is just one component of the experience completed during the 14 weeks so that you can demonstrate, first, how you were able to synthesize knowledge gained and, second, how you have applied this new knowledge (ACOTE, 2023). Let us step back for a moment to reflect on where you are in the process of designing your doctoral capstone. In Chapter 4, you utilized identity and empathy mapping to align with and procure a site for your capstone experience. Hopefully, by this point in time, you have secured your capstone site and are beginning to develop a relationship with the site through communication with your content expert. In Chapter 5, you began precursory steps of the needs assessment through the literature review and finding the gap at the site or population to begin to develop a project plan to mutually meet the site needs and your learning needs. You dug deeper into the needs assessment process within Chapter 6. As you begin this chapter, you are now approaching the point in which you are ready to outline your capstone experience objectives, determine a plan for supervision and mentorship, and develop your goals and objectives for your capstone project to create your experiential plan.

DEVELOPMENT OF THE EXPERIENTIAL PLAN

An experiential plan for the doctoral capstone is required per ACOTE (2023) standard D.1.4: "Ensure that there is a valid plan for the individual doctoral capstone experience, that, at a minimum, includes: individualized specific doctoral experience objectives, plans for evaluation, supervision, and mentoring, and responsibilities of all parties" (p. 43). The experiential plan must be signed by both parties (ACOTE, 2023, p. 43). It may be helpful to review some examples of experiential plans, and refer to these as you read this chapter for better clarity. (See 7.A and 7.B.)

As you review these examples provided in the appendices, note that these all show different structures for the student to identify the responsibilities of all parties; the objectives for their capstone experience; the plan for supervision, mentorship, and evaluation; and finally, the goals and objectives of their capstone project. Goals and objectives of the capstone project are not required by ACOTE to be on experiential plan; however, it is going to be a part of your experience. Documenting your project goals and objectives on your experiential plan ensures that everyone on the capstone team agrees and has collaborated on both the experience objectives and the project goal and objectives. Signatures are required by ACOTE to be on the experiential plan, and they have been removed from the examples for this publication. (See Text Box 7.1.)

TEXT BOX 7.1

Reflection Questions

As you begin to think about developing your capstone experience plan, it may be helpful to first answer these open-ended questions:

- I will be completing my 14-week capstone experience at the following site: _____.
- My capstone team consists of _____.
- I hope to be able to gain experiences in the following while at this site: _____.
- My goal at the site is to provide _____ to fill the following need of the site or population _____.
- I will feel successful when _____

When developing your capstone experience, you need to think broadly. What experience or experiences do you want to have, and what do you want to learn? You may have many opportunities during this 14-week period, so take advantage of what the site has to offer you and what experience may assist you in achieving your educational goals.

When developing your project, you need to think in more specific terms. You are trying to complete a project

that fills gap in services, training, curriculum, etc. This will be the gap you have identified through your needs assessment, which leads to the development of your specific capstone project. We will give you some examples to spark some inspiration later in this chapter.

Identification of the Capstone Team and Communication

The experiential plan outlines the members of the capstone team and responsibilities for all. Your capstone team will include your content expert, doctoral capstone coordinator, you (the capstone student), and a faculty mentor. You will work with your doctoral capstone coordinator to determine your team. Refer to Chapter 1 for specifics on the roles and responsibilities of each team member, as well as your program's handbook and/or capstone course syllabi. It will be your responsibility as the capstone student to communicate with your team and document responsibilities of all parties. As the capstone student, you are the leader of this team. During this planning stage, frequent and ongoing communication is critical among the capstone team to ensure success of the capstone experience and project. Figure 7-1 gives you a visual of the communication taking place between the capstone team as the capstone experience and project become finalized. You are the major communicator at this point in your doctoral capstone journey, and you are taking the initiative to remain in close contact with the content expert, doctoral capstone coordinator, and your faculty mentor. Most likely, your doctoral capstone coordinator will have developed a template for the experiential plan that outlines all parties' responsibilities. However, you will be the one to initiate and facilitate communication and make any adjustments to the template.

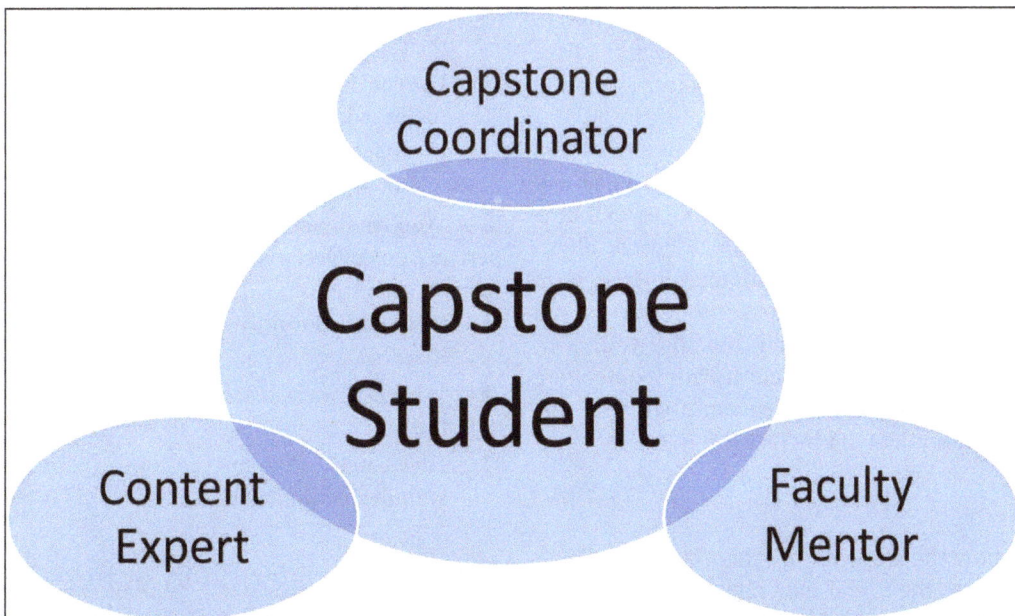

Figure 7-1. Communication with the capstone team.

Purpose

Through completion of the literature review and a detailed needs assessment, you will be able to establish a need or problem at the site to formulate the purpose of your doctoral capstone that is supported by evidence from the literature. It is important that the problem you want to address is a problem the site wants to address, so it can be a win–win for both you and the site. In this planning stage, before the start of the capstone experience and project, you are finalizing the overall purpose of your capstone, which will lead to the collaborative development of the goals and objectives for the experience and project. You may or may not include your specific capstone purpose on your experiential plan, but it is needed in order for you to begin planning development as your purpose "sets the stage" for your experience objectives and project goals and objectives. (See Text Box 7.2.)

Refer to Chapters 5 and 6 for more specifics on determining your problem statement and purpose based on the needs assessment.

TEXT BOX 7.2

This is a simple example of doctoral capstone purpose with the focus area of *program development and evaluation* that was developed from the problem identified at the site. The problem was an increase in falls at a senior living community, and their need was for falls prevention programming.

"The purpose of my doctoral capstone was to provide a multicomponent falls prevention program to residents of XXX." (Green, 2023, p. 6)

Student Objectives for the Capstone Experience

Once your purpose is determined, it is time to develop individualized capstone experience objectives (ACOTE, 2023. D.1.4) and capstone project goals and objectives (ACOTE, 2023. D.1.5). Your doctoral capstone objectives are individualized objectives that you want to achieve during your 14-week experience and align with your occupational therapy educational curriculum. (See Text Box 7.3.) In order to ensure alignment with your program's curriculum, you may want to begin with reviewing the curriculum, curriculum threads, and student learning outcomes of your program. While reviewing the student learning outcomes, think about how your experience can align with the outcomes as the student did in Text Box 7.3.

TEXT BOX 7.3

Here is how the student from the example in Text Box 7.2 framed the overall experience based on program educational outcomes and curricular threads and related to her capstone experience:

TEXT BOX 7-3 (continued)

Curricular Thread: Socially Responsive Health Care

Student Educational Outcome: Graduates will demonstrate entry-level competencies in providing client-centered, inclusive, equitable, and research-informed care in professional practice.

Student Learning Objective 1: The student will demonstrate the ability to provide equitable, evidence-based, and client-centered care through creating an evidence-based fall prevention program.

Curricular Thread: Critical Inquiry and Reflective Practice

Student Educational Outcome: Graduates will be prepared to apply principles of evidence-based and evidence-informed decision-making in professional practice to improve and expand the delivery and quality of occupational therapy services.

Student Learning Objective 2: The student will demonstrate the ability to evaluate and analyze study results as well as apply evidence-based decision-making in order to create/implement an evidence-informed fall prevention program.

Curricular Thread: Leadership and Advocacy

Student Educational Outcome: Graduates will demonstrate leadership and advocacy to promote health, well-being, and quality of life for people, populations, and communities.

Student Learning Objective 3: The student will demonstrate the ability to collaborate with and advocate for the target population to provide support and education that promote aging in place, health, and well-being.

After you have reviewed the objectives for the doctoral capstone experience within Text Box 7.3, answer the following questions:

1. How do you feel the experience objectives align with the program curricular threads and outcomes?
2. Do you feel the capstone experience objectives are too broad, too narrow, or about right?
   a. Based on your answer, how would you adjust the objectives?

As you think about individualizing **your** capstone experience objectives, it may be helpful to ask yourself these following questions:

1. Why did I choose this experience, and what do I want to learn?
2. What do I want to accomplish during my 14 weeks at the site?
3. How could I align my capstone experience objective with the learning outcomes of my OTD program?

Project Goals and Objectives

In order to demonstrate the learning and knowledge gained during your 14-week experience, you will need to develop and implement a capstone project and then synthesize and disseminate your outcomes. A collaborative effort needs to occur to develop the goals and objectives for the capstone project. The process of determining goals and objectives requires communication with the capstone team and should be directed by you, the capstone student. The process of goal development may require multiple iterations to ensure that the initial goals meet the needs of the site and meet your overall learning goals for the doctoral capstone. (See Text Box 7.4.)

TEXT BOX 7.4

Here are the project goals and objectives the student from the preceding examples formulated after determining an overall capstone purpose, followed by objectives for the experience:

Project Goal 1

The student will administer reliable/valid assessments and analyze results to measure program effectiveness.

Objective 1: The student will administer and analyze the Falls Efficacy Scale (FES) with all consenting participants.

Objective 2: The student will administer and analyze the Physical Activity Readiness Questionnaire (PAR-Q) with all consenting participants.

Project Goal 2

The student will demonstrate the ability to develop and implement a fall prevention program based on evidence-based practices and current research.

Objective 1: The student will demonstrate the ability to use pretest data to develop an evidence-based program to support this population.

Objective 2: The student will review XXX dimensions of wellness and current fall prevention initiatives in order to determine current barriers.

Project Goal 3

The student will ensure sustainability of program development initiatives by week 14 of the program to promote long-term health, independence, and well-being in this population.

Objective 1: The student will educate the target population on fall prevention strategies, proper footwear/community safety, home modifications, diet/medication, vision/vitamins, and home and community hazards.

Objective 2: The student will create educational handouts on the preceding topics listed.

Objective 3: The student will educate the target population on exercises that focus on balance, mobility, and strength training.

Objective 4: The student will educate about and advocate for this population through all future personal and professional encounters.

Source: Samantha Green, OTD, OTR, Indiana University (IU) OTD class of 2023.

Often, initial goals and objectives for a project will be developed to have a starting point when talking with a site but will then be reworked and refined based on collaborative, ongoing communication. (See Text Box 7.5.) It can be helpful to conceptualize the overarching goals for your project as a long-term goal (LTG), and your individualized objectives as short-term goals (STG), that is, the steps that you need to take to accomplish your LTG. Goals and objectives should be measurable so that you can tell when your goals have been met (Bonnel & Smith, 2018). Developmentally, you will have already had didactic curricula focused on establishing goals and objectives for clients through the occupational therapy process.

TEXT BOX 7.5

"While drafting my student learning plan, I went about writing my goals and objectives similarly to how I had learned to goal-set in my fieldwork experiences. Starting with three larger aims that I had for my project, I was then able to backward-plan stepwise objectives that would lead me to those bigger goals. It was helpful to have this well-thought-out plan to bring to my capstone mentor, who then provided me with feedback that led to some final editing of my learning plan. What started as a sloppy first draft of random brainstorming on a page in my journal became a clearly defined project to positively impact my community when I was able to apply the tools that I already had in my toolbox and to fill in the gaps with knowledge and insight from my mentor."

– Johnna Belkiewitz OTD, MAT, OTR, IU OTD class of 2023

A commonly used framework to create goals is the acronym SMART (Gateley, 2023). When creating goals using the SMART framework, you are writing goals for the project that are specific, measurable, action-oriented, realistic, and timely. As SMART goals are developed, then objectives for each goal can be written to give you action steps to meet the goals. (See Text Box 7.6.)

TEXT BOX 7.6

Two student examples of project goal and objectives that were documented on the experiential plan after collaboration with the student's content expert, faculty mentor, and doctoral capstone coordinator:

Project Goal 1

The student will develop a program for the role of OT in primary care and pain management through addressing the psychological impact of pain.

Objective 1: The student will develop evidence-based tools regarding acceptance commitment therapy and pain management for use by occupational therapists in the primary care setting.

Objective 2: The student will educate occupational therapists and physicians in the primary care setting on acceptance commitment therapy in relation to pain management for occupational participation.

Objective 3: The student will collect and analyze survey data regarding whether this program would benefit the primary care population.

(Dinwiddie, 2024, p. 19)

Project Goal 1

The student will develop an evidence-based aging-in-place program protocol/resources for patients at XXX Gender Health Clinic in order to decrease social isolation for the aging LGBTQ+ population.

Objective 1: The student will establish use of an evidence-based outcome measure to evaluate social isolation and social participation within the LGBTQ+ older adult population.

Objective 2: The student will communicate with referring providers of potential clients to attend aging-in-place program to try to aim for 7–8 spots filled.

Objective 3: The student will develop a screening protocol for clinicians to use for referral of LGBTQ+ older adults into the aging-in-place program with collaboration from social work for an interdisciplinary approach to the aging-in-place group.

Project Goal 2

OTS will implement an evidence-based aging-in-place program to increase social participation for the aging LGBTQ+ population.

Objective 1: The student will administer pre/post-test outcome measures assessing knowledge of aging-in-place measures and client learning along with perceived social participation.

Objective 2: The student will evaluate client needs within the scope of aging-in-place and make appropriate changes according to needs within the aging-in-place program.

Objective 3: The student will collaborate with other professions (medicine, social work, speech language pathologist, etc.) to implement an interprofessional frame of reference regarding the patient population and needs to be addressed.

– Shelley Gurevitz, IU OTD Student class of 2025

It is important to have these goals and objectives on the experiential plan because all capstone team members are signing the plan, and this will be verification that all parties agree. As you think about beginning your goals and objectives for your project, take a moment to answer the following:

For my capstone project, I hope to accomplish _____

Three overall capstone project goals I hope to accomplish are _____

What steps do I need to take to get started with my capstone project? _____

I will measure success of my capstone project by _____

_____

Another step in the development of the experiential plan is determining plans for supervision, mentoring, and finally, evaluation.

Plans for Supervision and Mentoring

Having a plan for supervision and mentoring is a requirement of ACOTE and must be documented on your experiential plan. By having a plan, you and the content expert are setting up an environment for success. Your content expert will most likely be your mentor and supervisor at the site. The conversation regarding expectations is important, and by writing out these expectations, all capstone team members will understand the plan. (See Text Box 7.7.)

Here are definitions from ACOTE that may be helpful as you begin thinking about a plan for mentoring and supervision:

Mentoring. A relationship between two people in which one person (the mentor) is dedicated to the personal and professional growth of the other (the mentee). A mentor has more experience and knowledge than their mentee.

Content mentor. Expertise in the content area of the project.

Faculty mentor. Person who meets the qualifications to support the objectives of the project and is familiar with the program's curriculum design.

Supervise. To direct and inspect the performance of workers or work.

Supervisor. One who ensures that tasks assigned to others are performed correctly and efficiently.

(ACOTE, 2023, p. 49, 52)

Table 7-1 gives suggestions for questions to ask your content expert and faculty mentor to consider as the supervision plan is developed.

You will want to develop statements for your experiential plan so the supervision and mentoring plan is clear to all capstone team members. Some ideas include:

- The student will be mentored and supervised by the content expert at the site.
- The student and content expert will meet once/week to review weekly progress and identify plans/goals for the next week.
- The content expert will complete a midterm and final evaluation of the student.
- The student will complete a final evaluation of the capstone site and content expert.
- The content expert will provide supervision as needed and as required by regulatory bodies.

Table 7-1. Items to Consider When Developing a Supervision Plan

- Roles and responsibilities for initial orientation?
- How often will we have formal face-to-face meetings?
- What is the best method of communication throughout the week?
- What is your learning style?
- What is the content expert's leadership and/or mentorship style?
- How will conflict be resolved?
- A midterm and a final evaluation are required – will there be other forms of evaluation?

As you are having these important conversations with your capstone team about plans for supervision and mentoring and your anticipated project outcomes, an initial discussion on a dissemination plan should occur. This will be addressed in further detail in Chapters 11 and 12, yet a brief introduction to authorship and intellectual property is provided here.

Statement of authorship. Because dissemination is a required part of the doctoral capstone, an initial discussion about authorship needs to occur. Authorship should be given to those that make considerable contributions to the project, and acknowledgments are given to those who offer a lesser contribution (American Psychological Association [APA], 2020, pp. 24–25). Therefore, it may be that the content expert and faculty mentor have authorship along with you on any dissemination presentations or publications. Depending on the level of involvement of the capstone coordinator, they may be given an acknowledgment or have authorship. Principal authorship is given to the person who is most involved (APA, 2020), and this most likely will be you, the capstone student. Initiating this discussion and making this determination at the start of the DCE will ensure that publication credit will be accurate and misconceptions will be avoided.

Statement of ownership of materials. If you are planning on developing materials for the site (such as new handouts or training modules that follow best health literacy principles), there needs to be an understanding of ownership and intellectual property. What is created for the site most likely will be owned by the site, and proper citations and permission for future use of materials will need to be followed. By having an ownership statement in the experiential plan, all parties agree, thus reducing any misunderstanding as to ownership of materials at the capstone completion. You may be noticing a theme in this chapter of the need to demonstrate good communication skills with your capstone team to improve the success of your doctoral capstone!

Additional resources and strategies to navigate conversations around authorship and ownership are provided in Chapters 11 and 12.

INSTITUTIONAL REVIEW BOARD

One final area to discuss as you finalize your experiential plan is the institutional review board (IRB). You will work with your doctoral capstone coordinator and faculty mentor on how to proceed with your IRB based on your capstone project. "To ensure that they [authors] meet ethical standards, before starting a research project, authors should contact the appropriate IRB or ethical review group for their institution or country for information on the kinds of research that require ethics approval" (APA, 2020, pp. 11–12). Your project may not be defined as research; however, the IRB is the board that determines whether your project is research or non-human subject research – this is not determined by you, the student (Bonnel & Smith, 2018). Your capstone coordinator will have more information specific to your program on the process you will go through to ensure you are in compliance with ethical standards. For example, your program might require you to engage in CITI (collaborative institutional training initiative), which is an online program that provides educational courses and certification in areas related to research ethics and compliance. It is widely used by universities, research institutions, and organizations to ensure that individuals involved in research understand the ethical, legal, and regulatory standards they must follow. Completion of the CITI courses helps ensure compliance with federal regulations, ethical standards, and institutional policies. Once completed, participants receive certificates that they may need to present to their institution's IRB board as proof of training.

STUDENT CHAPTER SUMMARY

This chapter described for you the components of the *experiential plan* that will guide your doctoral capstone experience and project. This is the final stage of your development phase. Know that when you do get on-site for your capstone based on the site needs and time that has elapsed since the completion of this plan, some adjustments to goals and objectives may need to happen. Stay optimistic and know that tweaks and adjustments to the experiential plan are likely inevitable and should be discussed with your capstone team. Text Box 7.8 gives a student perspective on how to keep a mindset of empathy and optimism. At this point in time, with your experiential plan developed and signed, you are ready to move into the implementation phase of your doctoral capstone.

TEXT BOX 7.8

"The goals I achieved during my DCE were quite different than the initial goals I created during the planning process. I'm sure that this information can even feel unsettling as you expend time and effort into building your plan. However, as occupational therapists, our greatest weapon is being a dynamic and client-centered professional. Just like planning for an OT session and paralleled in the DCE, creating a plan is necessary; it builds a foundation for preparedness and confidence. However, our ability to modify our methods and goals in order to best support the client will be your greatest tool during the DCE and as a practicing therapist. Feel free to potentially have to release commitment to your initial plans and move fluidly with your client, or in this case, program.

I also feel that working closely with my site mentor helped me feel successful. Don't be afraid to initiate check-ins with your site mentor and ask THEM questions on their goals, as it'll guide your (just like OT!).

Overall, my true guiding light throughout the DCE was staying client-centered instead of focusing on my own personal goals. I use this skill that I learned in the DCE process daily as a practitioner."

– Claire Havala, OTD, OTR/LIU, OTD class of 2023

Section 2: Educator Focus

Transformational Learning Phases and Framework for the Educator

One of the critical stages in Mezirow's theory of transformational learning is the "exploring options for new behavior," which is pivotal for OTD capstone students to reconsider their current actions and beliefs and to experiment with new ways of thinking or behaving. As your students are making their final preparations ahead of the start of their doctoral capstone, they are exploring alternative options, strategies, or actions to pilot during their doctoral capstone as they interact, think, or look at solutions. As an educator, be prepared that even though much preparation has occurred during the developing and planning phases, this stage is marked with experimentation, uncertainty, and gradual shifts in attitudes and behaviors (Mezirow,

(continued)

1997). This process of exploring and experimenting with new behaviors in Mezirow's theory is iterative, much like the trial-and-error approach within the human-centered design framework. The doctoral capstone involves cycles of action, assessment, feedback, and refinement – paralleling the trial-and-error nature of the exploration phase in Mezirow's model. Per Mezirow's theory, as your students explore these new behaviors, they feel a greater sense of empowerment and agency as they develop more awareness of their options.

INTRODUCTION FOR THE EDUCATOR

This chapter provides recommendations to guide you, the educator, in assisting the student to develop the *experiential plan* for their doctoral capstone. The term *experiential plan* is now a part of the 2023 ACOTE standards and has taken the place of the former memorandum of understanding (MOU) term. The experiential plan is the document designed to communicate an understanding of the students' individualized doctoral capstone experience objectives; plans for evaluation, supervision, and mentoring; and responsibilities of all parties. This chapter will provide you with teaching tips and learning strategies as you guide the students through the process of developing their experiential plans. During the development stage of the experiential plan, the student is planning their course of action and developing their strategy for learning, to include meeting the needs of their site, understanding new perspectives, and trying to solve problems. It is an exciting time for the student in their learning process, and as an educator, you will want to assist the student by providing the needed resources to help them plan, encourage reflection as they plan, and give them ongoing support as they address potential challenges that arise.

EDUCATOR OBJECTIVES

By the end of reading this chapter, the educator will be able to apply principles of transformational learning theory to structure learning activities, assignments, and/or assessments in order to promote the capstone's student's ability to:

1. Finalize the capstone purpose.
2. Collaborate with the faculty member and content expert to develop individualized specific doctoral capstone experience objectives.
3. Collaborate with the faculty member and content expert to create a plans for evaluation, supervision, and mentoring.
4. Determine responsibilities of the capstone student, faculty member, and content expert are identified and agreed upon.

5. Finalize the experimental plan and agreement for the doctoral capstone.
6. Create plan for the institutional review board process.

EDUCATOR REFLECTIVE QUESTIONS

1. What do I know about the experiential plan and how it is different from the former MOU?
2. What supports do I feel my students will need from me in my role as faculty mentor or doctoral capstone coordinator?
3. What active learning strategies might I bring into my coursework to assist the capstone students as they develop their experiential plans?
4. As a faculty group, how are we ensuring a link between our curriculum and the student capstone experiences?
5. Is there a template that is already created for the student to utilize as they build their individualized plan? If not, will it be helpful if I create a template for the students?

EXPERIENTIAL PLAN AND WRITTEN AGREEMENTS FOR THE DOCTORAL CAPSTONE

With you as the capstone coordinator and/or educator, it is important to understand that in the 2023 ACOTE standards, specifically D.1.4, there are two components. First, you must document that a process for ensuring valid written agreements between the organization and the program are in effect prior to and for the duration of the capstone experience (ACOTE, 2023, p. 43) and, second, that an experiential plan is in place. Let us discuss the differences between the two.

Written Agreements

This is an agreement that the students will not be involved in obtaining as it will be the "contract" or affiliation agreement that is signed between your university and the site where the student will be spending their 14 weeks. It will be best to collaborate with your academic fieldwork coordinator during this process of obtaining contracts or "written agreements" between the site and the university. Each program and university may have different procedures, and you will want to understand these procedures at your specific university to ensure you are following your contract management process at your institution. This process may take weeks to months to up to one year, so work on this early, as a written agreement must be in place PRIOR to the start of the students on-site 14-week experience (ACOTE, 2023). If your program uses a database to support clinical education processes, such as EXXAT, CORE, etc., contractual agreements necessary for the doctoral capstone experience can also be utilized with these.

Experiential Plan

The experiential plan outlines the members of the capstone team, which include the content expert, doctoral capstone coordinator, capstone student, and faculty mentor. Depending on the number of capstone students, most often the doctoral capstone coordinator will work with the program director or department chair to identify faculty mentors for the doctoral students and to serve as a capstone team member under the workload model of your institution. Depending on the number of students in the program and the number of faculty, workload may be calculated 1–2 credits of load for a small group of capstone students (3–4) during the semester the students are registered for their capstone experiences. ACOTE does not specify workload; however, ACOTE standard D.1.1 states the following: "Ensure that the doctoral capstone is designed through collaboration with the student, a faculty member in the occupational therapy educational therapy program who holds a doctoral degree, and an individual with documented expertise in the content area of the capstone" (ACOTE, 2023, p. 42). (Refer back to the education section within Chapter 1 for more examples of workload models.) Once the capstone team is in place, the student can begin working with the faculty mentor and content expert to design the *experiential plan*. (See Text Box 7.10.) Responsibilities of all parties must be stated and on the experiential plan. The content expert does not have to be an occupational therapist (ACOTE, 2023). The doctoral capstone coordinator will need to verify expertise, a professional résumé or curriculum vitae of the content expert should be obtained, reviewed, and verified to ensure expertise consistent with the student's area of focus. Documents such as the résumé to substantiate expertise and certifications or licensure verification obtained should be stored in electronic databases, such as EXXAT or CORE, or other electronic management systems that your institution utilizes.

TEXT BOX 7.10

It will be helpful to develop a template for the experiential plan paying close attention to the ACOTE requirements. (See Appendices 7.A and 7.B for examples.)

FINALIZING THE CAPSTONE PURPOSE

By this point in time, the student has their capstone purpose developed, and now it is time to solidify with the content expert and the faculty mentor so that the experiential plan can begin to be developed. Here are some ideas for classroom activities to assist the student in gaining confidence in communicating their capstone purpose:

- Create doctoral capstone purpose elevator speeches, and present in small groups to provide and receive peer feedback.
- Post on discussion boards their capstone purposes, and foster discussion and peer review of written capstone purposes.

- Post short videos on discussion boards for oral presentations of capstone purposes and have peer review.

Relationship of the Doctoral Capstone Experience Objectives to the Programs Curriculum Design and Professional Outcomes

The capstone experience needs to align with the curriculum design of the program (ACOTE, 2023). This allows the student to ensure that the plan for the experience and project aligns with the curriculum of the program and program mission and philosophy. It is essential that capstone students review and understand their program's curriculum design, mission, philosophy, and program outcomes during the initial development phase of the DCE.

How does the capstone experience and project plan match the program's curriculum? (Review the examples given earlier in this chapter in Text Box 7.3.) As the capstone student is in the final phase of planning, it is now time to collaborate with the doctoral capstone coordinator and faculty mentor to document this link between the curriculum design and the capstone site to ensure compliance to standard D.1.3 (ACOTE, 2023). (See Text Box 7.11.)

> **TEXT BOX 7.11**
>
> **Teaching Tip:** It will be important for the students to understand how the curriculum design is integral to the development of the doctoral capstone. Activities such as review of the curricular thread and educational outcomes will be important so the student can understand the link between their capstone and the curriculum. Refer to other suggestions that were covered in Chapter 1.

Development of Individualized Specific Doctoral Capstone Experience Objectives

The experiential plan requires the student to develop individualized doctoral capstone experience objectives. These are objectives for their overall 14-week experience. It may be helpful since these objectives will be linked to curricular design to share and review your program's curricular threads, educational outcomes, and any other pertinent information about your program's curriculum design with the students. To facilitate objective development, it will be important to take the time, during the doctoral capstone development course, to have students work on their individualized capstone experience objectives. Developing active learning strategies to allow students to engage with

program threads and educational outcomes will be helpful to the student. One idea could be to develop a Jeopardy-style trivia game that tests the student's knowledge in a fun atmosphere that facilitates engagement. Referring the students back to their student handbook on the curriculum design section, to then trying to link their objectives to the program's objectives, will be helpful – see student section of this chapter for examples. As the educator, you will want to determine how specific you would like the goals to be, and if you will utilize the SMART or COAST goal writing (Gateley, 2023).

Project Goals and Objectives

In order to demonstrate that learning has occurred and knowledge gained during the students' 14-week experience, they will need to develop a capstone project and disseminate the outcomes of the project. The experiential learning plan does not specify that the project goals and objectives need to be on the plan; however, ACOTE standard D.1.5 states that doctoral capstone experience must be a minimum of 14 weeks full-time and a minimum of 32 hours/week and consistent with the individualized objectives and capstone project (ACOTE, 2023, p. 44). It will be helpful to the student and the entire capstone team if the project goals and objectives are identified on the experiential plan to allow for everyone to have a clear understanding of the entirety of the experience. A collaborative effort needs to occur to develop the goals and objectives for the capstone project. The process of determining goals and objectives requires communication with the capstone team and should be directed by the capstone student. Refer to the student section for examples of project goals and objectives.

Plans for Evaluation, Supervision, and Mentoring

As stated in Chapter 1, assigning faculty mentors to capstone students is a process that will be different for each program. This will be dependent on the number of students and program philosophy. A faculty member in the occupational therapy educational program who holds a doctoral degree will be part of the capstone team (ACOTE, 2023 Standard D.1.1). It is required that the faculty mentor have documented expertise in the capstone student's area of focus for the capstone (ACOTE, 2023, standard D.1.1). The faculty mentor should be involved early in the development stage so they can be an active participant in goal development and assessment of site needs. The doctoral capstone coordinator will want to work with students to assist in the development of a supervision and mentoring plan. (See Table 7-1 in the student section.)

On the experiential plan, a plan for evaluation is also needed. Evaluation of the student and the site will be discussed in Chapter 10.

RESPONSIBILITIES OF THE CAPSTONE TEAM

Another area that is required on the experiential plan (ACOTE, 2023, D.1.3) are the responsibilities of the capstone team members. The student will need to identify the team and the responsibilities of each team member. It may be easiest for the student if, as the doctoral capstone coordinator, you put this on an experiential plan template for the student. Refer to Appendix A and B for examples. Also refer back to Chapter 1 for specifics on role delineations and responsibilities. (See Text Boxes 7.13 and 7.14.)

TEXT BOX 7.13

Teaching Tip: Questions for students to reflect upon as they think about the team member responsibilities:

- Who will be my primary mentor during the experience at the site, and will this be the person who is considered my content expert? Identify this person.
- Do I feel that I have communicated to the content expert their role on the team, or do I need more guidance from my capstone coordinator?
- What is the difference between the role of the faculty mentor and the content expert?

TEXT BOX 7.14

As the capstone coordinator, you will most likely work with your program director to assign students to faculty mentors based on areas of specialty and workload. The content expert needs to have documented expertise in the content area of the capstone (ACOTE, 2023, D.1.1), and it is recommended you develop a policy for how this expertise is determined.

INSTITUTIONAL REVIEW BOARD

A final step in the development of the experiential plan is the consideration of the institutional review board (IRB) policies at your university. A determination will need to be made as to whether the capstone project is considered research and if the capstone student will need to go through the institutional review board (IRB) at the capstone student's institution and/or capstone site. The US Department of Health and Human Services (2018) definition of *research* is "a systematic investigation, including research development, testing and evaluation, designed to develop or contribute to generalizable knowledge" (U.S. Department of Health and Human Services, 2017, n.p.). An IRB is in place to protect human participants who take part in research, and each institution will have policies on

what constitutes the need for approval. Some capstone projects may not be considered research or do not meet the research criteria. The IRB may consider a capstone project not to be research if, when students disseminate the information, they disseminate what they did during the capstone experience and the outcomes and do not make suggestions on replication of the methodology and are not suggesting generalizing the results. In both instances, it is the IRB that determines whether the project is research, not the student. If the student is interested in publishing the results of the capstone project, it will be important to go through the IRB to obtain a letter stating an IRB review has taken place. An IRB that considers a capstone project to be research may deem it to be exempt or expedited based on minimal risk to research participants. Minimal risk is, where the probability and magnitude of harm or discomfort anticipated in the research are not greater in and of themselves than those ordinarily encountered in daily life or during the performance of routine physical or psychological examinations or tests. (U.S. Department of Health and Human Services, 2018). This, however, is determined by each IRB at the various institutions and not the researcher (Bonnel & Smith, 2018). See Text Box 7.15.

TEXT BOX 7.15

Teaching Tip: It is recommended that occupational therapy programs proactively work with their IRB to determine if these capstone projects are considered research and need IRB approval. The capstone coordinator may first want to meet with the IRB chair when developing the capstone experience and project protocols. The IRB committee at the academic institution will want to be aware if there will be an increase of proposals submitted. This will enable the IRB committee to determine the best way to handle a large number of students submitting applications. Appendix 7.C gives an example of what is being utilized by the Department of Occupational Therapy at Duquesne University to expedite the process.

EDUCATOR CHAPTER SUMMARY

This chapter took you through the steps in assisting your doctoral students in the development of their experiential plans. Initially, the students are in the transformational phase of exploring options as they identify needs of the sites and explore a meaningful capstone experience and project. Students move into the phase of planning a course of action as they develop their experiential learning plans prior to the implementation of their experiences. In this phase, you, as the educator, are providing learning experiences to ensure success of the student as they build their experiential plan to include the experience objectives, the development of their capstone team, and the plans for supervision, mentorship, and evaluation.

ADDITIONAL LEARNING ACTIVITIES TO USE WITH STUDENTS

1. Have each student draw a tree on a large piece of paper. Make sure you draw roots, a large trunk, branches, leaves, and fruit. Once the outline of your tree is drawn, complete the tree as follows:
   - The roots: your values
   - The trunk: your mission statement, the program's mission statement, the site's mission statement
   - The branches: your DCE purpose.
   - The leaves: your capstone experience objectives, your project goals and objectives
   - The fruit: the proposed outcome/results

   Once they have completed your picture, have students share with another peer and discuss the meaning of your tree. You can also do this in digital form rather than with pencil and paper.

2. Have the students think about their DCE, and write one potential goal with two objectives. Share with a partner, and provide feedback to each other:
   - Is the goal measurable?
   - Does it sound doable?
   - Is it clearly written?
   - Does it have the components of a SMART or COAST goal?
   - Discuss recommendations.

REFERENCES

Accreditation Council for Occupational Therapy Education. (2023). *2023 Accreditation Council for Occupational Therapy Education (ACOTE) standards and interpretive guide.* https://acoteonline.org/accreditation-explained/standards

American Psychological Association. (2020). *Publication manual of the American Psychological Association* (7th ed.). American Psychological Association.

Bonnel, W., & Smith, K. V. (2018). *Proposal writing for clinical nursing and DNP projects* (2nd ed.). Springer.

Dinwiddie, J. (2024). *Unwavering occupational therapy: Acceptance and commitment therapy for chronic pain in geriatric primary care* [Doctoral capstone, Indiana University]. ScholarWorks Indianapolis. https://scholarworks.indianapolis.iu.edu/server/api/core/bitstreams/7d9a222c-6e26-4af9-9755-017d72d67eb9/content

Gateley, C. A. (2023). *Documentation manual for occupational therapy* (5th ed.). Routledge. https://www.perlego.com/book/4440924/documentation-manual-for-occupational-therapy-pdf

Green, S. (2023). *Rise up for fall prevention* [Doctoral capstone, Indiana University]. ScholarWorks Indianapolis. https://scholarworks.indianapolis.iu.edu/items/252ae24c-e753-4ebd-84b3-cf83bad1ef2f

Mezirow, J. (1997). Transformative learning: Theory to practice. *New Directions for Adult and Continuing Education,* (74), 5–12. https://doi.org/10.1002/ace.7401

U.S. Department of Health and Human Services. (2017, January 19). *Code of federal regulations.* https://www.gpo.gov/fdsys/pkg/CFR-2016-title45-vol1/pdf/CFR-2016-title45-vol1-part46.pdf

U.S. Department of Health and Human Services. (2018, revised). *Federal policy for the protection of human subjects.* Revised Common Rule. https://www.hhs.gov/ohrp/regulations-and-policy/regulations/finalized-revisions-common-rule/index.html

APPENDICES

Appendix 7.A Example of Experiential Plan

Appendix 7.B Example of Experiential Plan

Appendix 7.C Sample Abbreviated IRB Summary

Appendix 7-A

INDIANA UNIVERSITY DOCTORAL CAPSTONE EXPERIENTIAL PLAN

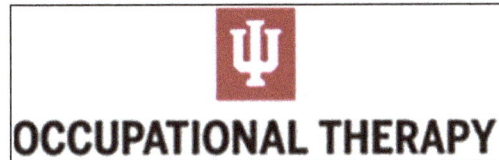

OCCUPATIONAL THERAPY

OTD Capstone Student: Grace Gillen (OTD class of 2025)

Primary Area of Focus: Education/research

Secondary Area of Focus (may or may not have this secondary area): N/A

OTD Capstone Student Roles and Responsibilities:

- Being **self-directed** throughout the entire doctoral capstone process, including developing, planning, and completing the capstone experience and project
- Working collaboratively with the content expert/site mentor and capstone coordinator and faculty mentor to create individual learning objectives for the doctoral experience that are in alignment with the OT program student outcomes
- Working collaboratively with the site mentor and capstone coordinator/faculty to create specific goals and objectives for the capstone project
- Completing a needs assessment, literature review, and evaluation plan that aligns with the curriculum design prior to the start of the capstone experience
- Collaborating with the content expert/site mentor on a plan for supervision and mentorship
- Ensuring that the doctoral capstone experiential plan is collaboratively developed and signed by student, content expert/site mentor, faculty mentor, and capstone coordinator
- Obeying all policy and procedures of the facility unless exempted, including prompt notification of absences
- Fulfilling all duties and completing all assignments made by the content expert/site mentor, unless exempted, within the time limit specified
- Completing all assignments per T880 and T830 course syllabi, including biweekly online discussions, synthesizing knowledge as demonstrated by submission of final capstone report to IUI Scholarworks, and at minimum, dissemination of project at the IU OT Doctoral Capstone Poster Presentation Showcase
- Completing 560 hours during the 14-week doctoral experience and documenting these hours on CORE; at least 80% on-site, all absences made up
    - **Prior fieldwork or work experience may neither contribute nor be substituted for these requirements.**
    - Time spent off site may include independent study activities, such as research and writing.
- Evaluating the content/site mentor and site to help continue to improve educational outcomes
- Keeping open lines of communication with the content expert/site mentor, faculty mentor, and doctoral capstone coordinator

Site Name and Address: Indiana University Indianapolis, Health Sciences Building: IU OT's T643 Children and Youth Practice Course, 1050 Wishard Blvd., Indianapolis, Indiana 46202

Content Expert/Site Mentor Name and Contact Information: Dr. Leah Van Antwerp: learvana@iu.edu

Content Expert/Site Mentor Credentials and Area of Expertise (ACOTE D.1.2): OTD, MS, OTR, PMH-C; pediatrics

Content Expert/Site Mentor Roles and Responsibilities:

- Providing expertise in the student's area of focus (**the site mentor does not have to be an OT**)
- Providing résumé to IU to verify expertise
- Providing orientation to the site, site personnel, and stakeholders
- Collaborating with the student to develop individual learning objectives for the DC experience and specific goals and objectives for the DC project
- Evaluating the student at the midpoint and the conclusion of the DC experience
- Working collaboratively with the student on developing a plan for mentorship and supervision as agreed upon in experiential plan.

- Verifying student hours completed on CORE
- Notifying the doctoral capstone coordinator if problems arise and collaborating with the student, doctoral capstone coordinator, and faculty mentor on plan of correction

Faculty Mentor: Julie A. Bednarski, OTD, MHS, OTR

Faculty Mentor Roles and Responsibilities:

- Collaborating to ensure the DC experience and project are consistent with the IU OT program curricular design and reflect the mission and philosophy of our program
- Collaborating with the student and capstone coordinator to ensure the doctoral capstone experiential plan is developed and includes individual student learning objectives for the DC experience and specific goals and objectives for the DC project
- Grading the final capstone report in preparation for the student to submit to IUI Scholarworks
- Keeping in biweekly contact via an on-line discussion board during the DC experience
- Providing feedback to the student as it relates to the development and presentation of the capstone project poster
- Collaborating with the content expert/site mentor as needed
- Being available to the student as a resource and consultant
- Notifying the doctoral capstone coordinator if problems arise and collaborating with the student, doctoral capstone coordinator, and site mentor on plan of correction

Capstone Coordinator: Annie L. Derolf, OTD, OTR

Capstone Coordinator Roles and Responsibilities:

- Ensuring the DC experience and project are consistent with the IU OT program curricular design and reflect the mission and philosophy of our program
- Ensuring a contract is signed between IU and each site
- Working collaboratively with the student to create individual learning objectives for the doctoral experience that are in alignment with the OT program student outcomes
- Collaborating with the student to ensure the capstone experiential plan is developed and includes individual learning objectives for the DC experience, specific goals and objectives for the DC project, plan for evaluation, plan for supervision and mentoring, and that it is signed by all appropriate parties
- Educating faculty mentors and content experts/site mentors on roles and responsibilities
- Ensuring the length of the DC experience is 14 weeks (560 hours) and that no more than 20% of the time is completed outside the mentored practice setting
- Being available as a resource and consultant to the student, content expert/site mentor, and faculty mentor during the doctoral capstone experience
- Reviewing résumés of the site mentors to ensure expertise in the students' area of focus and verifying appropriate licensure and/or certifications
- Working with student to match to sites and identify a site mentor
- Working with the OT program director to assign appropriate faculty mentors
- Developing course syllabi for T880 and T830 and creating online discussion prompts for T880

Overall Student Learning Objectives for the Doctoral Capstone Experience: Designed by the OTD student in collaboration and aligned with the IU OT program educational outcomes and curriculum design (ACOTE D.1.3 and ACOTE D.1.4)

Curricular Thread: Socially responsive health care

Outcome: Graduates will demonstrate entry-level competencies in providing client-centered, inclusive, equitable, and research-informed care in professional practice.

Student Learning Objective 1: The student will demonstrate the ability to apply client-centered, inclusive, equitable, and evidence-informed care principles to the T643 course development and implementation.

Curricular Thread: Critical inquiry and reflective practice

Outcome: Graduates will be prepared to apply principles of evidence-based and evidence-informed decision-making in professional practice to improve and expand the delivery and quality of occupational therapy services.

Student Learning Objective 2: The student will demonstrate the ability to evaluate research studies and apply results to develop and implement evidence-based T643 course content.

Curricular Thread: Leadership and advocacy

Outcome: Graduates will demonstrate leadership and advocacy to promote health, well-being, and quality of life for people, populations, and communities.

Student Learning Objective 3: The student will demonstrate leadership skills in planning and leading T643 labs and lectures and will advocate for occupational therapy's role in promoting health, well-being, and quality of life for the pediatric population through the creation and implementation of relevant course materials.

Goals and Objectives for the Doctoral Capstone Project: Designed by the OTD student in collaboration with the capstone coordinator, faculty mentor, and content expert/site mentor (ACOTE D.1.4). *Number of goals and objectives will vary based on the student project.*

Project Goal 1: The student will develop an evidence-based curriculum to facilitate maximal learning outcomes among IU OTD students in the T643 course.

Objective 1: The student will collaborate with the site mentor/content expert to learn about existing evidence-based curriculum in the T643 course.

Objective 2: The student will collect research, using AJOT, PubMed, and Google Scholar to learn about current evidence in pediatric occupational therapy practice.

Objective 3: The student will collect feedback regarding the curriculum from the site mentor/content expert and utilize the feedback to modify the curriculum and course content prior to implementation.

Project Goal 2: The student will develop an updated T643 course syllabus, which will include occupation-based curriculum, applicable ACOTE standards, and best curricular design practices.

Objective 1: The student will research updated ACOTE standards and understand their application to the T643 course.

Objective 2: The student will gather and analyze information regarding current, occupation-based practice in pediatrics and synthesize this information for current T643 students.

Objective 3: The students will develop course content, with best curricular design practices, which will be outlined in the updated syllabus.

Project Goal 3: The student will facilitate sustainability of implementation of the evidence-informed T643 curriculum by developing and uploading accessible course content on IU's Canvas learning management system (LMS).

Objective 1: The student will designate accessible digital locations, on Canvas LMS, for the site mentor/content expert to retrieve and utilized the updated course content, evidence-informed curriculum, and educational materials for future T643 classes.

Objective 2: The student will develop physical copies of updated, evidence-informed curriculum and resources for current T643 students and designate a physical location for future T643 students to access the material.

Project Goal 4: The student will gain fundamental skills related to planning, teaching, and evaluating the effectiveness of their teaching of higher-level occupational therapy content to graduate students.

Objective 1: The student will utilize site mentor/content expert input to create evidence-based lectures, labs, and weekly content to address student learning needs.

Objective 2: The student will teach at least one lecture and one lab session, independently, for the T643 course.

Objective 3: The student will implement a pre- and post-survey check to students to evaluate their learning, for review of the student as an instructor, and to gather their feedback regarding revised course content and delivery.

Plan for Evaluation of the Evaluation, Supervision, and Mentorship (D.1.4)

1. The student will be supervised by the content/site mentor.
2. The student will only participate in activities as approved by the content/site mentor.
3. If the student is providing skilled occupational therapy services, the supervision guidelines for the provision of occupational therapy services by students for each particular state are required.
4. If the content/site mentor is not available to supervise the student for a particular time frame (i.e., vacation), the site and mentor will identify a replacement supervisor for that particular time period.
5. The student may spend additional time at other locations within the site organization as assigned by the site mentor.
6. This is a 560-hour doctoral experience. At least 80% of those hours must be spent at the doctoral experience site. Any absences must be made up to get to 560 hours to ensure successful completion of the doctoral experience. The content expert/site mentor will verify hours in CORE.
7. The content expert/site mentor will complete a midterm and final evaluation of the student in CORE (D.1.7).
8. The student will complete an evaluation of the site in CORE at the completion of the capstone experience.
9. The student and site mentor will determine a plan for the supervision/mentoring meetings

10. The student and content expert/site mentor plan for mentorship is as follows:
    - The student and content expert will meet each Monday to plan for the week.
    - The student will attend all lectures and labs T643 with gradual increase of responsibilities.
    - The content expert will be available to meet after T643 lecture and lab on a weekly basis to provide mentorship.

Plan for Measuring/Reporting Outcomes: The student is required to collect data to demonstrate the effectiveness of their chosen project. Data collected may be qualitative, quantitative, or a mixed-method study. *There is no stated requirement of scale of data to be collected, simply a requirement that the data collected directly support or refute the expected outcomes of the study.* A departmental research coordinator will review and certify this plan is feasible, appropriate, and methodologically sound.

Plan for Dissemination and Authorship: The student is required to present the results of the capstone project that relates to the capstone experience in order to demonstrate how knowledge was gained and synthesis of knowledge occurred (D.1.6). The student will publish their capstone report in IUI Scholarworks and also complete a poster presentation in May at the IU OTD Capstone Presentation Showcase. If the student plans to disseminate beyond this, the student is required to complete the *document of capstone authorship* (DCA) with appropriate signatures and attach to this document. Note: Materials developed for the site during the capstone experience (i.e. handouts, program protocols, etc.) by the student are the property of the site unless otherwise noted here.

By signing and dating below, you are agreeing with this student learning plan (ACOTE D.1.4)

Student:

Director of Research:

Content Expert/Site Mentor:

Faculty Mentor:

Capstone Coordinator:

Appendix 7-B

EXPERIENTIAL PLAN AND WRITTEN AGREEMENT FOR THE OCCUPATIONAL THERAPY DOCTORAL (OTD) CAPSTONE

SECTION I

OTD Student Name: _____

Area of Primary Focus:

☐ Clinical Skills   ☐ Advocacy   ☐ Program Development/Evaluation

☐ Research Skills   ☐ Policy Development   ☐ Leadership

☐ Administration   ☐ Education   ☐ Other (please describe): _____

Area of Secondary Focus (If Applicable):

☐ Clinical Skills   ☐ Advocacy   ☐ Program Development/Evaluation

☐ Research Skills   ☐ Policy Development   ☐ Leadership

☐ Administration   ☐ Education   ☐ Other (please describe): _____

Faculty Chair Name:

Name of DCE Site: _____

DCE Setting: _____

Primary Content Expert for the Doctoral Capstone (Name, Title, and Credentials):

_____

Content Expert Preferred Email Address: _____

Content Expert Preferred Phone: _____

Description of Qualifications of Content Expert Aligned With the Focus Area: Please also attach a current curriculum vitae (CV), résumé, or document informing of your expertise in the focus area of the doctoral capstone.

General Overview of Doctorate Capstone Experience (DCE) and Project (100 words or less):*

*This may be subject to change based on the completion of the needs assessment but is meant to ensure the content expert and OTD student are considering the capstone project in similar ways. Please attach a Word document to this form providing this general overview.

*Page 1 should be completed by the OTD student.

SECTION II: RELATIONSHIP TO DUQUESNE UNIVERSITY CURRICULUM DESIGN ACKNOWLEDGMENT OF THE DUQUESNE UNIVERSITY OCCUPATIONAL THERAPY DOCTORAL PROGRAM BEHAVIORAL OBJECTIVES

Following are the OTD DCE learning objectives aligned with the curriculum design at Duquesne University (https://www.duq.edu/academics/schools/health-sciences/academic). You will see that there is space provided for the OTD student and you, the content expert, to mutually decide upon three student-specific objectives that would be achievable within the 14-week experience. These should align with the student's chosen area of focus. Once the three objectives are agreed to, students should continue to collaborate with you to outline action steps, activities, or strategies to help achieve their goals (see action plan and weekly schedule template provided).

1. Demonstrate effective communication skills and work interprofessionally with those who receive and provide care/services.
2. Display positive interpersonal skills and insight into one's professional behaviors to accurately appraise one's professional disposition strengths and areas for improvement.
3. Exhibit the ability to practice educative roles for consumers, peers, students, interprofessionals, and others.
4. Develop essential knowledge and skills to contribute to the advancement of occupational therapy through scholarly activities.
5. Apply a critical foundation of evidence-based professional knowledge, skills, and attitudes.

6. Apply principles and constructs of ethics to individual, institutional, and societal issues, and articulate justifiable resolutions to these issues and act in an ethical manner.

7. Perform tasks in a safe and ethical manner and that adhere to the site's policies and procedures, including those related to human subject research, when relevant.

8. Demonstrate competence in following program methods, quality improvement, and/or research procedures utilized at the site.

9. Learn, practice, and apply knowledge from the classroom and practice settings at a higher level than prior fieldwork experiences with simultaneous guidance from site mentor and DU OT faculty.

10. Relate theory to practice and demonstrate synthesis of advanced knowledge in a specialized practice area through completion of a doctoral field experience and scholarly project.

11. Acquire in-depth experience in one or more of the following areas: clinical practice skills, research skills, administration, leadership, program and policy development, advocacy, education, and theory development.

12. (Student-identified objective.)

13. (Student-identified objective.)

14. (Student-identified objective.)

Content Expert Signature: _____ Date: _____

OTD Student Signature: _____ Date: _____

Section III: Content Expert Acknowledgment of Supervision/Mentorship

I, _____, agree to:
(Content expert name)

1. Serve as a content expert to _____ during a 14-week DCE placement, which includes regular (at least weekly) communication.

2. Collaborate with the OTD student to create three individualized student learning objectives to customize this capstone experience.

3. Provide guidance and mentorship to the student's action plan to support accomplishment of the student learning objectives over the 14-week placement.

4. Complete a midterm and final evaluation of the OTD student using the DCE evaluation of the OTD student.

5. Communicate with the doctoral capstone coordinator regarding any concerns or needs during the experience.

6. Collaborate with the OTD student and be listed as a contributing author (as appropriate) regarding scholarly products, including, but not limited to, manuscripts, presentations, and posters.

7. Provide documentation of expertise in the OTD student's chosen focus area(s) by submitting a copy of a résumé, CV, or continued education in the area(s).*

8. Review content expert materials and supplemental materials provided by the doctoral capstone coordinator.

This may include years of experience, certifications, workshops, etc. Please contact the doctoral capstone coordinator with any questions regarding this.

Content Expert Signature:_____Date:_____

Section IV: OTD Student Acknowledgment of Supervision/ Mentorship with the Content Expert

I, _____, agree to:
(OTD student name)

1. Initiate a discussion with the content expert to create three individualized student learning objectives to customize this capstone experience using the DCE behavioral objectives form.

2. Collaborate with the content expert on an action plan designed to accomplish the individualized student learning objectives.

3. Work together with the content expert to create a schedule that will consist of at least 32 hours of on-site activity per week over the course of 14 weeks.

4. Create and implement a capstone project informed by evidenced and based upon a needs assessment at the DCE site.

5. Complete the student evaluation of the DCE site form at the completion of the DCE.

6. Proactively communicate with the content expert regarding any questions during the experience.

7. Proactively communicate with the doctoral capstone coordinator regarding any concerns or needs during the experience.

8. Collaborate with and include my content expert, faculty chair, and any other appropriate parties as contributing authors on scholarly products, including, but not limited to, manuscripts, presentations, and posters.

9. Demonstrate respectful interaction and communication with the student cohort, faculty, mentors, doctoral capstone coordinator, and other individuals who may be a part of the capstone.

10. Utilize constructive feedback from faculty, the content expert, my faculty chair, and the doctoral capstone coordinator for personal and professional growth.

11. Take responsibility for his or her own skills and professional development. (This can include professional writing skills, knowledge of IRB application process, maintaining my AOTA membership, updating all clearances as required before expiration within EXXAT, etc. . . .)

12. Complete and disseminate a culminating capstone project in a format and forum within the time frame determined by the academic program.

OTD Student Signature: _____ Date: _____

SECTION V: COLLABORATION FOR DESIGNING THE DOCTORAL CAPSTONE

The following signatures ensure that the doctoral capstone is designed through collaboration with the student, a faculty member in the occupational therapy educational program who holds a doctoral degree, and an individual with documented expertise in the content area of the capstone.

Please sign in what follows and attach a copy of the mentoring compact:

Faculty Chair Signature: _____ Date: _____

OTD Student Signature: _____ Date: _____

Submit this form into EXXAT and within Canvas assignments with supporting documentation to the doctoral capstone coordinator within the course-designated due date after completion of the needs assessment:

Michelle McCann, OTD, OTR/L, C/NDT, CBIS, PPSC

Duquesne University, #224 Health Science Building

600 Forbes Ave, Pittsburgh, PA 15282

Department Phone: 412–396–4216

mccannm2@duq.edu

Appendix 7-C

> DUQUESNE UNIVERSITY Rangos School
> of Health Sciences Department of
> Occupational Therapy

Sample Abbreviated IRB Protocol

Instructions:
The Protocol Summary is limited to 3–6 single spaced pages using a 12-point font. Appendices may include but are not limited to items such as a consent form, data collection tools or recruitment flyers and these are not included in the page limits. Each appendix must be submitted to in a separate file and named accordingly (e.g. Recruitment Flyer.docx). Similarly, instruments for data collection may be submitted in WORD or PDF and included as an appendix. The page limitation does not include appendices or attachments. You are provided the specific content guidelines below. Once reviewed and approved by your capstone coordinator and/or faculty (or capstone chair), you will be asked to submit this protocol summary to the IRB Board.

SPECIFIC CONTENT: The following sections with headings MUST be addressed. Each of these components are evaluated by the Institutional Review Board. If you do not use these specific headings, your protocol summary may be rejected

1) **Statement of the research question:** You must use this heading, but you may not have a specific research question. It is appropriate to make this section only a sentence or two and to qualify your content by identifying the focus of your capstone, i.e.program development, program evaluation, quality improvement or staff training nature of your capstone project. When your capstone has multiple parts, you are encouraged to focus on any one of these. That is, even though your project may have many parts choose one component. In particular, choose a part of the project that may most lend itself to preparing for formal dissemination, such as presentation or publication.

2) **Purpose and significance of the study:** Use language like, "the purpose and significance of this program evaluation or this staff training project or this quality improvement project is . . . ". In this section you should draw directly from the earlier capstone drafts you have created. You are not providing and the IRB board does not want to see a full-blown literature review. A synopsis and summation will suffice. Bear in mind that you are not trying to convince the reader of your knowledge of all the relevant background literature. Your purpose in this section is to provide a context for the program or training that you are describing in the protocol. You are encouraged to judiciously choose statements from your needs assessment that helps you make strong arguments, e.g., a preliminary needs assessment revealed that the staff at this community facility had a strong interest in improving programming for adults with IDD and in improving their own skill sets for increasing participation with individual consumers - OR - a preliminary needs assessment revealed that parents and teachers alike identified several areas where communication in IEP meetings might be improved.

3) **Research design and procedures:** Use language like, "this project is designed as a program evaluation or this project is designed as a staff training project or this project is designed as a quality improvement project to . . . ". The work you have already completed to describe project implementation can inform this section. Again, remember in a project that may have many component parts choose one or a few related parts that go hand in hand most effectively and which can be described efficiently

4) **Instruments:** Be matter of fact. If the tool is a published tool, then your descriptions in your earlier capstone propsoal will suffice. If you created the tool, describe the tool BRIEFLY. You will need to upload each tool that your use and describe in your appendices section. Remember, don't load tools for components of your project that you are not including in this protocol summary submission.

5) **Sample selection and size**: Be matter of fact. Most of you are working with convenience samples. You are encouraged to not identify protected populations as your sample as this invited the highest level of scrutiny by the IRB. For example, many of you are working in programs that directly impact children while others are looking at adults with cognitive limitations such as IDD or dementia. These are protected populations for human subjects research. However, you all are also including the parents, caregivers, teachers or staff working with these protected populations and you want to emphasize that group as your sample.

6) **Recruitment of subjects**: Be matter of fact. How will you identify and recruit? If you use a flyer or some other mechanism like this, include a copy in your Appendices and write a short, succinct but clear description of your procedures.

7) **Informed consent procedures**: Be straightforward and define the process. Include the who, what, when and how. You will need to include a copy of the consent form in your appendices.

8) **Collection of data and method of data analysis:** Be specific and state what data will be collected and by what means. Again, only discuss the tools you will use that correspond to the parts of your project that you are describing in this protocol. Any tools you describe need to be loaded as appendices. You do not have to go into critical details of your data analysis plan but do provide a description of what you will do.

9) **Emphasize issues relating to interactions with subjects and subjects' rights**: The critically key element in your descriptions is DE-IDENTIFICATION. Only collect information that you absolutely need should be collected and human subjects concerns are all about confidentiality. I've included I've included an example of "template language" that has worked in previous proposals. You should feel free to delete what does not apply and to change titles of tools to consistently and accurately reflect what you will do.

CHAPTER 8

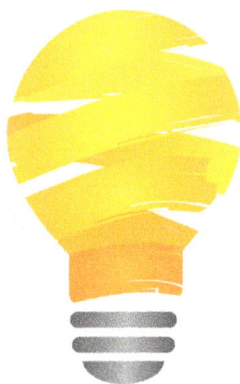

Create a Plan to Evaluate Project Outcomes and Sustainability Considerations

Amy Mattila and Elena V. Donoso Brown

Section 1: Student Focus

Human-Centered Design Mindsets for Doctoral Students

Human-centered design mindset concepts of optimism and creative confidence are important for doctoral students to embrace as they begin to problem-solve the sustainability of their project.

Optimism. As you think through how your project can be sustained, keep a positive focus. Be optimistic that your project can continue. Determine how you can overcome barriers, and limit constraints that might be preventing your project from being carried on after you are no longer at the site.

Creative confidence. You gained confidence in your ability to find solutions and create a meaningful project at your site; now, keep up that creative confidence as you think about your project sustainability. Trust yourself; trust that you will find a solution.

INTRODUCTION FOR STUDENTS

The concept of sustainability is gaining importance in all aspects of health care, from project design and management to service delivery. *Sustainability* can also often refer to the health of the clients that are served – for example, how programs designed around prevention or evidence-based practice ultimately led to sustained independence and quality of life. To ensure sustainability in a doctoral capstone project that is delivered in this current system, students need to be well-versed in the feasibility of the project, the desirability from all stakeholders, and in the end, the viability of the program long term. For successful implementation of a doctoral capstone project, you need to be knowledgeable in not only these design-centered concepts but also the evaluation processes that should occur in each phase of planning, implementation, and finalization of the doctoral capstone experience (DCE). This chapter begins with the overarching theme of sustainability and uses this as a frame to explore the evaluation of processes and outcomes and the development of a data analysis plan.

DOI: 10.4324/9781003541813-10

STUDENT REFLECTIVE QUESTIONS

During the implementation phase of the doctoral capstone, you may find it helpful to reflect on the following questions:

1. How can you consider sustainability, feasibility, and desirability in each stage of your capstone project?

2. How does program evaluation used during the capstone project support evidence-based practice?

3. Using the tables available in this chapter, what study design and statistical analysis would be most useful to you in establishing whether you have achieved statistically or clinically significant capstone project outcomes?

STUDENT OBJECTIVES

By the end of reading this chapter and completing the learning activities, the reader should be able to:

1. Describe processes that will support the sustainability of the doctoral capstone project.

2. Identify three ways that sustainability is supported through program evaluation.

3. Define the purpose of a logic or conceptual model in the program evaluation process.

4. Compare and contrast outcome and process evaluations and their corresponding research methods.

5. Describe methods for planning, implementing, and analyzing data from a program evaluation.

6. Identify characteristics that will support success in managing unexpected challenges in the program evaluation process.

SUSTAINABILITY

The sustainability of the capstone project should be a key outcome of the overall doctoral capstone experience. *Sustainability*, a term often used in project and health-care management, can be defined as "a component that ensures preservation of resources, is practical from ecological, social, and economical perspectives, and meets the interests of different stakeholders" (Molero et al., 2021). In project management (PM), *sustainability* also often refers to continuity planning and stakeholder engagement, two concepts that are particularly important in the DCE, where the capstone student is often the "outsider" in the organization. The understanding of *sustainability* from a PM perspective will be further explored in this section of the chapter.

The Substance Abuse and Mental Health Services Administration (SAMHSA, 2023, para. 4) defines *health-care project sustainability* as part of their Strategic Prevention Framework (SPF) model as "the process of building an adaptive and effective system that achieves and maintains desired long-term results." In many cases for the DCE, community engagement and buy-in are an extremely important part of whether the program remains stable, particularly for students placed at a role-emerging or community-based practice setting.

Having the goal of sustainability in mind throughout the planning, implementation, and finalization of the DCE process will help ensure that successful programs are supported not only at the occupational therapy level but also for the organization and even community as a whole. Fostering a mindset of sustainability and understanding the concept of capacity building can help you increase the organization's ability to respond to the changes put in place with innovative solutions created by the DCE and capstone project.

Capacity building is the idea that organizations can use a range of activities to expand or change directions that add to the functioning or "health" of the organization. The United Nations was one of the first organizations to develop the term and defines *capacity* as "the ability of individuals, institutions, and societies to perform functions, solve problems, and set and achieve objectives in a sustainable manner" (United Nations, 2006, p. 7). The two concepts can go hand in hand to allow you, the capstone student, to infuse sustainability and capacity building practice into your DCE and capstone project.

FRAMEWORKS OF SUSTAINABILITY

As mentioned earlier, *sustainability* and *capacity building* are used in many practices, from business and PM to health-care systems, and even in environmental design and development. Three key frameworks of sustainability are discussed in this chapter: PM models, the Substance Use and Mental Health Services Administration (SAMHSA) model, and the Occupational Therapy Intervention Process Model (OTIPM). Each of these models can provide a blueprint for a capstone student to continually plan, reflect, and respond to sustainable project practices.

PM is gaining interest with many health-care managers, including occupational therapists. With ever-increasing costs, waste, and diversity in the health-care system, a growing number of practitioners are taking courses in PM, such as Lean Six Sigma, or the Project Management Academy (Palm & Fischier, 2021). There is also a rising number of stakeholders in the health-care environment. It is no longer a simple "therapist–client relationship," but often, it is the provider, client, insurance, organization, or even government who can dictate how, why, and when the care can occur. For example, for occupational therapy practitioners to be successful in their clinical reasoning of an individual post-stroke, they need to understand the complex relationship between the client, the authorized length of stay, the continuum of care, and the interdisciplinary plans, to name just a

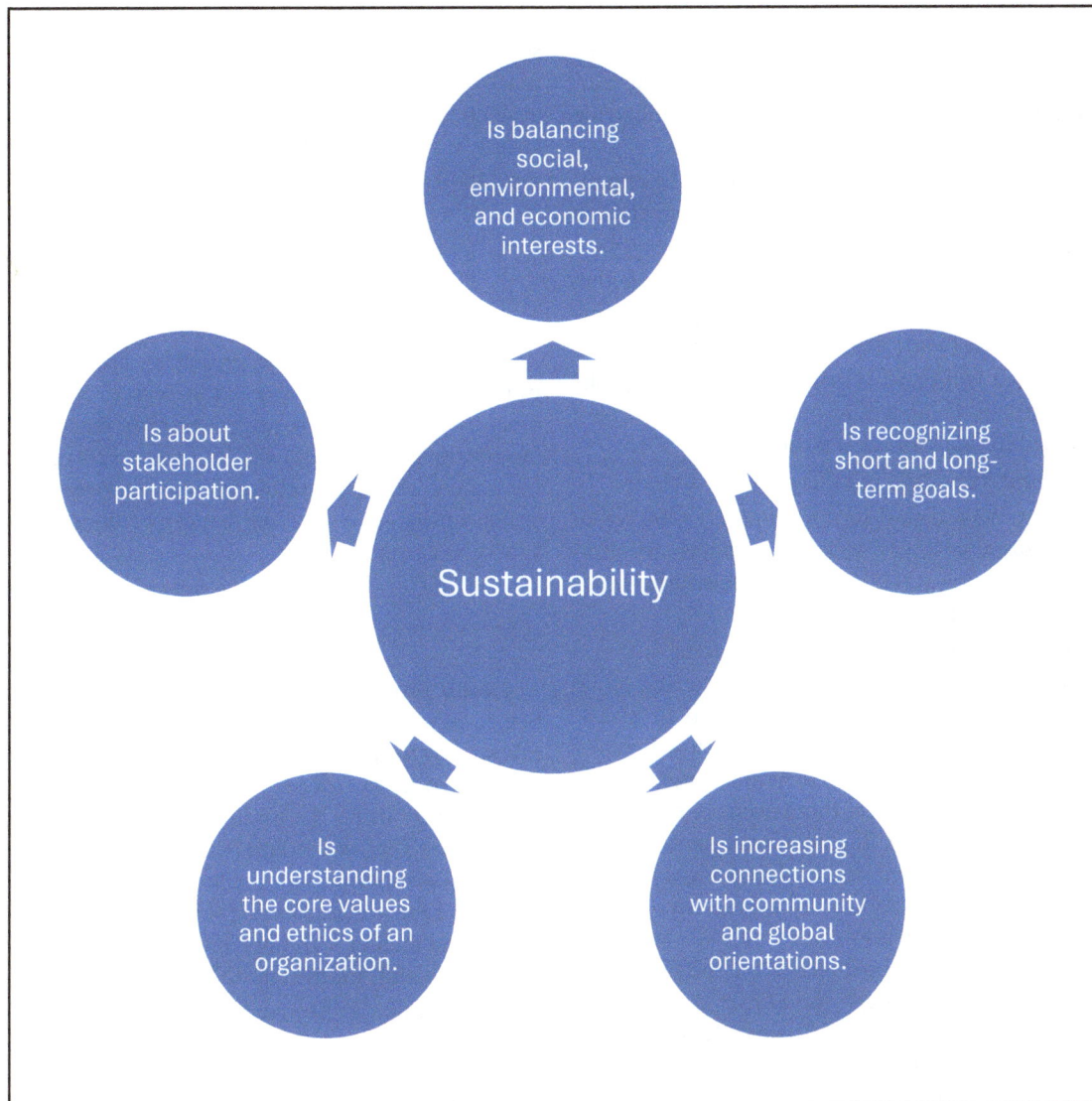

Figure 8-1. Dimensions of sustainability. *Source:* Adapted from Silvius, A. J. G., and Schipper, R. (2012). Sustainability in the business case. *Proceedings of the 26th IPMA world congress*, Crete, Greece, pp. 1,062–1,069. fig8–1.jpg.

few of the important factors at hand. As you learn about the greater impact of your potential project, it is more apparent than ever that you will need to have the skills to identify and work, from conception to completion, with all parties involved.

In addition to the stakeholders, PM provides a framework for understanding the social, economic, and environmental consequences associated with the design and execution of projects, such as the capstone (Thomson et al., 2011). Considering each of these concepts in the early stages of the doctoral capstone can allow you as a capstone student to obtain the necessary models, metrics, and tools that will ultimately allow for sustainable outcomes, which are further described later in this chapter. Figure 8.1 provides an overview of some of the key PM-based dimensions of sustainability that should be reflected on throughout the capstone experience.

The ideas of sustainability and capacity building are also heavily present in health-care prevention and community services, such as the World Health Organization (WHO) and SAMHSA. These concepts have a great fit in these organizations because their primary roles are to respond to the needs and resources of communities and populations as a whole. According to SAMHSA's Strategic Prevention Framework (SPF), the organization uses *capacity building* to "understand various types and levels of resources available to establish and maintain a community prevention system that can identify and respond to community needs" (SAMHSA, 2023, para. 1). Capstone students can utilize the logic model set forth by this organization as a step-by-step guide to developing relationships, including stakeholders, and becoming champions for their projects and roles. Logic models will be defined and discussed in detail later in this Chapter.

SAMHSA's (2019) SPF has suggested a five-step process using a data-driven, change-based model that capstone students could potentially use for ensuring the sustainability of their project. The model includes the following stages:

1. *Assess needs.* What is the problem within the organization or population? How can I learn more and dig deeper into this issue?
2. *Build capacity.* What are the resources available that I have to work with? Are there ways I can acquire further resources to help my mission and vision?
3. *Plan.* What is it that I actually hope to accomplish? How should I carry this out and ensure I have included the appropriate stakeholders?
4. *Implement.* How can I put this plan into action?
5. *Evaluate.* What data-driven tools have I gathered to ensure sustainability? Can I define whether my project is succeeding as well as meeting the original needs of the organization or population?

One of the distinctive features of this model is that it encourages assessment as more than just a starting point. As you use this framework, they will return to assessment repeatedly throughout their project because it allows them to recognize that as the needs of their organization changes, their capacity to meet those needs or create programming will also evolve. The additional benefit of this model is that it goes beyond simply identifying stakeholders but also encourages a team-based approach, consistent with most health-care environments where you will work beyond graduation. Additional resources, online courses, and tools are available through the SAMHSA Center for the Application of Prevention Technologies and are listed in the "Resource" section of this chapter.

The final framework explored in this chapter is unique to occupational therapy: the OTIPM. This model, originally introduced in 2002 by Anne G. Fisher and Kristin Bray Jones (Fisher & Jones, 2009), has been practiced more recently as a framework for long-term improvement projects by Sirkka et al. (2014). The authors of this study aimed to understand how the OTIPM could drive long-term improvement work on an occupational therapy unit and found it to be a meaningful process to support sustainable improvements in practice. Capstone students could potentially use a similar framework as they evolve their project and ensure sustainability and long-term improvement outcomes are met in all phases of design. Table 8.1 provides an example of how aligning the components of the OTIPM with factors to consider in a sustainable capstone project could potentially benefit an organization.

The use of this occupational therapy model of practice can guide capstone students in an improvement process that ensures sustainability is infused throughout each phase of the DCE and capstone project.

Regardless of what framework is chosen to guide sustainability and capacity building, having the tools to make a lasting impact at the capstone site will be an invaluable skill for the entry-level doctoral student. Sustainability practice requires constant planning, reflection, and re-evaluation. The plan needs to be practical and feasible to ensure not only student success but also buy-in and implementation on the part of the capstone site.

EVALUATION OF PROCESS AND OUTCOMES

For a doctoral capstone project to sustain itself over time, it is imperative, as noted in several of the models described here, that the project provide data to support how it was implemented, as well as the benefit of its implementation. This next section provides an overview of the types of program evaluation that can be done with corresponding examples.

OVERVIEW OF EVALUATION METHODS

Health program evaluation is a cyclical process that begins with understanding what the program is and does, followed by the generation of questions and well-designed methods to answer those questions, and circles back to the beginning by using the findings to change the program (Centers for Disease Control [CDC], 2024). Therefore, the following sections present the process of program evaluation, from the initial planning stages, through implementation, and ending with data analysis, interpretation, and program modifications (Figure 8.2).

Before walking through the three stages of program evaluation, understanding the different categories of program evaluation is critical. The CDC (2024) outlines a total of five different types of program evaluations: formative, process, outcome, impact, and economic evaluations. The three most likely to be used in a capstone project are formative, process, and outcome. A *formative evaluation* is beneficial for new programs because it looks at new programs' feasibility and acceptability (CDC, 2024). As you may be starting something new at your site, this type of evaluation could be useful in identifying if you were able to recruit people to the program and if they were satisfied with the experience. The next type of evaluation that could be highly relevant as part of a capstone project is a *process or implementation evaluation.* This type of evaluation can focus on a variety of topics, including reach, attendance, use of materials or resources, as well as areas, such as quality of the program (CDC, 2024; Suarez-Balcazar et al., 2024). This type of evaluation is helpful if you are augmenting a program that is already running or identifying key areas that contribute to program success or failure (CDC, 2024; Suarez-Balcazar et al., 2024). Both formative and process evaluations can use quantitative or qualitative methods to answer their evaluation questions. Finally, an *outcome evaluation* as

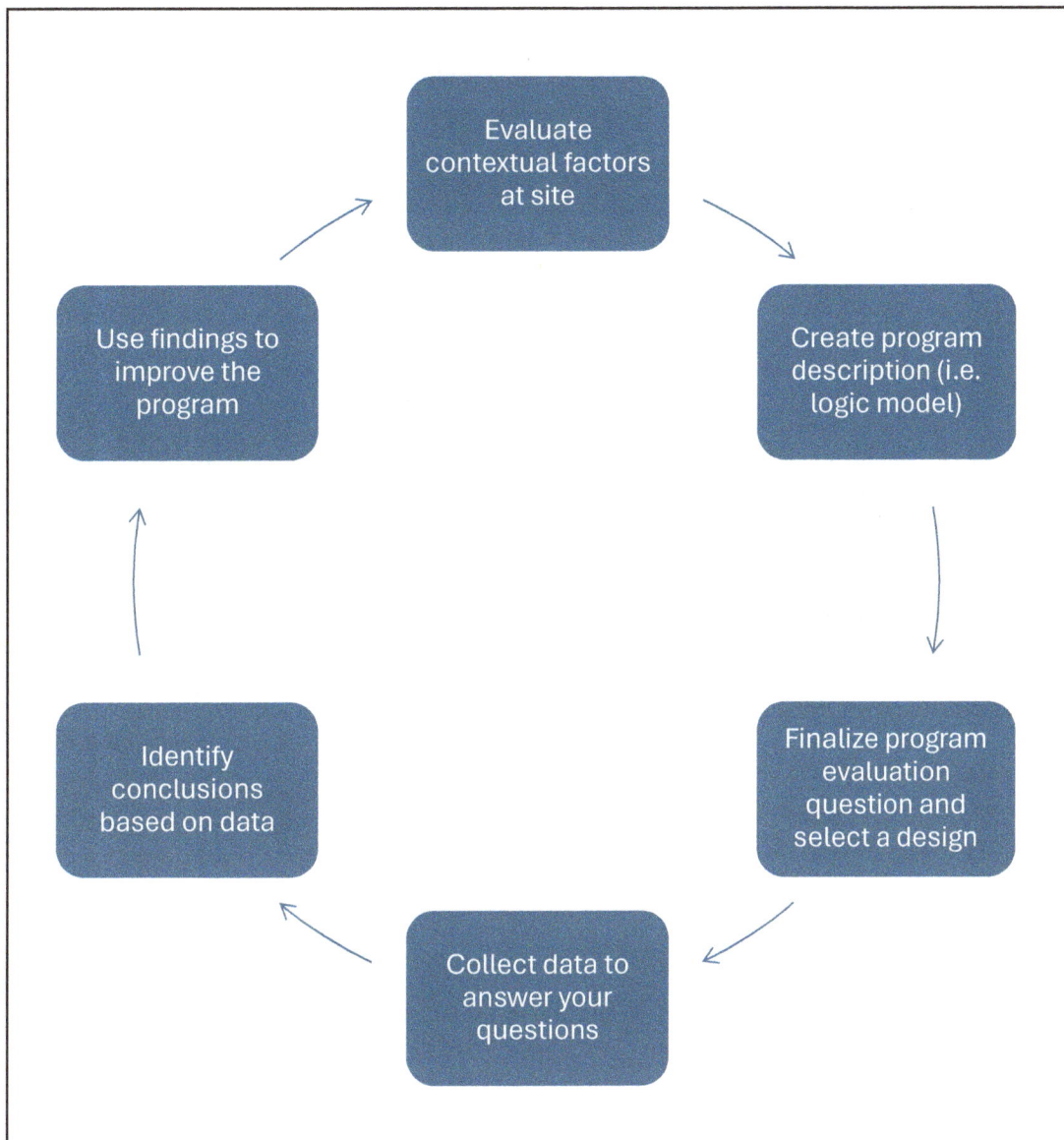

Figure 8-2. Cyclical process of program evaluation. *Source:* Adapted from CDC (2024). fig8–2.jpg.

defined by the CDC (2024) could be of value in identifying if the program is achieving its intended results. This type of evaluation typically uses a quasi-experimental research design to determine whether the program resulted in an effect on the target outcome areas (CDC, 2024; Suarez-Balcazar et al., 2024).

Doctoral Capstone Program Evaluation Planning

In many of the models described here, the concept of evaluation is presented as the last step, but the process of how you will evaluate the doctoral capstone project should be planned in concert with the project itself. (See Text Box 8.1.)

This begins with an understanding of how you think your program works (Suarez-Balcazar et al., 2024). This is often represented in the form of a logic model. This concept is common throughout program development and is a key element of not only planning your program but also planning the evaluation (Suarez-Balcazar et al., 2024). Logic models contain information on resources, activities, outputs, and outcomes at the short-term, midterm, and long-term time points. The development of the logic model will be informed by the needs assessment, epidemiological information about the population to be served through the program, and information from various forms of evidence, including peer-reviewed research. Inputs are needed to run the program and goes in the first column (CDC, 2024), this includes elements like the participants, environment, and materials needed. Next is the activities column, which outlines what would be done in the program, which should draw from the peer-reviewed literature to ensure that effective practices are being integrated into the program but also consider the characteristics of the site. Next, the logic model outlines both outputs and outcomes (CDC, 2024). Outputs are direct results of the program that will indicate the feasibility of a program, such as the number of family members who use the iPad to access materials. Outputs are often measured as part of a process evaluation. Outcomes are the areas in which change is anticipated, given the selected interventions, such as agitation.

For example, Figure 8.3 is an example of a logic model for a doctoral capstone project at a skilled nursing facility that was designed to address the issue of agitation for residents with dementia through the use of technology with both residents and their families. This example illustrates that a solid understanding of how the doctoral capstone

project is expected to work can support an understanding of what to measure in a program evaluation.

It is also possible to integrate the guiding theory into the logic model to ensure that the project remains directly connected to a guiding theory. See Appendix 8.A for a more updated logic model with theory. Once you have used a logic model to gain an understanding of how the program should work, the next step is developing a program evaluation plan.

PROGRAM EVALUATION PLAN

Once a logic model has been developed, you can begin to identify which questions are of the greatest importance to the site. Depending on the project, this may be an outcome-focused question, such as, "Do the comprehensive therapy services provided through interaction with and caring for animals in a farm context result in changes to social participation skills for children with autism spectrum disorder?" In this case, the program is already established, and the capstone student's focus may be more on supporting rigorous outcome measurement to use in future grant applications for the program. At the other end of the spectrum, a capstone student may be working with a site that has noted challenges with transition services and wishes for the doctoral student to complete a process

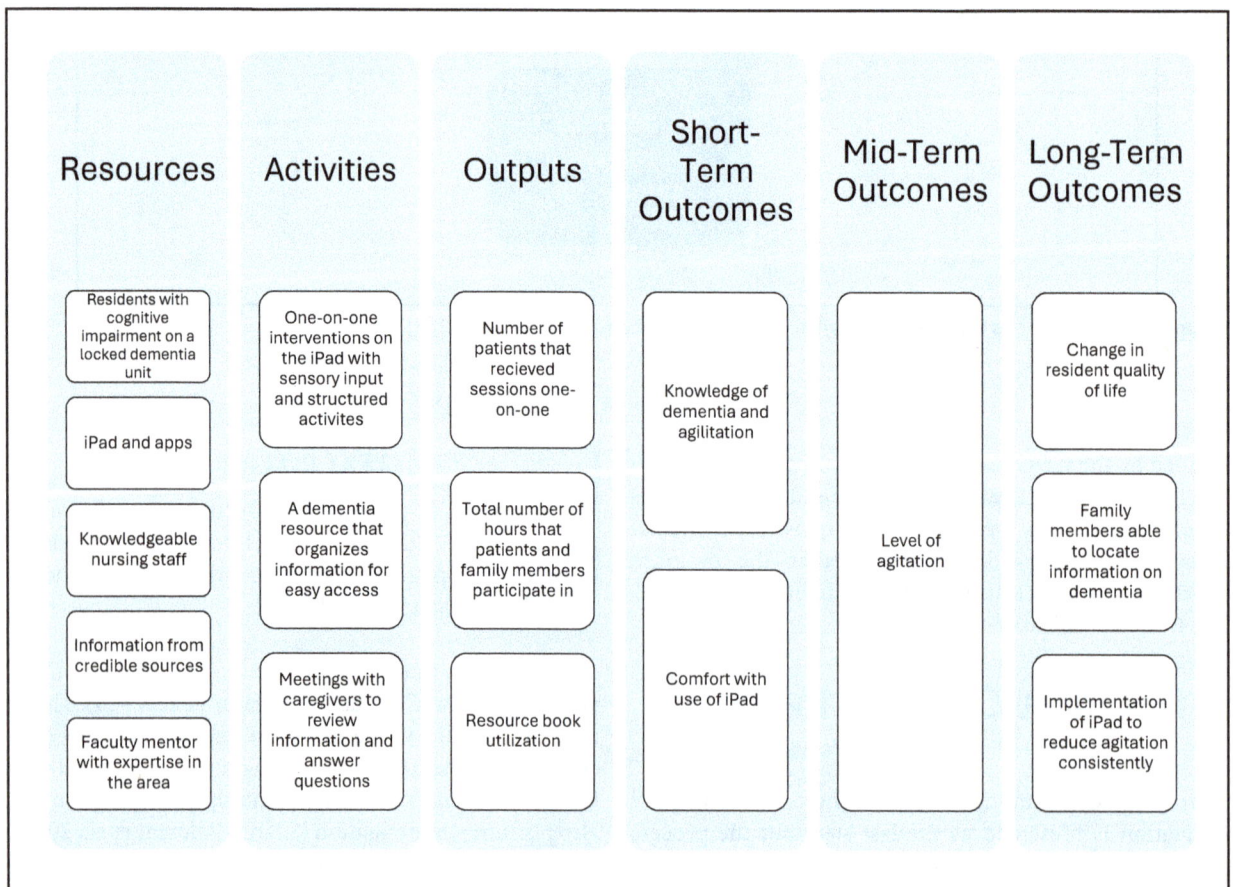

Figure 8-3. DCE logic model of the interpersonal approach to dementia program. *Source:* Reprinted with permission from Anna Olexsovich, OTD class of 2016, Duquesne University.

Table 8-1. Phases of the Occupational Therapy Intervention Process Model with Capstone Student Examples

PHASES	STEPS WITHIN THE PHASE*	POTENTIAL QUESTIONS AND CONSIDERATIONS FOR THE CAPSTONE STUDENT
Evaluation and goal-setting phase	Establish the client-centered performance context.	• What are the organization's values, mission, interest, and goals? • What roles are important to the organization? What does the organizational leadership look like? What is the expertise of the staff? • Does the organization have connections and relationships with others in the community or other health care context? • What are the daily routines of the organization? • What are the economic factors (funding) that influence the organization? • What are the rules, regulations, and policies that impact the organization? • What other conceptual models within occupational therapy will allow me to better understand the organization's perspective?
	Identify the organizations reported, and prioritize strengths and problems with occupational performance.	• Conduct a SWOT analysis. • On the basis of the needs, what occupation-focused tools can be used to gather to prepare for the next step in this process?
	Observe organizational performance.	• Engage in observation, interviews, focus groups, surveys, or other data-collection methods to gain a holistic picture of the organization and its needs. • Ensure these assessments are occurring within the natural context of the organization, and allow for multiple vantage points.
	Define and describe task actions the organization does and does not perform effectively.	• Using collected data, create a list of all task actions within the organization that are effective, and another list of those that are ineffective. • Select no more than 10 task actions from each list that best "capture" the performance of the site.
	Establish, redefine, or finalize goals of the organization.	• In this final step of the evaluation process, consider what might be the reasons for the gaps in services, decreased performance, or other organizational issues. • In direct collaboration with the organization, sustainable program development should be considered only from what is on this list.
Intervention phase	Select the goals to plan and implement a capstone project that addresses either educational programs, collaborative consultation, development of occupational skills, or acquisition/restoration of person factors and body functions.	In terms of sustainability and feasibility, the capstone student should consider the following factors for capstone project implementation: • Effective marketing • Price or funding for services • Length of project/timeline • Available resources (staff, equipment, time, etc.)

continued

Table 8-1. Phases of the Occupational Therapy Intervention Process Model with Capstone Student Examples (continued)

PHASES	STEPS WITHIN THE PHASE*	POTENTIAL QUESTIONS AND CONSIDERATIONS FOR THE CAPSTONE STUDENT
Re-evaluation phase	Re-evaluate for enhanced and satisfying performance of the organization.	• What was the effectiveness of my project/program? • What is my lasting relationship with the organization or community? • How will funding affect the sustainability of this project? • Do the staff have the expertise to continue, or should an occupational therapy practitioner be part of the organization? • What are opportunities for additional program integration?

Note: SWOT = strengths, weaknesses, opportunities, threats.

*In this example, the client is the organization.

evaluation that would answer the question "What are the barriers to addressing transition services?" and, possibly, "How do their clients, staff, and stakeholders want to address these challenges?" It is also possible for a capstone student to create and run the first iteration of a new program, for which a formative evaluation might be most relevant, as the questions could be, "Will this program be attended by our clients?" or "Are the content and activities in the program acceptable to the clients?"

It is possible to combine types of evaluation simultaneously, answering questions about the outcomes, experience, or feasibility of the program that was implemented. Using two types of designs may allow for the most robust picture of the program, which could support future sustainability. Once program evaluation questions have been determined, an appropriate design to answer these questions should be selected.

OUTCOME EVALUATION

As noted previously, outcome evaluations are typically quantitative in nature and are intended to measure whether a program made changes in the anticipated outcome areas (CDC, 2024; Suarez-Balcazar et al., 2024). As you may recall from prerequisite didactic courses in evidence-based practice and research methods, one of the strongest types of research designs is a randomized controlled trial (Portney, 2020). In this design, participants are prospectively assigned at random to either the control group or the experimental group. This design is strong because it reduces threats to internal validity, such as selection bias, through the process of randomization (Portney, 2020). It also increases the ability of a researcher to determine whether any observed change is due to the program. Despite the strengths of this type of design, it is generally impractical for implementation during a capstone project, due to time and resources needed to complete this design well. Given that you will

have limited time and resources to complete an outcome evaluation, it is strongly suggested that one of the following designs be considered in the doctoral capstone project: (1) pretest/posttest, (2) pretest/posttest with comparison group, (3) repeated measures design, or (4) single-subject design. The strengths and weakness of each design, as well as examples of use in capstone projects, are outlined in Table 8.2. These types of designs, although limited in their ability to demonstrate whether a change in outcome is due directly to the program, are feasible to complete within the time frame and resources most capstone students will have available to them for their projects.

FORMATIVE AND PROCESS EVALUATIONS

As formative and process evaluations answer different kinds of questions, designs for these types of evaluations span both quantitative and qualitative methods. For quantitative investigations, designs are generally descriptive in nature and may use direct observation or survey methods to obtain the desired information. Qualitative methods can also be useful in gathering process evaluation data, as interviews and focus groups allow participants and other stakeholders involved in the program to provide feedback on experiences and perceived strengths and barriers to the program. (See Table 8.3 for process evaluation examples.)

Selecting Measurement Tools and Methods

After program evaluation questions have been finalized and an appropriate design to shape your evaluation has been selected, it is time to identify the outcomes and process areas that will be measured. Again, this is where reference to the logic model is helpful because it was through that process that you identified short-term, midterm, and

Table 8-2. Doctoral Capstone Project Outcome Evaluation

DESIGN	STRENGTHS	CHALLENGES	EXAMPLE
Pretest/posttest: Single group receives the intervention. Data collection occurs at two times points, before and after intervention.	• Ease of implementation. • Can measure a change over time (Suarez-Balcazar et al., 2024).	Changes observed could be due to several other factors, including time passing, an outside external event, the measurement tools used, or retesting (Suarez-Balcazar et al., 2024).	First iteration of a program for schoolchildren with sensory processing issues could measure changes on participation in the classroom before and after implementation.
Pretest/posttest with comparison group: two groups. One receives the intervention; one does not. Data collection occurs at two time points, before and after intervention.	• Increased rigor of design means more confidence in results potentially being attributed to your program. • Provides a reference group to compare results of program (Portney, 2020; Suarez-Balcazar et al., 2024).	• Selection bias main threat to internal validity as groups are not randomized. • Need to locate a reasonable non-equivalent comparison group. • Increased demand for data collection (Portney, 2020; Suarez-Balcazar et al., 2024).	A rehabilitation facility has two outpatient locations, but a new assessment protocol for clients post-stroke is implemented at only one site, creating a naturally occurring non-equivalent comparison group that did not receive the program, for which outcomes could be measured in both.
Repeated measures: single group with measurements at multiple times (i.e., three or more).	• Can establish a baseline level of performance for participants before intervention, which can reduce threats due to maturation. • Evaluates simple behaviors well (Portney, 2020).	• Requires the establishment of a baseline, which, given the 14-week timeline, will require advanced planning. • Vulnerable to threats related to instrumentation if new instruments are added at the same time as the intervention. • Also requires increased time for assessment as data collection points are greater (Portney, 2020).	A home program to support upper-extremity motor recovery post-stroke measured outcomes upon entry to the study, prior to the beginning of the home program, halfway through the home program, and immediately following the completion of the program.
Single-subject: experimental design with one or more cases completed across time. Several designs could be applied, including reversal (A-B-A-B) and alternating treatment (A-B-C) (Deitz & Lin, 2024).	• Decreases threats to internal validity, such as change due to the passing of time or occurrence of outside events. • Good for populations with high variability and initial investigations (Deitz & Lin, 2024)	• Depending on the number and diversity of cases, limited generalizability. • Requires specific definition of operationalized outcomes, often of behavior (Deitz & Lin, 2024).	In an outpatient hand therapy clinic, an alternating treatment design could be used to compare the effectiveness of different modalities to decrease pain and increase duration of participation in functional activities in a client with complex regional pain syndrome.

Table 8-3. Doctoral Capstone Experience Process Evaluation

DESIGN	STRENGTHS	CHALLENGES	EXAMPLE
Observation	• Can provide quantitative data that informs understanding of how program was implemented and/or how program resources were used. • Feasible implementation in the timeline provided. • Ecologically valid as it will occur in the context the DCE is delivered (Bhatt et al., 2024).	• Vulnerable to other variables impacting observation. • Dependent on the rigor and neutrality of the observer. • Behavior could be different if individuals know they are being observed (Bhatt et al., 2024).	Implementation of a program to address falls on the orthopedic unit, tracking the use of fall safety measures after two in-service sessions.
Survey	• Provides descriptive information that can help identify areas of need or measure patient satisfaction. • Can be administered via questionnaire or interview. • Allows for correlational analysis if characteristics of respondents are collected. • Can feasibly be implemented in the time frame of the DCE (Johnson & Kapousouz, 2024).	• Requires consideration of the sample and how they are gathered. • Individuals who may respond are different from those who do not, or if administered in person, participants may not feel comfortable being honest. • Individuals may interpret questions differently, not recall information, or may not have a choice that represents their opinion (Johnson & Kapousouz, 2024).	Capstone student in a state political action committee uses a cross-sectional survey to gain information from state association members about areas of concern related to policy. Could also use a survey to gain insight into participant satisfaction with the program or use of program materials after the conclusion of the program.
Interview	• Can provide narrative data that clearly describes participants' experience (Suarez-Balczar et al., 2024).	• Time-consuming to complete with a large number of individuals. • Response bias, especially if interviewer is the student who completed the project (Johnson & Kapousouz, 2024; Suarez-Balczar et al., 2024).	In a higher education setting, after a mentoring program is implemented, one-on-one interviews are completed to understand the benefits and key elements to the program as perceived by the students.
Focus group	• Allows for social component in responding to questions. • Provides narrative understanding of experience from more people in a single setting (The & Magasi, 2024).	• Requires competent moderator to facilitate. • Fewer questions can be asked as time to respond from the group increases (The & Magasi, 2024).	After the completion of a 6-week social participation program for families with children with intellectual development disorder, a focus group could be held with parents to support a better understanding of their experience of the program and what were the perceived supports and barriers to program participation.

long-term outcomes. Given that the capstone project is implemented over a short period (14 weeks), when thinking of outcome areas, it is important to focus on short-term outcomes that are closest to the intervention. For example, imagine a capstone student has implemented a patient education program for individuals with multiple sclerosis in an acute inpatient rehabilitation hospital. The short-term outcome identified was change in knowledge, and the long-term outcome identified was quality of life. It would be most appropriate to focus measurement on the change in knowledge because it may take a longer duration of program implementation and follow-up to see changes in quality of life. This example illustrates the challenging nature of selecting outcome measures for the capstone project; however, this process, in many ways, parallels the selection of assessment tools for the evaluation of clients because many of the same key pieces of information are considered. To select appropriate outcome measures, it will be beneficial for the capstone student to answer the following questions:

1. Who is being evaluated?
2. What type of measurement tool would be best to capture this outcome or process area?
3. What tools can be implemented in this setting?
4. Can these measures provide a consistent and accurate picture of the desired area?

Who Is Being Evaluated?

This may be a challenging question to answer precisely because, until you move on-site and begin the implementation phase of your doctoral capstone, the exact mix of people in your program may fluctuate. For example, capstone students may know that the clients at their site all have a diagnosis of an eating disorder, but the specific disorder may vary, as does the age, gender, and comorbidities of each client. However, regardless of the specifics of the population, selecting an outcome measure can be supported by knowing their site population's general diagnostic category because it is best practice to first look at tools that have been validated with your population of interest.

The additional details about the individuals who actually attend your program should be collected through the completion of a demographics form. This form should contain information that would help describe to others key characteristics about your sample that could influence how they understand and apply the findings of your program evaluation.

What Type of Measurement Tool Would Best Capture This Outcome or Process Area?

As occupational therapists, we are trained to have a unique skill set to assess a wide variety of areas, and numerous strategies and methods to evaluate them. We will look at selecting outcome areas and process areas separately, although there can be overlap between the two. When selecting an outcome measure, it is critical that you consider the best way to capture information on this outcome. For example, if you want to understand a program participant's perceived performance and satisfaction on personal goal areas, use of the Canadian Occupational Performance Measure or Goal Attainment Scale (GAS), despite some measurement limitations, may be a good option, as both of these tools are patient report measures that look at goal areas identified by the client (Doig et al., 2010; Logan et al., 2022; McColl et al., 2023). However, if you are creating a community-based activity program that is intended to improve motor function of the impaired upper extremity for persons post-stroke, you may want to use a tool that evaluates performance through observation, such as the Fugl–Meyer Upper Extremity Subtest or Chedoke Arm and Hand Activity Inventory (Barreca et al., 2006; Lin et al., 2009). In some cases, standardized assessment tools may not be available for an outcome area. For example, in staff or patient education programs, standardized knowledge tests are not often readily available for all areas of content. Therefore, capstone students may need to develop their own tools or adapt tools found in the literature. With the creation or adaptation of a measurement tool, it is important for the capstone student to recognize the limitations that come from the tool's lack of previous use. These limitations include limited reliability and unknown validity (Portney, 2020). When considering methods to measure process areas, you will need to match the method with what you want to know and also consider logistical factors (CDC, 2024). For example, if you wish to evaluate use of a community resource book provided at a staff training, you have several measurement options, including observation of the number of times staff members are observed using the book, to administering a survey that asks staff members for this information. Deciding how to measure any given area will involve several factors and collaboration with the capstone team, but once you have a set of possible measures and methods, you can begin to compare them.

What Tools Can Be Implemented in the Setting of the Doctoral Capstone Experience?

Once possible assessments and methods have been identified for implementation within the program evaluation, capstone students will need to refer back to their knowledge of the site and the expertise of their capstone team to determine which of the identified measurement tools are most feasible for implementation. This is known as *utility* and considers the time to complete the assessment or method, the materials and space needed, as well as any potential staff training that might need to occur to use that measurement tool (Chisholm, 2020). This is important to consider because, although an assessment or data collection method may look at your desired area in your population, if it is not practical to complete in the setting, a capstone student may become discouraged at the time of implementation.

CAN THESE MEASURES OR METHODS PROVIDE A CONSISTENT AND ACCURATE PICTURE OF THE DESIRED AREA?

After feasibility is ensured, it is important to consider which of the remaining choices has the strongest profile related to consistent and accurate measurement. For standardized assessments, this would include a review and consideration of psychometric properties, including test–retest reliability, responsiveness, standard error of measure, content validity, and criterion validity or construct validity (Grampurohit & Mulcahey, 2020; Portney, 2020).

1. Again, it is noted that assessment tools in some areas of practice may have limited psychometrics data available. This does not mean that such assessments cannot be used for a capstone project; however, it does mean that the limitations and negative impact on the strength of the evaluation need to be reflected in the data analysis and interpretation phase of the project. For example, if an outcome measure has not been evaluated for test–retest reliability, it needs to be noted that any change observed in a pretest/posttest design could be due to measurement error from the assessment and not change due to the intervention (Portney, 2020).

For process evaluations, to generate a consistent and accurate data set, considerations of bias and influence are often in the forefront. For instance, when evaluating participant satisfaction, one can consider either an interview or an anonymous survey. A capstone student would need to reflect on whether data collected via an interview would be unduly influenced if the capstone student who ran the program was also completing the interview (Johnson & Kapousouz, 2024; Suarez-Balcazar et al., 2024). Therefore, students will want to identify the method for collection that will be least vulnerable to these types of influences. Another method that can increase the trustworthiness of the qualitative findings is the use of triangulation. *Triangulation* is the "use of multiple methods to document and confirm observations related to a phenomenon" (Portney, 2020, p. 654), and by doing so, the credibility of the findings increases (Portney, 2020). For example, if a staff education program on how to prevent falls on an orthopedic unit instructs staff to use a resource book, both observation of the number of times the book is used and interviews of staff on the use of the book can

be triangulated to determine the value of this piece of the program. Triangulation can also occur in analysis and will be described later in the chapter.

PROGRAM EVALUATION PLANNING LOGISTICS

After selection of program evaluation design and measurement tools, the capstone student can begin to define logistics around data collection. This begins with a continued discussion of who will be included in the capstone project. For instance, will the doctoral capstone project be something that all persons who are admitted to a facility go through, or will participants need to be gathered from the community? Depending on the mode of recruitment, different levels of marketing will be required. It is best to go into this with an agreed-on plan to ensure that your doctoral capstone project is successful in gaining participants.

In addition to planning how participants will be recruited, creating a timeline and processes for implementation of assessment measures will support implementation. When developing a timeline, it is important to recognize that this is a guide and that it may need to change, as unexpected circumstances arise during the DCE and adjustments may need to be made. This will be discussed further in Chapter 9. The importance of having a timeline for the implementation of the program evaluation will support communication between the capstone student and the context expert, thus increasing the likelihood for seamless implementation.

DEVELOPING A DATA ANALYSIS PLAN

In preparation for the start of the DCE, the capstone student should revisit the overarching program evaluation questions and components of their project, as outlined in the logic model. It is imperative to the success of the project that the student create alignment between their program evaluation questions, program components, data collection, and analysis. It is highly recommended that a student develop not only a data collection plan but also a data analysis plan before DCE implementation in an effort to guide organization of outcome measures, data entry, summarization of data, and testing of program evaluation hypotheses through data analysis and to minimize unexpected changes during capstone project implementation.

A data analysis plan typically consists of (1) the identification of key dependent (a.k.a. outcome) and independent (a.k.a. predictor) variables to be measured during the DCE, (2) the definition of the levels of measurement of each variable measured, (3) the consideration of the number of participants needed to detect a clinically significant change or reach saturation of themes with program evaluation quantitative and qualitative data (discussed later in this chapter), and (4) the quantitative and qualitative analyses and software the student intends to use to make sense of data collected and test program evaluation hypotheses (CDC, 2024). *Variables* are "a characteristic that can be manipulated or observed and that can take on different values, either qualitatively or quantitatively" (Portney, 2020, p. 654). *Independent variables* are those that are manipulated in a doctoral capstone project and typically represent the "intervention" or "comparison" (no-intervention) in a program evaluation project, whereas *dependent variables* are the outcomes or observed results of a project, which potentially occur in response to the manipulation of one or more independent variables. Drawing on foundational research knowledge, variables can be classified generally as categorical (i.e., nominal or ordinal variables) or continuous (i.e., interval or ratio variables). When creating their own measurement tools (e.g., demographic surveys, satisfaction surveys), capstone students should make every effort to gather variables from participants at the highest level of measurement possible (continuous data). One way to organize this information is in a table, as modelled by the CDC (2024). This table could contain the specific program evaluation questions, the type of program evaluation that will be used to answer the variables of interest, the method of collecting those variables, how and when they will be captured, and the plan for analysis (CDC, 2024).

For example, a capstone student implementing a social skills program for school-age children with autism spectrum disorder may seek to evaluate the program participants' social skills pre- and post-program implementation using the social profile (Donohue, 2013). The capstone student may also want to create a survey to gather valuable process evaluation data on the number of children who participated in her program and their demographic characteristics. In this example, the social skills program or intervention is considered the independent variable, as well as the personal, social, and environmental characteristics of each child, their parents, and their home/school life. The dependent variable is the change in social skills observed in the children and measured over a given period of time. In gathering demographic characteristics for each child, rather than asking parents to place their children in a given age bracket (which would represent categorical data), gathering their actual age (a continuous variable), would provide more meaningful information about each child and allow for more advanced statistical analyses to be conducted using this demographic information.

ORGANIZATION AND IMPLEMENTATION OF THE DOCTORAL CAPSTONE EXPERIENCE PROGRAM EVALUATION

The strength of a doctoral capstone project's program evaluation is only as good as the quality and completeness of the data collected from its participants. Each capstone project is individualized to the capstone student and site.

Therefore, program evaluation data will vary; however, to maximize the quality of data collected, initial steps should be undertaken to ensure organization of the data collection and data entry process and to avoid missing data and errors on the back end.

Capstone students are encouraged to first locate and obtain the assessment tools and outcome measures they intend to use to collect data on participants and program outcomes as part of their doctoral capstone project. Because capstone students may not have funds available to purchase new assessment tools and outcome measures, there are a variety of other sources where tools can be sought, including the occupational therapy doctoral program's assessment library, academic institution's library, or online through open-access channels or free digital resources. For example, two frequently used occupational therapy assessment tools that are located online and have copyrights that allow permission for clinical use include the Montreal Cognitive Assessment (MoCa; Nasreddine et al., 2005) and Modified Interest Checklist (Kielhofner & Neville, 1983).

Capstone students who choose to create their own outcome and process evaluation measures, such as knowledge tests, demographic surveys, or program satisfaction surveys, are encouraged to pilot-test these measures before the start of their DCE, with special consideration given to the health literacy and readability of these tools. *Health literacy* refers to a person's ability to obtain, process, and understand health information so that he or she can make informed decisions about his or her care (Walters et al., 2020). The highest prevalence of low health literacy is observed in men, the elderly, racial and ethnic minorities, and individuals with low socioeconomic status (Ayotte et al., 2009; Rikard et al., 2016). When creating patient education materials or new outcome measures, capstone students should consider principles for improving health literacy – for example, create materials at or below a sixth-grade reading level, avoid medical terminology and abbreviations, include ample white space on the page, use pictures, and check readability statistics using Word processing systems (e.g., Microsoft Word's Flesch-Kincaid Readability tool).

Once all assessments and outcome measures have been obtained or created, a schedule of administration of these measures should be developed in concert with the faculty mentor (or capstone chair) and content expert. This assessment schedule should strike a balance between ensuring that enough data is collected to answer program evaluation questions and adequately test hypotheses but that the capstone student can still manage DCE time effectively and that program participants are not subject to overassessment or assessment fatigue.

A critical step in collecting and organizing high-quality program evaluation data is setting up database(s) for data entry, confidential security, and storage of records. A data spreadsheet can be created in software, such as Microsoft

Excel, as soon as assessment tools and outcome measures have been identified for use in the capstone project, and independent and dependent variables defined. A common method used in establishing a data spreadsheet involves organizing independent and dependent variables as column headers and entering one program participant's assessment data per row. It is recommended that you create a data spreadsheet, document and enter data on a regular basis throughout the capstone project because it is easy to fall behind in data entry and management. Human error is also common in data entry and management. Therefore, as the capstone student, you should take the lead in managing the data spreadsheet, providing limited access to others involved in the capstone project. High attention to detail is necessary when entering program data to minimize the amount of missing data gathered for independent and dependent program evaluation variables. For example, when entering pairwise data for program participants, pre-assessment data should be entered and matched to the same participant's post-assessment data.

To protect the confidentiality of doctoral capstone project program participants, all data collected while on the DCE should be de-identified, coded numerically, and recorded in a password-protected data spreadsheet (Benson & Taylor, 2024). One solution to increasing security of participant data is the upkeep of a separate password-protected code sheet, in which numeric identifiers are assigned to each program participant and their demographic characteristics. These numeric identifiers are the only link between individual-level demographic information and assessment data for the program participants. It is also recommended that you and your content expert/faculty mentor have sole access privileges to these files and to any locked filing cabinets where hard copies of assessment data are stored.

Subsequently, identification of statistical analysis software that interfaces well with a student's data spreadsheet is equally as important. (See Table 8.4 for a list of statistical analysis software systems that may be available to capstone students, with a special focus on health and

Table 8-4. Review of Quantitative Statistical Analysis Software Systems

STATISTICAL SOFTWARE PACKAGE	BASIC FEATURES	STRENGTHS	WEAKNESSES
Excel (Microsoft, n.d.)	• Point-and-click software • Can be used for descriptive statistics (median, mean, standard deviation, frequencies, and percentages), correlations, t-tests, ANOVA, regression	• Inexpensive • Easily accessible • Widely used in many workplaces as part of Microsoft Office • Can easily create databases for data entry	• Decreased ease of use (e.g., Excel formulas not intuitive and require macro downloads) • Creating tables and figures and exporting them challenging
R (The R Foundation, n.d.)	• Code-based software • Can be used for descriptive statistics, correlations, bivariate analyses (chi-square test), X tests, ANOVA, regression	• Free software • Can be used to analyze large data sets • Creates high-quality tables and figures	• Learning code/syntax requires increased time (can be ameliorated by R Studio) • Limited/no customer support; can seek help only via online forums
Statistical Package for the Social Sciences (SPSS) 25.0 (IBM, n.d.)	• Point-and-click software with a coding option • Can be used for descriptive statistics, correlations, bivariate analyses (chi-square test), X tests, ANOVA, regression	• Choice for user to use point-and-click and/or write syntax • Increased ease of use for health-care professionals and other social scientists • Tables and figures can be easily created, modified, and exported from SPSS	• SPSS license more expensive than for other statistical software • Few workplaces purchase SPSS license(s) • Memory-intensive, thus difficult to manage large data sets and run other programs

continued

STATISTICAL SOFTWARE PACKAGE	BASIC FEATURES	STRENGTHS	WEAKNESSES
jamovi (The Jamovi Project, 2024)	• Code-based software with a point-and-click interface • Can be used for descriptive statistics, correlations, bivariate analyses (chi-square test), X tests, ANOVA, regression	• Free to use • Highly intuitive point-and-click interface • Analysis output shown directly adjacent to the data for increased understanding of processes; many available resources created by members of the community (e.g., online guides, manuals, textbooks)	• Updates occur at the rate of the community • Ability to edit certain elements of graphs limited

Table 8-4. Review of Quantitative Statistical Analysis Software Systems (continued)

Note: ANOVA = analysis of variance.

social sciences.) When selecting a software, it is important to consider factors such as the type of data collected (quantitative vs. qualitative), usability (point-and-click vs. code-based programming), cost, level of customer support available, interface with other programs and operating systems, amount of memory needed to run the program, types of statistical analyses that can be conducted using the software, and quality of tables and graphs produced to choose the best statistical processing system for the doctoral capstone project and data analysis.

PROGRAM EVALUATION DATA ANALYSIS

Analysis of data collected over the course of a doctoral capstone project is one of the most important steps of the capstone process, as it allows the student to generate answers to their program evaluation questions and test hypotheses set at the beginning of the capstone planning process.

Whether you collect quantitative, qualitative, or mixed data, descriptive statistics should be used to summarize and describe the main features and patterns that emerge from participants included in the program evaluation (Portney, 2020). (See Table 8.5 for a sample descriptive statistics table used to present demographic data gathered from participants with intellectual and developmental disabilities [IDD]).

QUANTITATIVE DATA ANALYSIS

In determining the statistical tests that can be used to analyze quantitative data collected in the capstone project, capstone students must, first and foremost, understand whether the data they have collected meets the assumptions

of normality. A normal distribution represents a symmetrical distribution of scores on either side of the mean, or a "bell curve," in which the majority of scores fall in the middle of a scale and fewer scores fall at the extremes of a scale (Portney, 2020). Parametric tests assume that a sample is drawn from a population with a distribution that approximates a normal distribution; therefore, to use a parametric statistical test, such as a t-test or analysis of variance (ANOVA), the sample data must meet the assumptions of normality. To assess for normality, you can use statistical analysis software to create a histogram, or bar graph that displays all assessment scores for a given sample of program participants, and then visually inspect the graph for a normal distribution curve. However, a more precise method for assessing normality would be to run a formal test using statistical analysis software (Bishara et al., 2021). The Shapiro–Wilk test is recommended as one of the best tests for assessing normality in small samples that will be seen in many capstone projects (Portney, 2020). If a data set meets normality assumptions, *parametric tests*, such as independent samples t-tests, paired samples t-tests, between-subjects ANOVA, mixed ANOVA, and repeated-measures ANOVA, can be used in analyzing participant data. However, if this normality assumption is not met, then equivalent nonparametric tests, such as a chi-square test, Mann–Whitney U test, Wilcoxon signed rank test, or Krukal–Wallis, will need to be used instead.

DETERMINING THE SIGNIFICANCE OF PROGRAM EVALUATION FINDINGS

At the end of the doctoral capstone experience, you will ultimately want to be able to use the data they have collected to answer questions such as, "What did we

Table 8-5. Sample Demographics

INDIVIDUAL-LEVEL CHARACTERISTICS TOTAL SAMPLE (N = 597)
Age, mean (SD), years, n(%)
Youth: 18 to 24
Young adult: 25 to 44
Midlife: 45 to 64
Later life: 65 and older
Gender, n(%)
Female
Male
Transgender
Other
Type of developmental disability, n(%)
Autism spectrum disorder
Cerebral palsy
Down syndrome
Neurological disorder
Other(s)
Level of intellectual disability, n(%)
None/unspecified
Mild
Moderate
Severe
Profound
Self-identified race/ethnicity, n(%)
American Indian or Alaska Native
Asian
Black or African American
Hispanic/Latinx
Native Hawaiian or other Pacific Islander
White
Other
Living arrangement, n(%)
Institution
Group home
Family home
Supported apartment

learn about running this program?" or "Did this program achieve the desired outcomes?" Determining the significance of the findings will be dependent on the capstone focus and type of doctoral capstone project.

Determining the clinical significance of program evaluation findings can also be accomplished by analyzing changes in occupational performance that are deemed meaningful to a client or treating clinician. A *minimally clinically important difference* (MCID) is the "amount of change in a measured variable that signifies an important rather than trivial difference" (Portney, 2020, p. 646). At the heart of measuring the MCID for an outcome, capstone students must use their professional and clinical judgment to estimate how much meaningful change they would expect to see in an assessment of occupational performance to make it "clinically significant." For example, a capstone student who is working with adolescents with psychiatric disabilities who are "at risk" may choose to use GAS to measure achievement of vocational outcomes before and after implementation of a 14-week vocational training program. The student might identify a change from "somewhat less than expected" (−1) to "expected level of outcome" (0) on the GAS pre- to post-training program to be an MCID for her adolescent client.

Although there may be certain doctoral capstone projects that implement qualitative methodologies, such as phenomenology or ethnography, which require complex analysis, most capstone projects are likely to use qualitative analysis for responses to open-ended questions on a survey or as a part of process evaluation interviews or focus groups. In this case, a content analysis approach that aims to summarize the information into categories and possibly implement counts (Stanley, 2024) is often sufficient to determine the perspectives of the participants related to program processes or key ingredients. While the goal in most qualitative research is to reach data saturation or the point at which no new information is being gathered (Portney, 2020), reaching this point may not be feasible given the short timeline of the DCE unless the sole focus of the project is to complete a qualitative investigation. Therefore, it is important for the capstone student to consider other ways to increase the trustworthiness and rigor of their findings. One way to do this is for the capstone student to consider ways to triangulate the data through the use of multiple analysts who analyze the data separately at first and then join and compare coding structures to decrease the influence of bias (Portney, 2020). Another way to increase the trustworthiness of the qualitative findings is to complete member checking, in which the initial interpretation of the findings is sent to those who participated to determine if it represents their perspectives (Portney, 2020). Use of these strategies can support the validity of the qualitative findings but does require advanced planning and additional resources.

Managing the Unexpected

Although the PM principles outlined here, as well as the use of a logic model and the development of data collection and data analysis plans, are meant to minimize the myriad problems that can occur during program implementation and evaluation, a variety of unexpected changes can still occur. For example, DCEs and projects conducted in community-based mental health settings can be affected by low funding streams and thus decrease participant recruitment to the program. A low census on an acute care unit in the hospital can have an impact on a capstone student's sample size and change the data analysis plan. When sample sizes vary from what is anticipated,

it will require considerations and advisement from the capstone team as to what approach to take. If a project does not yield a sufficient sample for parametric or non-parametric statistics, considerations for the use of case study or case series reporting of outcomes with comparisons to values like the minimally clinically important difference or minimal detectable change may be what is most appropriate. In addition, utilizing visualization as a key component to describe the observed changes but not generalize them is another method that can be utilized (Hopkin et al., 2015). Changes to the initial program evaluation and data analysis plans are inevitable, and it is important to remain flexible and collaborative.

To minimize unexpected modifications to the DCE and capstone project and problem-solve through unexpected changes, you must maintain open lines of communication with your faculty and content expert, drawing on the resources within the capstone team. The capstone team should be engaged in every step of the planning process, project implementation, and evaluation to support appropriate selection of methods that will work effectively with the capstone site's current organizational processes. Capstone students who remain flexible and communicate regularly with their faculty mentor to actively solve problems will produce successful capstone project results, despite unexpected changes.

Drawing Conclusions and Disseminating Program Evaluation Findings

Findings from the doctoral capstone project can and should be disseminated to a broader audience to contribute evidence-based practice knowledge to the field of occupational therapy and to the capstone site so that they can receive valuable information on the impact of the services provided at their organization. Program evaluation findings can be used to advocate for much-needed policy change, procure additional funding for occupational therapy services, or inform future iterations of the program, making any necessary changes to the logic model should the capstone student choose to continue to implement the program moving forward. Chapters 11 and 12 review best practices and recommendations on how and where to disseminate capstone findings.

Student Section Chapter Summary

The doctoral capstone is an optimal opportunity for occupational therapy students to create sustainable, meaningful projects in diverse settings. To achieve this goal, it is imperative that you have a solid understanding of program evaluation and appropriate data analysis throughout each stage of the experience. Having a well-thought-out process in place will allow you to not only experience a successful capstone experience but to also potentially have a direct impact on populations in the health-care system. If doctoral programs can place an emphasis on skills such as sustainable design, assessment, measurement, and evaluation, capstone students can confidently work through human-centered design phases of feasible and desirable projects.

STUDENT LEARNING ACTIVITIES

1. Think about a program you consider to be "sustainable." Reflect on why you think the program has outlasted others. What resources do they have? What does their leadership and staffing look like? What makes this program important to its community or organization? What lessons can you learn from the program's mission, vision, funding structure, staffing, or other factors that have led to its sustainability?

2. Think of a program. This could be one that currently exists at your DCE site or one you are hoping to create. Use a logic model to identify the resources, activities, outputs, and short-term outcomes from this program.

Section 2: Educator Focus

Link Between Human-Centered Design Mindset for Student and Transformational Learning for the Educator

As capstone students begin to think through methods to support the sustainability of their capstone projects and design their program evaluation processes, they further embark into the transformational learning phase of planning for a course of action (Mezirow, 1997). In this phase, capstone students are envisioning their path forward as they prepare to move on-site for their doctoral capstone experience. As their educator, you will want to guide your students to anticipate potential challenges and pitfalls that might occur, as well as strategies to overcome them. You will want to ensure that your students begin to formulate concrete steps and lay groundwork ahead of the actual implementation. Specifically, your students will be developing a plan of action for program evaluation. As their faculty or doctoral capstone coordinator, you must acknowledge how important it is to facilitate this learning phase by creating an educational structure that will facilitate students' abilities to develop and execute a sound evaluation plan for their capstone project in order to ensure sustainability. Facilitating the mindsets of optimism and creative confidence within the student so that they can create and problem-solve components of program evaluation will be important.

INTRODUCTION FOR EDUCATOR

Sustainability is a critical factor in ensuring the long-term success and impact of doctoral capstone projects within occupational therapy education. As the field of occupational therapy continues to evolve, it is essential that educators ensure that capstone projects not only address site objectives but also possess the capacity to endure and adapt over time. One of the key mechanisms for achieving sustainability is program evaluation, which allows students and educators to assess the effectiveness, efficiency, and long-term viability of their projects.

The remainder of this chapter explores the role of the educator in fostering sustainable capstone projects, emphasizing its importance for doctoral capstone coordinators, faculty members, and students alike. By integrating structured evaluation methods, such as logic models and outcome assessments, educators can guide students in developing projects that are responsive to stakeholder needs, evidence-based, and adaptable to future challenges. Additionally, practical strategies for teaching program evaluation, engaging stakeholders, and utilizing data-driven decision-making to support sustainable initiatives will be discussed.

By equipping students with the tools and knowledge to conduct meaningful evaluations, occupational therapy educators play a vital role in preparing future practitioners to implement impactful, long-lasting programs.

EDUCATOR REFLECTIVE QUESTIONS

1. What challenges or barriers do you anticipate students may face to create sustainable programming at their capstone sites?

2. What type of skills or abilities are essential for implementing program evaluation?

3. What assignments or action steps can you facilitate to develop skills in planning, implementing, and analyzing data in program evaluation?

EDUCATOR OBJECTIVES

By the end of reading this chapter, the educator will be able to design teaching methods to meet the stated student learning objectives:

1. Describe processes that will support the sustainability of the doctoral capstone project.

2. Identify three ways that sustainability is supported through program evaluation.

3. Define the purpose of a logic or conceptual model in the program evaluation process.

4. Compare and contrast outcome and process evaluations and their corresponding research methods.

5. Describe methods for planning, implementing, and analyzing data from a program evaluation.

6. Identify characteristics that will support success in managing unexpected challenges in the program evaluation process.

OVERVIEW FOR THE EDUCATOR

Sustainability is one of the hallmarks of a successful doctoral capstone project. In the dynamic and ever-evolving landscape of occupational therapy practice and education, projects must not only address immediate goals of capstone sties but also demonstrate their capacity to endure and adapt over time. The student portion of this chapter has explored the processes and tools essential for ensuring sustainability, with a focus on program evaluation as a critical mechanism for achieving this goal.

From the perspective of the doctoral capstone coordinator or occupational therapy faculty member, teaching program evaluation should provide a structured approach to assessing the effectiveness, efficiency, and impact of a program or project (Carrion et al., 2021). It supports sustainability in three key ways. First, it identifies areas where the project generates measurable impact, ensuring that resources are allocated to interventions that matter most. Second, it aligns the project's activities and outcomes with the needs and expectations of stakeholders, fostering continued support and investment. Finally, educating doctoral students on program evaluation facilitates evidence-based decision-making, enabling the project to evolve in response to new challenges and opportunities. (See Text Box 8.2.)

TEXT BOX 8.2

Teaching Tip: Help Students Build Capacity and Raise Community Awareness

The following ideas may help capstone students better understand their role and increase readiness for their capstone projects to occur:

- Meet one-on-one with public opinion or community organization leaders.
- Submit articles to local newspapers, club newsletters, and other resources to spread the word on ideas and services.
- Convene focus groups to get input on capstone project ideas and plans.
- Go to the stakeholders in their own environments to share information on wants and needs. As a capstone student, think holistically about this process. If the capstone project is in a community or large organization, the capstone student should seek feedback from other providers, local government, neighborhood and cultural organizations, law enforcement, or even local university or research institutions that could ultimately form a sustainable partnership.

A logic or conceptual model is a powerful tool within the program evaluation process. These models offer a visual representation of the relationships between inputs, activities, outputs, and outcomes. By facilitating students in clearly articulating the connections between these elements, logic models help stakeholders maintain a shared understanding of the project's purpose and how its goals will be achieved. Educators can use these models to guide students in mapping their projects, ensuring that the pathways to sustainability are well-defined and grounded in evidence. (See Text Box 8.3.)

TEXT BOX 8.3

Utilizing Logic Models for Program Planning and Program Evaluation

The following ideas are strategies used to help capstone students organize their thoughts and ideas around how their program is anticipated to work.

- The logic model template is best used as an iterative living document. It is helpful to have students draft their logic model after having completed a literature review or annotated bibliography. In addition, the students should think about what theories best align with their program. This can be fostered through discussion and course assignments.
- Initial drafts should be revised after feedback from the instructor and peers. Often, students will need support in properly categorizing outputs versus outcomes or may need to better integrate their guiding theory into the logic model.

Logic models can be further developed to include not only outcome areas but also anticipated measures for each outcome, which then can be incorporated into a subsequent table that outlines the program evaluation plan.

Selecting measurement methods for use in program evaluations is an important step in the planning process. This activity builds on knowledge of assessments and methods gained throughout the earlier phases of occupational therapy training and often applies it to a larger programmatic perspective. Again, conversation with the capstone team, and especially the content expert, will support the selection of measures that will be sustainable after the DCE and capstone project is completed, to allow for continued program evaluation.

Understanding the different types of evaluation is another critical step in the process for students. While there are many types of program evaluation, the three focused on in this text due to their relevance to most students are formative, process, and outcome evaluations. Formative evaluations are often used to see the acceptability of a new program (CDC, 2024). Process evaluation can look at the manner in which a program is functioning, how activities are carried out, the resources utilized, and if it could be a good fit for an existing program that is being modified. Outcome evaluations focus on measuring the results of a project, its tangible impacts, and whether it achieves its intended objectives (CDC, 2024). Each approach offers valuable insights, but they require distinct research methods and serve different purposes. It is important to guide students first to what questions they hope to answer and then to the type(s) of program evaluation(s) that are best suited for the project that they are completing.

(See Text Boxes 8.4 and 8.5.)

TEXT BOX 8.4

Occupational therapy educators and students can refer to other prominent resources regarding research methodology by referring to the following texts that are rated as most frequently used according to the National Board for Certification in Occupational Therapy's OTR Curriculum Textbook and Peer-Reviewed Journal Report (retrieved from http://www.nbcot.org):

- DePoy, E. (2026). Introduction to research: Understanding and applying multiple strategies (7th ed.). Elsevier.
- Taylor, R. R. (2024). Kielhofner's research in occupational therapy: Methods of inquiry for enhancing practice (3rd ed.). F.A. Davis.
- Portney, L. G. (2020). Foundations of clinical research: Applications to practice (4th ed.). F.A. Davis.

TEXT BOX 8.5

Another Teaching Tip

A capstone project with a focus on research may use quantitative data to measure program outcomes and statistical significance as an indicator of success.

Statistical significance is a measure that expresses the likelihood that program outcomes or findings are due to chance (Brown, 2022). A significance level of 0.05 is used by most researchers and program evaluators to indicate a statistically significant effect.

Drawing on foundational statistics knowledge, a *p* value, or probability value, is typically used to decide whether the result obtained reflects true differences between groups of participants (Portney, 2020). If the *p* value derived from a statistical test is less than the established level of significance (0.05), there is sufficient evidence that the findings are not due to chance.

EDUCATOR CHAPTER SUMMARY

Planning, implementing, and analyzing data from a program evaluation are skills that require careful consideration and strategic thinking. Ensuring your students think

through effective planning involves setting clear objectives, selecting appropriate evaluation methods, and engaging their stakeholders in the process. The CDC's (2024) action framework provides an excellent resource with tables that can help organize all the components needed for a program evaluation. The skills for implementation of the project and evaluation require attention to detail, adherence to ethical and curricular standards, and flexibility to adapt as needed. Finally, data analysis must be thorough and aligned with the evaluation's goals, ensuring that findings provide actionable insights to support the project's sustainability.

No program evaluation process is without challenges. Unexpected obstacles, such as shifts in stakeholder/site priorities, resource limitations, or unforeseen external factors, can disrupt even the most well-planned capstone project. Success in these situations requires key characteristics: adaptability, collaboration, and a problem-solving mindset. By fostering these traits emphasized within Chapter 3, educators can prepare students to navigate uncertainties with confidence and resilience.

Through program evaluation, you and your students alike can develop a deeper understanding of what makes a doctoral capstone project successful and sustainable. By applying structured processes, utilizing tools like logic models, and balancing outcome and process evaluations, students can create projects that not only fulfill academic requirements but also generate lasting, meaningful impact. In doing so, they contribute to a legacy of practice and innovation that stands the test of time.

REFERENCES

Accreditation Council for Occupational Therapy Education. (2023). *Standards and interpretive guide, effective January 21, 2025.* https://acoteonline.org/accreditation-explained/standards/

Altimier, L., & Phillips, R. (2016). The neonatal integrative developmental care model: Advanced clinical applications of the seven core measures for neuroprotective family-centered developmental care. *Newborn and Infant Nursing Reviews, 16*(4), 230–244. https://doi.org/10.1053/j.nainr.2016.09.030

Ayotte, B. J., Allaire, J. C., & Bosworth, H. (2009). The associations of patient demographic characteristics and health information recall: The mediating role of health literacy. *Neuropsychology, Development, and Cognition. Section B, Aging, Neuropsychology and Cognition, 16*(4), 419–432.

Barreca, S. R., Stratford, P. W., Masters, L. M., Lambert, C. L., & Griffiths, J. (2006). Comparing 2 versions of the Chedoke arm and hand activity inventory with the action research arm test. *Physical Therapy, 86,* 245–253.

Benson, J., & Taylor, R. R. (2024). Ensuring ethical research. In R. R. Taylor (Ed.), *Kielhofner's research in occupational therapy: Methods of inquiry for enhancing practice* (3rd ed., pp. 186–205). F.A. Davis.

Berry, J. O., & Jones, W. H. (1995). The parental stress scale: Initial psychometric evidence. *Journal of Social and Personal Relationships, 12*(3), 463–472. https://doi.org/10.1177/0265407595123009

Bhatt, T., Taylor, R. R., & Kielhofner, G. (2024). Collecting data: Now and into the future. In R. R. Taylor (Ed.), *Kielhofner's research in occupational therapy: Methods of inquiry for enhancing practice* (3rd ed., pp. 421–445). F.A. Davis.

Bishara, A. J., Li, J., & Conley, C. (2021). Informal versus formal judgment of statistical models: The case of normality assumptions. *Psychonomic Bulletin & Review, 28*(4), 1164–1182. https://doi.org/10.3758/s13423-021-01879-z

Blasco, P. M., Acar, S., Guy, S., Saxton, S., Duvall, S., & Morgan, G. (2020). Executive function in infants and toddlers born low birth weight and preterm. *Journal of Early Intervention, 42*(4), 321–337. https://doi.org/10.1177/1053815120921946

Brown, C. (2022). *The evidence-based practitioner: Applying research to meet client needs* (2nd ed.). F.A. Davis.

Carrion, A. J., Miles, J. D., Thompson, M. D., Journee, B., & Nelson, E. (2021). Program evaluation through the use of logic models. *Currents in Pharmacy Teaching and Learning, 13*(7), 789–795.

Centers for Disease Control and Prevention. (2024). *CDC's program evaluation framework action guide.* https://www.cdc.gov/evaluation/media/pdfs/2024/12/FINAL-Action-Guide-for-DFE-12182024_1.pdf

Chisholm, D. (2020). Practical aspects of the evaluation process. In P. Kramer & N. Grampurohit (Eds.), *Hinojosa and Kramer's evaluation in occupational therapy: Obtaining and interpreting data* (5th ed., pp. 123–133). American Occupational Therapy Association.

Crump, C. (2020). Preterm birth and mortality in adulthood: A systematic review. *Journal of Perinatology, 40*(6), 833–843. https://doi.org/10.1038/s41372-019-0563-

Deitz, J. C., & Lin, T. (2024). Single-case research. In R. R. Taylor (Ed.), *Kielhofner's research in occupational therapy: Methods of inquiry for enhancing practice* (3rd ed., pp. 507–522). F.A. Davis.

Doig, E., Fleming, J., Kuipers, P., & Cornwell, P. L. (2010). Clinical utility of the combined use of the Canadian occupational performance measure and goal attainment scaling. *American Journal of Occupational Therapy, 64*, 904–914.

Donohue, M. V. (2013). *Social profile: Assessment of social participation in children, adolescents, and adults.* American Occupational Therapy Association.

Fisher, A. G., & Jones, K. B. (2009). Occupational therapy intervention process model. In J. Hinojosa, P. Kramer & C. Brasic Royeen (Eds.), *Perspectives on human occupation: Theories underlying practice* (pp. 237–286). F.A. Davis.

Grampurohit, N., & Mulcahey, M. (2020). Scoring and interpreting results. In P. Kramer & N. Grampurohit (Eds.), *Hinojosa's and Kramer's evaluation in occupational therapy: Obtaining and interpreting data* (5th ed., pp. 123–133). American Occupational Therapy Association.

Hopkin, C. R., Hoyle, R. H., & Gottfredson, N. C. (2015). Maximizing the yield of small samples in prevention research: A review of general strategies and best practices. *Prevention Science, 16*(7), 950–955. https://doi.org/10.1007/s11121-014-0542-7

IBM. (n.d.). *IBM SPSS statistics [software].* https://www.ibm.com/products/spss-statistics

The Jamovi Project. (2024). *jamovi (version 2.5) [computer software].* https://www.jamovi.org

Johnson, T. P., & Kapousouz, E. (2024). Survey research. In R. R. Taylor (Ed.), *Kielhofner's research in occupational therapy: Methods of inquiry for enhancing practice* (3rd ed., pp. 522–548). F.A. Davis.

Kielhofner, G., & Neville, A. (1983). *The modified interest checklist.* Model of Human Occupation Clearinghouse, Department of Occupational Therapy, University of Illinois Chicago. https://www.moho.uic.edu/products.aspx?type=free

Lemola, S. (2015). Long-term outcomes of very preterm birth. *European Psychologist.* https://doi.org/10.1027/1016-9040/a000207

Logan, B., Jegatheesan, D., Viecelli, A., Pascoe, E., & Hubbard, R. (2022). Goal attainment scaling as an outcome measure for randomised controlled trials: A scoping review. *BMJ Open, 12*(7). https://doi.org/10.1136/bmjopen-2022-063061

Lin, J. H., Hsu, M. J., Sheu, C. F., Wu, T. S., Lin, R. T., Chen, C. H., & Hsieh, C. L. (2009). Psychometric comparisons of 4 measures for assessing upper-extremity function in people with stroke. *Physical Therapy, 89*, 840–850. https://doi.org/10.2522/ptj.20080285

McColl, M. A., Denis, C. B., Douglas, K. L., Gilmour, J., Haveman, N., Petersen, M., Presswell, B., & Law, M. (2023). A clinically significant difference on the COPM: A review. *Canadian Journal of Occupational Therapy, 90*(1), 92–102. https://doi.org/10.1177/00084174221142177

Merryman, M. B., Shank, K. H., Reitz, S. M. (2020). Theoretical frameworks for community-based practice. In M. E. Scaffa & S. M. Reitz (Eds.), *Occupational therapy in community and population health practice* (pp. 38–58). F.A. Davis.

Mezirow, J. (1997). Transformative learning: Theory to practice. *New Directions for Adult and Continuing Education,* (74), 5–12. https://doi.org/10.1002/ace.7401

Microsoft. (n.d.). *Microsoft excel [software].* https://products.office.com/en-us/excel

Molero, A., Calabrò, M., Vignes, M., Gouget, B., & Gruson, D. (2021). Sustainability in healthcare: Perspectives and reflections regarding laboratory medicine. *Annals of Laboratory Medicine, 41*(2), 139–144. https://doi.org/10.3343/alm.2021.41.2.139

Nasreddine, Z. S., Phillips, N. A., Bédirian, V., Charbonneau, S., Whitehead, V., Collin, I., Cummings, J. L., & Chertkow, H. (2005). The Montreal Cognitive Assessment (MoCA): A brief screening tool for mild cognitive impairment. *Journal of the American Geriatric Society, 53*, 695–699.

Palm, K., & Fischier, U. P. (2021). What managers find important for implementation of innovations in the healthcare sector–practice through six management perspectives. *International Journal of Health Policy and Management, 11*(10), 2261.

Pineda, R., Guth, R., Herring, A., Reynolds, L., Oberle, S., & Smith, J. (2017). Enhancing sensory experiences for very preterm infants in the NICU: An integrative review. *Journal of Perinatology, 37*(4), 323–332. https://doi.org/10.1038/jp.2016.179

Pineda, R., Raney, M., & Smith, J. (2019). Supporting and enhancing NICU sensory experiences (SENSE): Defining developmentally-appropriate sensory exposures for high-risk infants. *Early Human Development, 133*, 29–35. https://doi.org/10.1016/j.earlhumdev.2019.04.012

Pineda, R., Wallendorf, M., & Smith, J. (2020). A pilot study demonstrating the impact of the supporting and enhancing NICU sensory experiences (SENSE) program on the mother and infant. *Early Human Development, 144.* https://doi.org/10.1016/j.earlhumdev.2020.105000

Portney, L. (2020). *Foundations of clinical research: Application to evidence-based-practice* (4th ed.). F.A. Davis.

The R Foundation. (n.d.). *The R project for statistical computing [software].* https://www.r-project.org/

Ricci, D., Romeo, D. M., Haataja, L., van Haastert, I. C., Cesarini, L., Maunu, J., Pane, M., Gallini, F., Luciano, R., Romagnoli, C., de Vries, L. S., Cowan, F. M., & Mercuri, E. (2008). Neurological examination of preterm infants at term equivalent age. *Early Human Development, 84*(11), 751–761. https://doi.org/10.1016/j.earlhumdev.2008.05.007

Rikard, R. V., Thompson, M. S., McKinney, J., & Beauchamp, A. (2016). Examining health literacy disparities in the United States: A third look at the National Assessment of Adult Literacy (NAAL). *BMC Public Health, 16*(975), 1–11.

Silvius, A. J. G., & Schipper, R. (2012). Sustainability in the business case. *Proceedings of the 26th IPMA world congress,* Crete, Greece, pp. 1062–1069.

Sirkka, M., Zingmark, K., & Larsson-Lund, M. (2014). A process for developing sustainable evidence-based occupational therapy practice. *Scandinavian Journal of Occupational Therapy, 21*, 429–437.

Stanley, M. (2024). Qualitative descriptive a very good place to start. In S. Nayar & M. Stanley (Eds.), *Qualitative research methodologies for occupational science and occupational therapy* (2nd ed., pp. 57–62). Routledge.

Suarez-Balcazar, Y., Braveman, B., Rockwell-Dylla, L., Taylor, R. R. (2024). Program evaluation research. In R. R. Taylor (Ed.), *Kielhofner's research in occupational therapy: Methods of inquiry for enhancing practice* (3rd ed., pp. 566–581). F.A. Davis.

Substance Abuse and Mental Health Services Administration. (2019). *A guide to SAMHSA's strategic prevention framework.* Center for Substance Abuse Prevention. https://library.samhsa.gov/sites/default/files/strategic-prevention-framework-pep19-01.pdf

Substance Abuse and Mental Health Services Administration. (2023). *What is the SPF? An introduction to SAMHSA's strategic prevention framework.* https://www.samhsa.gov/technical-assistance/sptac/framework

Supporting and Enhancing NICU Sensory Experiences (SENSE). (2017). Washington University. https://chan.usc.edu/research/clinical-tools/sense. (Available to be licensed from the University of Southern California, Chan Division of Occupational Science and Occupational Therapy)

The, K., & Magasi, S. (2024). Gathering qualitative data. In R. R. Taylor (Ed.), *Kielhofner's research in occupational therapy: Methods of inquiry for enhancing practice* (3rd ed., pp. 291–316). F.A. Davis.

Thomson, C. S., El-Haram, M. A., & Emmanuel, R. (2011). Mapping sustainability assessment with the project life cycle. *Proceedings of the ICE – Engineering Sustainability, 164*(2), 143–157.

United Nations. (2006). *Definition of basic concepts and terminologies in governance and public administration* (UN Publication E/C.16/2006/4). United Nations Economic and Social Council.

Walters, R., Leslie, S. J., Polson, R., Cusack, T., & Gorely, T. (2020). Establishing the efficacy of interventions to improve health literacy and health behaviours: A systematic review. *BMC Public Health, 20*, 1–17. https://doi.org/10.1186/s12889-020-08991-0

DePoy, E., & Gitlin, L. N. (2020). *Introduction to research: Understanding and applying multiple strategies* (6th ed.). Elsevier.

Jacobsen, K. (2020). *Health research methods: A practical guide* (3rd ed.). Jones & Bartlett.

Taylor, R. R. (2024). *Kielhofner's research in occupational therapy: Methods of inquiry for enhancing practice* (3rd ed.). F.A. Davis.

Websites

Centers for Disease Control and Prevention Program Evaluation Framework. https://www.cdc.gov/evaluation/php/evaluation-framework/index.html

Provides a framework informed action guide that can support each step of the process.

SAMHSA Center for Application of Prevention Technologies (CAPT). https://www.samhsa.gov/capt/

Offers tools, resources, funding, and online courses related to projects that focus on practicing innovate and effective prevention.

RESOURCES

Brown, C. (2022). *The evidence-based practitioner: Applying research to meet client needs* (2nd ed.). F.A. Davis.

APPENDICES

Appendix 8.A Logical Model With Theory Example

Appendix 8.A

Logic Model

Feasibility Study Exploring the Utilization of a Modified SENSE Program for Preterm Infants

Setting: Neonatal Intensive Care Unit (NICU)

Inputs	Activities	Outputs	Outcomes – Impact		Data Sources	Description of Program Evaluation
			Short (During DEC)	*Medium (After DEC)*		
Capstone Team: OTDS, DS, Neonatologist, Capstone chair	**Doing:*** **Consistent positive sensory exposure** will vary by infant age; up to 1 hour delivered by OTDS each weekday (Pineda et al., 2020).	**Logbooks** that can continue to be used to record sensory exposure and promote carryover.	**Becoming:*** Eight families will demonstrate increased knowledge of sensory exposure and role of occupational therapy by using sensory exposure techniques during all (100%) visits in the NICU.	The **long-term benefits** of sensory exposure could be explored in a future prospective study similar to Blasco et al. (2020); Lemola (2015); Altimier and Phillips (2016); and Crump (2020) through the NICU follow-up developmental clinic within **two years** of study completion by the **DS**.	**Logbooks** stored at infants' bedside to record details of sensory exposure	OTDS will **record in logbooks daily** and **monitor family logbooks weekly**.
Education Materials: SENSE program: parenting, sensory system, NICU environment, delivering sensory exposure, monitoring infant status, logbooks (Supporting and Enhancing NICU Sensory Experiences [SENSE], 2017)	**Weekly infant assessment** by OTDS (SENSE, 2017)	**Educational materials** for other NICU families or health-care providers beyond the study.	Eight families will demonstrate an understanding of appropriate dosages of sensory exposure for preterm infants by accurately adhering to the SENSE program **75% of the time.**	**Consistent, positive sensory exposure** will continue to be delivered by nurses, DS, families, and/or volunteers so that **70% of preterm infants in the NICU** receive consistent positive sensory exposure **within one year.**	**HNNE** to be administered by the OTDS when the infant has **reached full term**	OTDS will **perform weekly infant assessment** (SENSE, 2017).
	Data collection to monitor elements of feasibility.	Introduce a **standardized assessment** to evaluate infant development to be used in the future.	Eight families will show **positive trends regarding parental stress** by scoring a **54 or less** on the PSS (Berry & Jones, 1995).	The OTDS will share findings with the NICU team regarding our understanding of the role of parental stress in the NICU by December 2021, as indicated by **scores on the PSS.**	**PSS and exit questionnaire** to be completed by the infant's parent when the infant has reached full term.	Administer HNNE, PSS, exit questionnaire when the infant has reached full term (37 weeks or greater).
Sensory Input Tools: SENSE program, Music, books, toys	**Being and Belonging:*** **Family education** on SENSE to increase knowledge of **perceived benefits**** and establish cues for action** (Pineda et al., 2017, 2019, 2020)	Increased **staff knowledge** of the benefits of sensory exposure and OT role.	Eight infants will demonstrate **positive trends in neurodevelopment** on the HNNE by achieving an optimal score, as defined by Ricci et al. (2008) for preterm infants, depending on their gestational age at birth.		**Weekly infant assessment** completed by OTDS following the SENSE program guidelines (SENSE, 2017).	(Variables to evaluate feasibility): **Demand Feasibility:** Recruitment rate
	Staff education about SENSE and OT role	**Established guidelines** for implementing SENSE.				**Process Feasibility:** Retention rate; Responses on exit questionnaire; Types of sensory exposure
Data Collection Tools: Logbooks, Initial data form, Weekly infant assessment		**One fully trained staff member** on implementing SENSE (DS).				**Management Feasibility:** Trends in family and infant demographics; Frequency and duration of parent education
Assessments: HNNE, PSS, Exit questionnaire		**Eight NICU families** increase **knowledge and adhere** to SENSE.				**Scientific Feasibility:** Trends on HNNE scores; Trends on PSS scores
						Resource Feasibility: Delivery of sensory exposure by OTDS (time commitment)
						Fidelity: Adherence to SENSE. Rate of parent presence; Duration of sensory exposure

Note: *As defined by Wilcock's Framework for Health, these four categories (doing, being, belonging, becoming), which align with the activities and outputs of SENSE, are occupation-based approaches to be utilized by the parents of preterm infants, OTDS, and NICU staff to improve population health within the NICU (Merryman et al., 2020). **As defined by the health belief model, cues to action can help people begin a new behavior that they believe will result in positive outcomes; perceived benefits are a person's thoughts about how an action will decrease a negative health experience (Merryman et al., 2020). Both of these terms support the goals of SENSE via parent education and involvement in infant care. *Source:* Template adapted from http://templatelab.com/logic-model/.

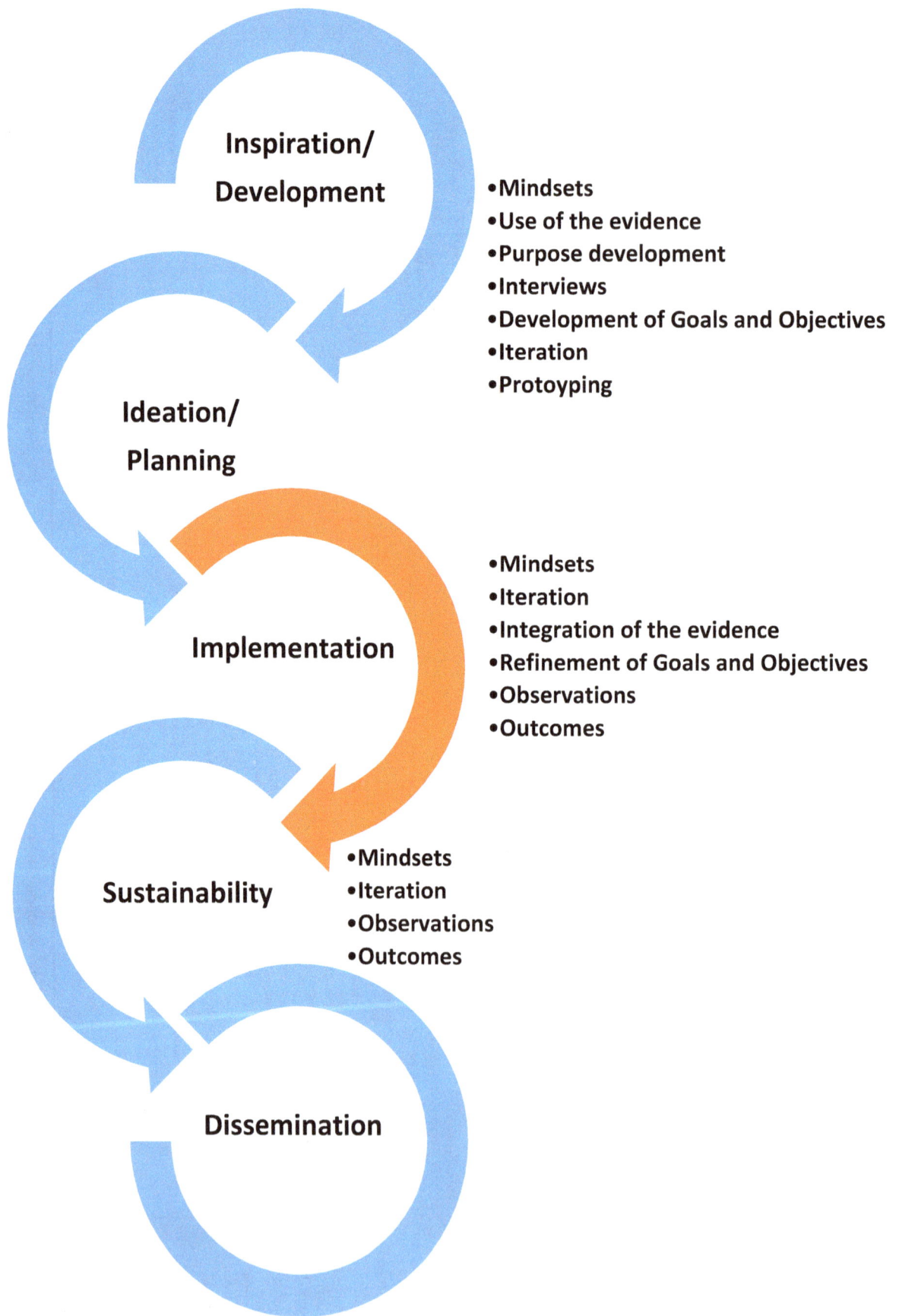

Inspiration/ Development

- Mindsets
- Use of the evidence
- Purpose development
- Interviews
- Development of Goals and Objectives
- Iteration
- Protoyping

Ideation/ Planning

Implementation

- Mindsets
- Iteration
- Integration of the evidence
- Refinement of Goals and Objectives
- Observations
- Outcomes

Sustainability

- Mindsets
- Iteration
- Observations
- Outcomes

Dissemination

PART III.
IMPLEMENTATION

The third step in the capstone process is **implementation and sustainability,** of the doctoral capstone experience and project and aligns with the **implementation** process of human-centered design. This phase allows capstone students to bring all their ideas and planning to life. Capstone students will continually be making adjustments during the implementation phase as they work with their specified client. Assessing and adjusting the planned solutions is important throughout the implementation of the capstone project. To be a human-centered designer means you are client-centered. Interacting and communicating with the client for feedback and adjusting goal and objectives as needed is important in this stage of the capstone. During the implementation phase, capstone students are determining how their doctoral capstone project affects their identified client, group, or population and how the project will be sustained.

DOI: 10.4324/9781003541813-11

CHAPTER 9

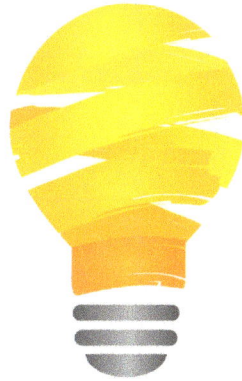

On-Site Implementation of the Capstone Experience and Project

Cambey Mikush and Sara J. Stephenson

Section 1: Student Focus

Human-Centered Design Mindsets for the Implementation Phase

Human-centered design (HCD), like the occupational therapy process, is not linear. You move between the inspiration and ideation phases early in your capstone experience to ensure your work and project align with your site's expectations, needs, *and* occupational therapy. As you begin the implementation phase, it is important to embrace the following HCD mindsets – iterating, embracing ambiguity, building collaborative relationships, and conscientiously advocating.

Iterating requires you to frequently refine your plan and work based on feedback and collaboration. The needs of a capstone site, mentor, and population change rapidly, which can impact your capstone proposal and objectives. That's okay! Revisiting the literature and updating your capstone needs assessment will help you iterate on your initial proposal to develop a mutually beneficial plan for your capstone project and 14-week experience.

Embracing ambiguity is just as critical in the implementation phase of human-centered design as it is in the inspiration and ideation phases. Because mentorship and the HCD process are iterative, embracing ambiguity allows you to approach challenges with innovation, curiosity, and open-mindedness.

Being a curious researcher requires that you lead with curiosity over judgment (Ahmed & Stafford, 2022). You are open to listening to and seeking diverse perspectives to inform each phase of your project and experience.

Building collaborative relationships is a central tenet of the OTD capstone and is essential to creating a mutually beneficial project and experience that is desirable, feasible, and viable (Ahmed & Stafford, 2022). Using this mindset, you view collaborators, such as clients, caregivers, mentors, staff, and faculty, as partners in the project.

Conscientiously advocating means you work to balance power in your collaborative capstone relationships (Ahmed & Stafford, 2022). Reflecting on your own positionality and power in the project helps you and your team identify solutions that center the authentic needs of the community you hope to support.

DOI: 10.4324/9781003541813-12

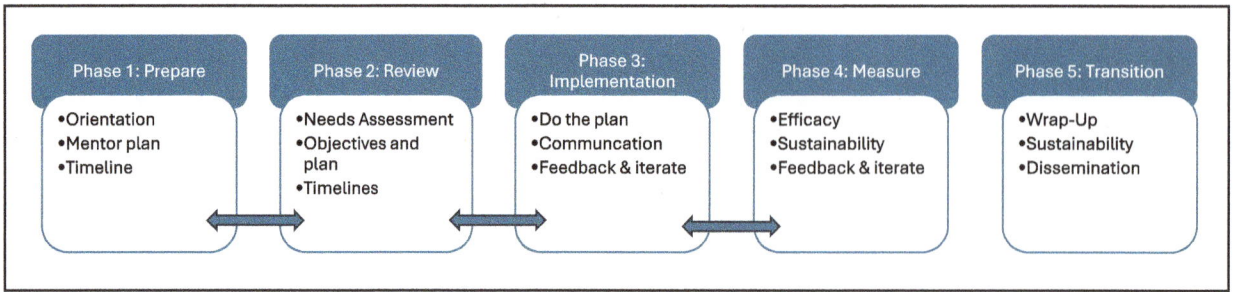

Figure 9-1. Overview of the capstone development process for students.

INTRODUCTION FOR STUDENTS

Prior to the implementation phase, you may spend up to 18 months in the inspiration and ideation phases planning and developing your capstone project and experience (DeIuliis & Bednarski, 2019). The specifics of the development and planning process will vary based on your occupational therapy program's curricular design. However, the standards for a doctoral capstone experience are consistent across all entry-level degrees, as outlined by the Accreditation Council for Occupational Therapy Education ([ACOTE], 2023). This chapter moves you through the five suggested phases of capstone implementation, as depicted in Figure 9.1.

STUDENT REFLECTIVE QUESTIONS

1. How does your capstone project align with your program's mission, values, and the current trends and evidence in OT practice?
2. What ethical considerations have you accounted for in your project, and how do these influence your scholarly work?
3. What steps can you take to ensure your project is feasible within the timeline and resources available?
4. How are you using feedback from your program, content expert, mentors, peers, and population to refine and improve your project?
5. How prepared do you feel to navigate a mentor–mentee relationship?
6. What strategies can you use to foster and maintain effective communication with your mentor?
7. How will you demonstrate that you are actively engaging in reflective practice throughout your capstone to monitor your growth and progress as a mentee?

STUDENT OBJECTIVES

By the end of reading this chapter and completing the learning activities, the student should be able to:
- Develop a site orientation plan for the capstone experience.
- Revise the needs assessment to reflect updates once on-site.
- Modify the capstone experience goals and objectives as needed once on-site.
- Create a timeline and implementation plan for the capstone experience and project.
- Implement and actualize best practices for communication with mentors (on-site and the faculty).
- Advance skills to navigate problems and address barriers.

PHASE 1: PREPARE

Human-Centered Design Mindset: Building Collaborative Relationships

Whether they are mentors, peers, clients, or community members, it is important to create space to build authentic, collaborative relationships with those you, the capstone student, plan to work with and learn from.

Key Takeaways

The *prepare phase* of your capstone includes activities that need to be completed prior to initiating your capstone experience (i.e., onboarding and compliance requirements) and the orientation tasks that take place in the first couple of weeks. Orientation is important to help you acclimate to your site, nourish relationships with your collaborators, and situate your capstone project and experience in context. Each capstone site will have different expectations for orientation. Some sites, for example, may have a consistent formal training plan for student collaborators. Other sites may have less formal orientation procedures, requiring you to draw on your self-directed learning skills to fill your knowledge gaps. Developing an orientation plan and sharing it with your context expert and site for feedback ensure all collaborator expectations are aligned.

Once you understand the expectations of your site, you can develop a collaborative orientation plan. At a minimum, an orientation plan should include activities addressing:
- Site environment and space
- Site policies and procedures

- Collaborators and employees
- Experience logistics
- Mentorship plans

Table 9.1 offers suggested questions to consider as you build your capstone experience orientation plan.

Tips for Students

- While your project is self-directed, it does not mean you need to work in isolation. Identify a small group of peers within your cohort and meet regularly (in-person or virtually) as accountability partners. In these meet-ups, share celebrations and work together to problem-solve challenges. Seek feedback on your email drafts, assignments, deliverables, or capstone activities.
- To prepare for meeting new people at your capstone site, consider crafting a brief pitch about why you are there and what your project entails. Here are a few activity ideas:

Table 9-1. Questions to Consider When Developing a Capstone Orientation Plan

QUESTIONS TO CONSIDER WHEN DEVELOPING A CAPSTONE ORIENTATION PLAN
Site Environment and Space
• Will you be working virtually, in person, or hybrid?
• What rooms, equipment, and spaces do you have access to?
• Where can you sit to work?
• Which computers can you use?
• Do you need to reserve rooms for capstone activities? If so, how do you do this?
• If you are driving to the site, where should you park?
Site Policies and Procedures
• What compliances are required prior to initiating the capstone (i.e., immunization records, fingerprinting, background checks, or drug screenings)?
• What certifications are required (i.e., CPR, first aid, population-specific certifications)?
• Is there a policy and procedure or onboarding manual to review?
• What trainings are required to initiate the 14-week experience (i.e., HIPPA, electronic medical record training, or modules)?
• Are there policies around virtual or telehealth communications (i.e., specific platforms used for communication)?
• If you are completing a research or quality improvement project, what additional training or requirements are necessary? When should they be completed? For example, you may need to complete a series of Collaborative Institutional Training Initiative (CITI) modules and submit an Institutional Review Board (IRB) application for project approval prior to beginning your capstone. (Refer back to Chapter 7).
Collaborators and Employees
• Who are the primary partners and collaborators at your site?
• Who are you most likely to collaborate with and how? Be sure to consider the many people who support the success of the system, organization, or program you are supporting.
• How will you introduce yourself and your project?
• Explaining your capstone, "what's your pitch"?
Experience Logistics
• Is there a dress code? For example, at some sites, it will be appropriate to wear scrubs, while others expect business attire.
• Should you wear a name tag or badge? Is there a specific place you are expected to wear your badge?
• What are the work hour expectations?
• How many (and which) days during the week are you expected to be in person (or logged on)? How many days will you work remotely?

continued

Table 9-1. Questions to Consider When Developing a Capstone Orientation Plan (continued)

Mentorship Plan

While the plan for mentorship should be established upon the initiation of the capstone in the experiential plan (ACOTE D.1.4), it is critical to collaboratively revisit the plan with your content expert and site mentor(s). This information could be included in your mentor compact (see Chapter 3). Consider the following as you review and revise the plan:

- How have you prepared yourself to be a mentee?
  - What specific skills or knowledge are you hoping to gain from your mentor?
  - How will you ensure your mentor understands how to support you?
  - How will you balance seeking guidance with being self-directed?
  - What actions will you take to uphold your responsibilities as a mentee?
  - What tools, methods, or resources will you use to stay accountable in your capstone work and mentoring relationship?
- Who is your primary mentor? Who is responsible for reviewing your work and signing off on your time logs, for example?
- What are your communication needs and plan for the 14-week experience? Consider:
  - How will you communicate with your content expert and mentor?
  - Will you send weekly project updates via email?
  - What are the expectations of your faculty mentor and capstone coordinator in terms of communication?
  - What is the best method of communication for urgent needs?
- When, where, and for how long will you meet with your mentor(s)?
- What are the expectations for meetings (i.e., student sets an agenda, follows up with email action items)?
- How will you, as collaborators, address conflicts or challenges over the next 14 weeks?
- How do personal and professional differences influence your expectations for the capstone?
- What are mutually beneficial expectations you can set for the mentoring relationship? For example:
  - As a mentoring team, we will . . .
  - As a mentee, I will . . .
  - As a mentor, I will . . .

- Record a short video that can be sent out to employees.
- Tailoring a 1- to 2-minute pitch to different audiences helps address their unique interests and priorities. (See Table 9.2 for pitch examples that could be for a faculty member, parent, and a state agency.)
- Create a one-page flyer that explains what a *capstone* is, what your project entails, and what you envision for your capstone. See Appendix 9.A for a template and Appendix 9.B for an example.

PHASE 2: REVIEW

Human-Centered Design Mindset: Iteration, Curious Researcher, and Conscientious Advocate

As you update your needs assessment and revise your capstone experience plan, it is important to acknowledge the value of diverse experiences. Lead with curiosity, asking yourself whose perspective might be missing. These insights can help you iterate on your initial ideas and lead to the most impactful and innovative solutions.

Key Takeaways

Because level II fieldwork experiences must be completed prior to initiating the doctoral capstone experience, students might have a three- to six-month or more gap between the planning and the implementation phases (DeIuliis & Bednarski, 2019; Stephenson et al., 2020). The needs of a site, content expert, or population can shift dramatically during these months; thus, it is critical that you take the first one to three weeks of your experience to orient, get to know your collaborators and clients, update your needs assessment, and revise your objectives to reflect your site's current needs.

Table 9-2. Capstone Pitch Examples for Students

ACADEMIC MENTOR	PARENT OR CAREGIVER	STATE AGENCY REPRESENTATIVE
Hello, Dr. [Name]. My capstone focuses on occupational therapy's role in supporting youth aging out of foster care. Through surveys with house managers, I plan to examine their perceptions of behavioral challenges and emotional regulation needs in older teens, helping clarify which skills might benefit most from OT interventions. I will also be using the KELS-Y assessment directly with youth to understand their self-perceived support needs as they transition out of care. Finally, I will have meetings with my mentor(s) and the state Medicaid representatives to expand OT coverage for transition support services. This capstone not only explores the practical impact of OT in youth transitions but also opens pathways for state-level policy change, making it a significant area for future OT practice and research.	My capstone project focuses on helping foster teens gaining the skills they need as they transition to independence. Through surveys with house managers, I will learn about the challenges these teens face and how they manage their emotions in stressful situations. I will also speak with the teens transitioning out of the foster system using an assessment to understand their specific needs and how they think they could best be supported. Lastly, I am meeting with state Medicaid representatives to advocate for occupational therapy services that could help these young adults transition more successfully. OT could provide them with the skills they need to live independently and reach their goals, such as graduation, ongoing education, employment, and financial stability.	My capstone focuses on the role occupational therapy can play in supporting teens as they transition out of foster care. Youth transitioning into adulthood from the foster care system often face challenges which are exacerbated by trauma histories and disruptions of daily life experience (housing and school). This population has staggering statistics for homelessness, unemployment, substance dependence, and pregnancy before age 21, with less than half obtaining a high school diploma (Courtney & Dworsky, 2006; Armstrong-Heimsoth et al., 2020). My work is directly with the transitioning teens, using the KELS-Y assessment to evaluate their needs for independent living and develop interventions to ensure their success. By adding OT services, the state could better prepare these young people for success, which, in turn, could reduce long-term reliance on state support. I believe this collaboration could be a valuable investment in both the well-being of foster youth and the state's future resources.

Updating Your Needs Assessment

As you have learned, there are a variety of approaches that can be used to guide the needs assessment process (for example, SWOT, SOAR, SBAR, PDSA, Six Sigma). This book highlights the PRECEDE–PROCEED model and appreciative inquiry framework, as outlined in Chapter 6. No matter the format, carve out time in the first few weeks of your capstone experience to revisit and update your needs assessment to reflect the most current challenges and opportunities of your site and population. This crucial step will help you take what you learn from your mentors, clients, and collaborators and translate that into a meaningful experience and project that supports the community and site.

First, take a moment to reflect on your positionality in relation to your project and site. Acknowledging your social position, identity, privilege, and power within the context of your capstone allows you to reflect on how your experiences may influence the trajectory and outcomes of your project. At the very least, this reflection increases the conscious awareness of your own bias and assumptions, creating space for change. Consider using the questions in Table 9.3 as a guide. Alternatively, you may choose to create a social identity map to support your reflection. This flexible tool challenges you to name your social identities, consider how these identities influence your life, and reflect on the impact these identities have on your role in the project (Jacobson & Mustafa, 2019).

Table 9-3. Reflective Questions on Positionality in Relation to Capstone

Use the following questions to reflect on your social position, identity, privilege, and power within the context of your capstone.
How do my social identities (e.g., race, gender, ethnicity, socioeconomic status, ability, education, etc.) influence the way I understand and approach my capstone?
How does my personal worldview influence how I identify and interpret the needs of the site and objectives of my capstone?
What assumptions do I have about my capstone population and site? How might these be influenced by my personal biases?
What steps am I taking to minimize bias in my capstone work?

Next, consider how you might update your needs assessment sources to help you develop a deeper understanding of the needs and capacities of your site, population, and team. In many ways, you are developing an occupational profile for your capstone site. To do this, you may:

- Revisit the peer-reviewed literature and update your literature review and references accordingly.
- Consider whose perspectives might be missing from the literature. How might you capture those experiences?
- Explore open-access population-level data, such as the National Center for Health Statistics or US Census Data.
- Review site-specific documents, like strategic plans, program outlines, previous capstone and internship projects, etc.
- Shadow and interview with leaders, employees, and clients.
- Observe daily work activities and interactions.
- Explore existing community resources and how they serve as facilitators or barriers to your site's work.

Revising Your Capstone Objectives and Evaluation Plan

Based on the needs assessment outcomes, collaboratively update your capstone objectives and evaluation plan for both the project and the experience. Keep in mind the communication required for all mentors by referring to your mentor compact agreement (see Chapter 3). You may choose to use a form to track your progress, like the example provided in Appendix 9.C.

Your objectives are the foundation of your capstone project and experience. To support you in developing strong objectives that will inform the timeline and structure of your experience, consider the following:

- Are your objectives specific, measurable, achievable, relevant and time-bound ([SMART], Bowman et al., 2015).
- Is the role of occupation explicit in your objectives? Bringing occupation to the forefront is one way we demonstrate our value as OTs.
- Are your objectives within the scope of OT practice?
- Can you complete these objectives independently with input and mentorship from your content expert?
- Do you have a clear plan to evaluate the outcome of your objectives?

Remember that your objective and evaluation plan are a living document and will be revised throughout your capstone experience.

Creating a 14-Week Timeline

Now that you have updated your objectives, you can begin working backwards to think about specific action steps needed to meet these objectives. For this you may consider:

- What tasks need to be completed and by what week?
- What do you need to learn to complete those tasks?
- Where and how will you gain that knowledge?
- What support do you need to fill your gaps in knowledge?
- Are there logistical considerations you need to plan for (i.e., room reservations, HIPAA-compliant communication platforms, IRB approval)?
- How will you know you have achieved your objectives?

You will also want to consider program-specific requirements and expectations. For example:

- Do you have assignments due throughout your capstone experience?
- What is the dissemination requirement for your program?
- How often do you need your content expert to sign off on your time log?

This is where the self-directed learning component of the capstone is particularly important. The onus is on you to set your schedule, create a weekly plan, and identify the tools and resources you need to implement your plan. To reiterate, this does not mean you must work in silo without support in this process. See Table 9.4 for tips from former OTD capstone students. Remember to reach out to your capstone coordinator, faculty mentor(s), site mentor(s), content expert, and peers when you are stuck.

Table 9-4. Tips From Former OTD Capstone Students

TOPIC	IT HELPED ME TO . . .
Check-ins	"... have weekly check-ins with my mentor as protected time; if we didn't need to meet, we could cancel, but at least I knew we had something on the books." "... check in with my doctoral capstone coordinator and/or advisor to share wins and troubleshoot challenges." "... make a calendar that was shared with my mentor so we could both see what I was doing with the project and what was coming up. We put things like assignments, progress updates, interviews, deliverables, etc. on the calendar."
Organization	"... have my mentor sign off on my hours every Friday during our regularly scheduled meetings." "... keep track of all my activities. My mentor got a job in a different state 5 weeks into my capstone and left before signing off on my hours for weeks 4 and 5. Because I kept track of all my activities, the doctoral capstone coordinator was able to discuss my activities and sign off on my hours for those 2 weeks." "... make my plan (I did hour-by-hour) and stick to it the best I can. Do not expect to be told how to spend my time. This was a big difference from level II FW to capstone. Think of it like a scheduled caseload. I did this every Sunday night for the upcoming week. This allowed me to think critically about what needed to be accomplished, how, and when, and made it easier to collaborate with my mentor's schedule." "... start broad and think about what I wanted to accomplish. From there, I broke down this large goal into small tasks. Once I had the list of small tasks that needed to be completed, I wrote down the time and day I could tackle the task."
Collaborate	"... determine my work schedule. I liked getting my online research done in the morning and scheduling meetings later in the day. I found I was more productive with certain tasks in the morning and enjoyed collaborating with others in the afternoon." "... talk to someone when I got stuck (peers, mentor, family, friends, instructors). Many times my peers and I would discuss the progress of our projects to work through challenges, revise each other's drafts, and talk through where we were going next. It helped to surround myself with productive people."
Confidence	"... streamline our communication. I wanted a lot of time with my mentor at first. I was overwhelmed by capstone, was a little anxious, and wanted to be sure I was on track. As the weeks progressed, so did my confidence. I did not need as much time from my mentor." "... keep a journal of my process; it can be useful for future interviews! I find that employers like to hear how you navigated situations where things did not go perfectly."

continued

Table 9-4. Tips From Former OTD Capstone Students (continued)

TOPIC	IT HELPED ME TO . . .
Well-being	". . . take time to do the things that motivate me. For me, it was exercise and spiritual practice. Remind yourself of your 'why' on days you don't feel motivated."
	". . . be diligent about establishing good routines/habits right from the start in order to make the most of my capstone. This includes work–life balance routines to maintain my overall well-being throughout the 14-week experience."

Tips for Students

- Consider creating weekly practices that help you stay on track. You may, for example:
  - Set smaller weekly goals and review them with an accountability partner (i.e., a peer from your cohort) on Mondays.
  - At the end of each day, identify the specific task you will start on the following day. For example, "Tomorrow morning I will draft the email to schedule an interview."
  - Try using the "Pomodoro Technique" for self-directed work time (Cirillo, 2018). Students report that this is particularly helpful if you are having a hard time getting started or need to complete less-preferred tasks. You may, for example, set a timer to work for 24 uninterrupted minutes, followed by a required 6-minute break. This systematic process can lead to higher levels of concentration, productivity, and motivation (Biwer et al., 2023). When reflecting on planning their day, one student stated, "I used a focused, 25-minute timer on my computer to remind me to take movement breaks."
  - Send a wrap-up email to your mentor each week, outlining your accomplishments and articulating the following week's action items. (See Figure 9.2 for a template.)
  - Consider incorporating some movement into your schedule, like a daily stroll as a mid-morning break. Alternatively, try hosting a walking or movement meeting.

It is easy to get distracted by life activities and long to-do lists. Create a "parking lot" where you can write down divergent ideas to refer to later. (See Table 9.5.)

Designate a workspace for weekly activities, particularly those being completed remotely. Be thoughtful about your environment and where you work best. For example, if you are easily distracted by house projects when you work from home, you may consider working from a public library one day a week.

Weekly Wrap-Up Email Template

Good [*morning/afternoon*], [*mentor name*]!

I hope you are doing well. My focus this week was on progressing [*insert capstone objectives being addressed*]. Following is a summary of my work, with corresponding links, for your review. Please note that I need [*list specific things you need from your mentor, like a signature on your time log or feedback on a deliverable; be sure to link the documents*].

Accomplishments Towards Objectives	Actions in Progress	Priorities for Next Week

Figure 9-2. Example weekly wrap-up.

Please let me know what feedback, comments, or questions you have.

Thanks,
[*your name*]
[*Insert your professional email signature*]

Phase 3: Implement

Human-Centered Design Mindset: Iteration, Embracing Ambiguity

As you move into the *implementation phase* of your capstone experience, remember that your objectives and evaluation plan are a living document. It is to be expected that, as you learn more about your site and the community you are serving, the priorities and tasks will shift.

Key Takeaways

This is when your diligent and hard work in the preparation and review phases pay off. In this phase, your focus is on moving through your timeline, managing your project, and implementing your collaborative ideas. You

Table 9-5. Parking Lot Example – Got a Great Idea but Not Sure What to Do With It? Park Your Ideas Here!

TOPIC	IDEA/OUTCOME	ACTION
Example: Look at continuing education courses for car seat fit training	*Example:* Could partner with a local nonprofit for car seat checks,	*Example:* Find community partner and schedule a meeting.
Example: Curious about getting a certification during capstone	*Example:* Identify what courses or certification courses are available to students.	*Example:* Sign up and take the courses. How can you demonstrate understanding of the information?
Example: Caregiver education need identified	*Example:* Caregivers need information on back safety and body mechanics.	*Example:* Talk with mentor(s) to decide if this is a "right now" or future project (may be a good idea for the next capstone student.)

should continually refer to your capstone objectives and evaluation plan and update it as your project and experience unfolds.

The implement phase is a good time to consider what you will provide to the site. Some programs may require you to create a deliverable for your capstone site. Landfried et al. (2023) define *deliverables* as "tangible products produced by the student team that are mutually beneficial to student's professional development goals and partner organization needs" (p. 7). Examples of deliverables could be a group protocol or facilitation guide, grant proposal, scholarly paper or presentation, a comprehensive collection of resources, assessment tool, recommendation reports, white paper, training modules, etc. These are tangible products that can support the sustainability and viability of your project, and further discussion on this will occur in Chapters 11 and 12.

Feedback throughout the implementation phase is critical to ensure your work truly meets the needs of your site. Like level II fieldwork experiences, you will likely have a midterm and final evaluation with your mentor. However, to truly embrace the iterative and collaborative mindset necessary for a successful capstone project and experience, it is critical that you seek and incorporate feedback prior to these formal evaluations. This book will dive into the evaluation process in Chapter 10.

It can be challenging doing meaningful work with people whose perspectives and life experiences differ from your own. Conflicts can (and likely will) arise during your capstone. Seeking feedback early and often allows you to address issues or concerns early. Remember to use your resources and to reach out to your faculty advisor(s) and capstone coordinator for support.

Recommendations to Address Common Barriers During Implementation Phase

Because the capstone reflects the realities of practice, it is to be expected that you will experience some challenges along the way. This section offers suggestions to address or overcome common difficulties reported by students during the implementation phase of the capstone.

- *Difficulty fulfilling the hour requirement.* Because capstone is self-directed, you are often responsible for setting your own schedule. If you are struggling to fulfill the hour requirement for capstone, consider:
  - Reaching out to your capstone coordinator to brainstorm additional learning experiences to fill your time.
  - *Ideas.* Update your literature review and annotated bibliography, create a digital folder for all your literature and search strings, draft a proposal to submit a poster or presentation to AOTA or state conference, develop education materials, or create a journal club with peers.
  - Connect with professionals and experts in related fields. Think about how you might gain more in-depth knowledge on the topic.
  - Set up times to observe similar projects or work environments to gain a different perspective.

- Engage with community members and organizations by following your program's process for outreach.
- **A change in context experts or mentorship changing mentors.** It is possible for a mentor to change jobs, take a leave of absence, or transition into a new role. Do your best to stay open-minded to new perspectives, flexible with new working styles, and proactive in addressing challenges. Revisit the tips from phases 1–3 around communication and expectations to create a strong foundation with your mentor.
- *Scope of your project is too big.* You are here because you are ambitious and have big dreams. That is a strength. And your capstone needs to be feasible in a 14-week time frame. If your idea has gotten too big, collaborate with your mentor and break your ideas down into smaller, more manageable tasks. What elements are you able to address now, and which ones might be best carried out by the next student or colleague?
- *Personal challenges.* Balancing personal challenges amidst capstone can be difficult. Recognize that setbacks, personally and professionally, are normal. Keep in mind that:
  - It is important to take breaks and prioritize self-care to maintain your own sense of well-being. Incorporate brief movement or brain breaks, work in community (if this serves you well), and make space outside of work to engage in occupations that bring you joy.
  - Asking for help is a sign of strength. Reach out to your content expert, other mentor, capstone coordinator, trusted faculty advisors, or peers for support. Your community wants to see you succeed *and* appreciates the opportunity to be a part of your experience.
  - If personal challenges are impacting your capstone process, communicate your needs and concerns as soon as you can. Be open to creative solutions.
- *Divergent mentor–student ideas.* Professionals often have differing opinions and ideas in the work context. Some of the most innovative solutions come from these collaborations. Here are a few tips to support you in managing these tensions:
  - Lean into direct communication, open dialogue, and collaboration. Acknowledge your mentor's expertise while expressing your viewpoint with respect. What might it look like if you merged your ideas?
  - Invite feedback and broader discussions around solutions. Do not assume that your way is the one and only right way.
  - If a consensus cannot be reached, consult with your faculty mentor and/or your capstone coordinator for advice on how to navigate conflict in the workplace.
- *Self-advocacy.* It is important to clearly express your needs and set boundaries to support your capstone success. Communicating your goals, progress, and challenges with your mentor on a regular basis to provide you with space to address issues in the moment. Be assertive *and* respectful when discussing workload, timelines, and expectations. If necessary, advocate for additional resources or adjustments.

TIPS FOR STUDENTS

- Setting clear expectations around communication during the implementation phase of your capstone will support the student–mentor relationship while ensuring the work you are doing truly meets the needs of your site. Consider aligning with your content expert on the following:
  - Preferred method of communication (phone call, text, email, shared platform like Microsoft Teams, Slack).
  - When to communicate. For example, you may mutually decide you will send a weekly email on Mondays with plan and action items and a wrap-up email on Fridays with accomplishments and next steps (Figure 9.2).
  - How and when to obtain signatures. Consider looking at a calendar and marking when you will need to request signatures from your mentor.
  - Where documents will live to allow you to seek efficient feedback (i.e., shared drive, email). Be mindful of HIPPA policies and sharing protected health information (PHI) on unsecured shared drives and platforms like Google.
  - *Frequency and time of meetings.* Be sure to articulate who is responsible for setting the agenda, when it should be sent out, and who will typically lead the meetings. In most cases, these responsibilities will fall on the student.
- Remember that your project is one of many responsibilities for your mentor and collaborators. Consider sending a *brief* email to collaborators after important meetings that thanks them for their time, provides a quick overview of the discussion, and identifies clear action items for each person.
- Conflict is an inherent part of working and collaborating with others. It is also a part of program design and implementing projects. If you experience tension with your mentor or a colleague:

- Communicate the concern directly to your content expert or colleagues. Approach the situation with an open mind and a willingness to learn. Seek to understand their perspective.

- Contact your capstone coordinator to help you identify effective and thoughtful approaches to address the conflict. It can be helpful to role-play the conversation for feedback.

- It is hard to hear difficult feedback; try to depersonalize it. Remind yourself that the people around you are eager to see you succeed and are here to help move your project forward. Consider using and sharing a communication log with your mentor(s). A structure like this can help you outline objective feedback, responses, and next steps. This strategy can help keep feedback depersonalized (Appendix 9.D).

PHASE 4: MEASURE

Human-Centered Design Mindset: Iteration, Conscientious Advocate, Collaborative Relationships

As you enter the final weeks of your capstone, your focus shifts toward reflecting on the impact of your work and ensuring its sustainability. Although your active participation is concluding, your contributions can create lasting value for your site and its community. This is a key time to solidify collaborative relationships, advocate for future initiatives, and ensure that the outcomes of your project are meaningful and measurable.

Key Takeaways

Measuring the outcomes of your project helps you demonstrate your own learning *and* the impact of your capstone on your site. The final weeks of your capstone are a time for assessment – both of your personal growth and the project's effectiveness. Measuring outcomes allows you to demonstrate the impact on the site, its clients, and your own learning. This is also when you should consider how your project can continue to thrive after your departure.

Just like in level II fieldwork, formal evaluations such as midterm and final assessments will occur. These evaluations will capture how well you have met your objectives, what outcomes were achieved, and any areas for further growth and improvement. This is an opportunity for reflective learning and fine-tuning your deliverables. Consider what your program requires of you for capstone and how this can align with the site.

It is essential to consider what your work will look like after you complete the project. Collaborate with the site to identify next steps in maintaining and building upon the work you have initiated. Your goal is to leave behind resources, protocols, or frameworks that continue to provide value (see Chapter 8).

Tips for Students

As you approach your final weeks of the capstone experience, you move from being an active participant to a reflective practitioner. Your journey does not end here; it evolves as you carry forward the skills, insights, and relationships you have built into your future practice. A significant part of the measure phase is taking time to document your reflections. For example, you may:

- Take time to reflect on your role as an advocate for your project and the community you served. Ask yourself:

  - *When I leave capstone, I want . . .*
    Consider what you hope to leave behind and what outcomes you envision for your project.

  - *When I leave capstone, I want the site to . . .*
    Think about how you want the site to benefit from your contributions and how you can set them up for success.

  - Engage in personal reflection on your journey through the capstone. How have your experiences shaped you as a professional? How will you apply this learning to future projects and professional roles? What will you take with you to practice?

  - Value: Reflection is not just about assessing the outcome; it is about understanding the value your work has brought. Take time to reflect on both the personal growth you have experienced and the tangible outcomes that will continue to benefit the site.

- Acknowledge the hard work you have put in, and celebrate your achievements. This helps you and your site collaborators recognize the value of the partnership and progress made.

- Discuss with your content expert and other collaborators among your capstone what comes next for the project. Identify any follow-up actions or ongoing tasks that may be required and offer suggestions for who can take on these roles.

- As you think about the sustainability of your project, what other tools might be helpful to leave behind? For example, are there email or document templates or a list of helpful resources you could share to ease the transition?

PHASE 5: TRANSITION

Human-Centered Design Mindset: Collaborative Relationships

The HCD framework emphasizes the importance of solutions being desirable, feasible, and *viable*. True collaboration means that you are thoughtful about how your project will wrap up. Taking time to focus on transitioning the project is critical to ensuring your work has a long-lasting impact.

Key Takeaways

This phase of your capstone experience is a time where you transition your project to its next stage. For some students, the project has run its course, and once the outcomes are disseminated, it is complete. For other students, though, the project will live on in some way. Maybe another capstone student is expanding on your project, or a team member plans to take the next steps in implementing your work. Either way, articulating how your project will transition beyond your capstone is an important step toward sustainability.

While your program dictates how and when you disseminate your capstone outcomes, it is important to make time and space to share your experience and findings with your capstone site. Presenting your deliverables and project outcomes to your capstone site for final feedback supports the transition of the project to the next person. Be sure to leave space in your timeline to make revisions based on the feedback.

Tips for Students

- A significant part of successful collaborations is showing gratitude and acknowledging contributions. Take time to thank those who have supported your capstone work. Be sure to acknowledge people's efforts and in your disseminated materials.
- Remember to update your résumé, CV, or portfolio to reflect your capstone work.

STUDENT SECTION CHAPTER SUMMARY

Although it is a required assignment, your capstone is so much more than just an academic exercise. Your doctoral capstone is a comprehensive process and opportunity that integrates project management, critical thinking, reflection, and professional collaboration. You must practice adaptability and reflection and engage with mentors to ensure your project creates a meaningful, lasting impact. Your capstone represents a unique opportunity to bridge academic learning and real-world application, demonstrating your capacity to address complex challenges through a collaborative, evidence-based approach. Embracing this process not only enhances your professional skills but also prepares you to advocate for sustainable, impactful change in your future practice.

Section 2: Educator Focus

Transformational Learning Phases and Framework for the Educator

The actual engagement within a 14-week doctoral capstone experience aligns closely with Mezirow's phases of acquisition of knowledge, trying new roles, and building confidence from his theory of transformative learning (Mezirow, 1997). As the formal capstone experience begins, students move from theoretical learning to practical, hands-on application in real-world settings, which is essential for fostering transformative growth. An essential component for success during the implementation phase is ensuring our content experts and site mentors offer our students a *structured* learning environment where they can integrate theoretical knowledge, explore diverse professional roles, and develop confidence. This not only contributes to their professional identity development but also prepares them for success as future practitioners in the profession.

By facilitating strong mentorship and supervision, offering meaningful constructive feedback, fostering opportunities for reflection, and encouraging active engagement in new roles, as educators (or doctoral capstone coordinators), we can help students bridge the gap between theory (the classroom) and practice. This supportive learning environment will allow our students to develop the necessary knowledge, skills, and confidence to succeed in their doctoral capstone experience.

INTRODUCTION FOR EDUCATOR

This section builds upon preparatory work in the planning classes and provides a framework for educators guiding capstone projects, emphasizing the collaborative and iterative processes necessary to support capstone students. For educators, it is important to create an environment and curriculum that encourages ongoing feedback and helps students engage in self-directed learning. Figure 9.3 depicts the phases of capstone implementation from an educator's perspective. This section offers guidance on how educators can best support capstone students and mentors by adopting HCD mindsets, asking reflective questions, and implementing teaching strategies that encourage adaptability and transformative learning.

EDUCATOR REFLECTIVE QUESTIONS

1. **How will you prepare the context experts that will serve as mentors to your occupational therapy doctoral students?** Reflect on how you onboard these individuals, providing them with clear expectations, resources, and a structured support system.

    a. How can I ensure both students and context experts are aligned on goals and expectations from the start?

    b. What methods will I use to facilitate relationship-building between students, content experts, and other relevant stakeholders at the capstone site?

2. **How will you prepare students to function in a mentee role?** Consider how to prepare students to communicate effectively, seek feedback, and engage actively with mentors.

    a. Use of self-assessments, reflective assignments targeted to mentee skills.

3. **What portions of a student's capstone do you see as flexible, and how do you demonstrate this?** Reflect on areas where flexibility can be integrated, including modifying goals, timelines, and approaches as projects evolve.

    a. What frameworks can I introduce to help students evaluate and communicate changes in their project?

4. **What data do you want to collect throughout the implementation process?** Identify key data points to monitor student progress, mentor skills, mentor feedback, and the project's overall impact on the site.

EDUCATOR OBJECTIVES

By the end of reading this chapter, the educator will be able to apply principles of transformational learning theory to structure learning activities, assignments, and/or assessments in order to promote the capstone student's ability to:

1. Develop a site orientation plan.
2. Create a timeline and implementation plan for the capstone experience and project.
3. Modify the needs assessment to reflect updates once on-site.
4. Modify the capstone experience goals and objectives as needed once on-site.
5. Develop strategies to support the content experts in the role of mentor.

PHASE 1: PREPARE

Human-Centered Design Mindset: Building Collaborative Relationships

Collaboration is key during the preparation phase. Student activities should focus on understanding their site, team, and population while building strong communication skills.

Key Takeaways

The *prepare* phase focuses on the steps necessary to initiate the capstone experience. This includes orientation to the site, establishing and building relationships, and setting clear expectations.

Expecting students to automatically synthesize didactic education, engage independently in capstone, and lead a project may not be realistic without practice. For example, we would not teach someone to ride a bike on a residential street and then expect the same level of competence while mountain biking. Students need opportunities to practice managing the myriad expectations, such as completing onboarding processes and compliances, learning student management systems, and developing a capstone plan.

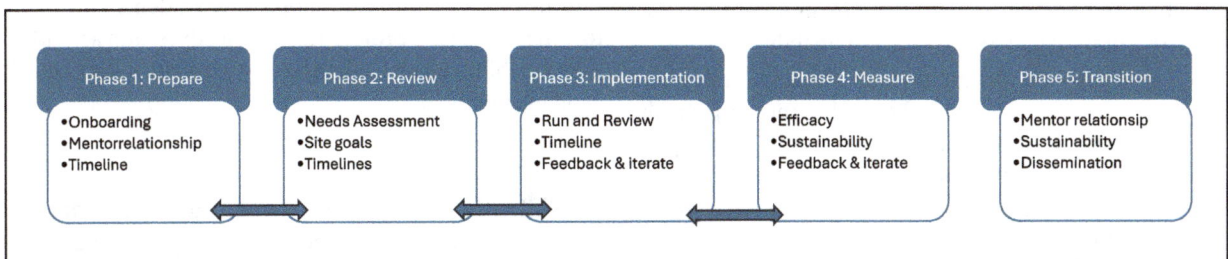

Phase 1: Prepare	Phase 2: Review	Phase 3: Implementation	Phase 4: Measure	Phase 5: Transition
•Onboarding •Mentorrelationship •Timeline	•Needs Assessment •Site goals •Timelines	•Run and Review •Timeline •Feedback & iterate	•Efficacy •Sustainability •Feedback & iterate	•Mentor relationsip •Sustainability •Dissemination

Figure 9-3. Overview of the capstone development process for educators.

Aligning orientation activities across the curriculum (i.e., for fieldwork experiences) will help students build confidence to independently complete preparatory tasks. The following are considerations for educators in the prepare phase:

- Prior to starting the capstone experience, ACOTE (2023) emphasizes that there must be a valid written affiliation agreement between the organization and program. Students should not be involved in the development of an affiliation agreement or contract between the university and capstone site.

- Students must also have an experiential plan that outlines specific doctoral capstone objectives and plans for evaluation, supervision, and mentoring. The experiential plan must be signed by all parties involved (e.g., capstone coordinator, student, capstone mentor; ACOTE, 2023).

- Support students in establishing clear expectations, with a focus on the site environment, policies (e.g., uniforms, TB testing, background clearances, résumé, references, drug testing, CPR, vaccination records, etc.), work culture, and logistical requirements (e.g., work hours, personal computer use, scheduling, holidays, parking, staffing, go-to personnel, etc.). Consider the use of existing time tracking systems (e.g., CORE or EXXAT), and embed them into the capstone class to ensure the capstone project and experience meet the ACOTE standards (2023).

- Mentoring in health care is a long-established activity that is an iterative and multifactorial process between mentor and mentee (Kemp et al., 2022; Stephenson et al., 2024). Problems may arise from misunderstandings about expectations. A critical element of an effective capstone mentoring collaboration is a shared understanding of what mentors and mentees expect from the relationship. Additionally, expectations may change over time. It is important to prompt students to engage in reflection and sustain clear communication throughout the capstone development and implementation process. See Appendix 9.E for activity and reflection prompt recommendations.

- Be thoughtful about how you are orienting and supporting mentors, particularly those outside of the academic context. Maintaining effective communication amongst the program and mentors can support long-term partnerships and sustainability.

- Use backward design to help students and mentors identify and outline key tasks, ensuring timely completion of objectives (Wiggins & McTighe, 2005). Ideally, this process mirrors one that students have been exposed to a capstone planning course or throughout their curriculum. This method of starting with the end in mind can help students and mentors set realistic timelines for capstone implementation.

Teaching Tip

- Collaborate with the academic fieldwork coordinator (AFWC) at your program to leverage existing onboarding systems and logistic strategies. For example, if fieldwork is already using a week-by-week or feedback tracking activity, how might you adapt it for the capstone context?

- During capstone courses, you may structure a course in a way that simulates the expectations of implementation. For example, ask students to develop a timeline to complete their literature review and needs assessment or develop outlines for program development and delivery.

- Provide mentors with an orientation to the expectations of capstone mentors and capstone generally. This may include FAQ's, self-assessment, mentor education opportunities, and templates they can use at their own site and to build their mentor resources.

- Create a community of practice for mentors. Here, mentors can share ideas and experiences, co-present at conferences, and share exemplary projects that highlight the student–mentor collaboration.

- Mentors may not feel confident in approving a student's hours engaged in capstone activities if the student is not with them or physically on-site. Be explicit about how much detail is expected in the time log, and encourage students to keep record of their activities on a weekly basis. This ensures that if a DCC needs to step in to sign off student hours, they can ethically rationalize why it was or was not approved.

PHASE 2: REVIEW

Human-Centered Design Mindset: Iteration

In the review phase, students are focused on updating their literature review, revisiting their needs assessment, and revising their objectives and evaluation plan. It is critical that educators emphasize the importance of iteration in capstone projects, supporting students and mentors in refining the project scope, objectives, and activities. This flexibility ensures alignment with a site and mentor's evolving needs.

Key Takeaways

While the capstone is self-directed, the educator supports students and mentors in progressing their projects through intentional assessments or checkpoints. For example, students are expected to update their needs assessment upon initiating the 14-week capstone experience. You can support mentors by explicitly articulating student expectations, like updating the needs assessment. Similarly, you may need to facilitate communicating academic requirements of the capstone to a site while helping students identify the most appropriate tools to use as they revise their needs assessment and objectives.

Teaching Tip

- Help students translate academic concepts into practice terms that fit the site's language and culture. For example, presenting a needs assessment in a format other than what your academic program uses may be indicated. On-site options may include:
  - PRECEDE–PROCEED model and appreciative inquiry framework (see Chapter 6)
  - SBAR (situation, background, assessment, recommendation)
  - SOAR (strengths, opportunities, aspirations, results) (Stavros & Hinrichs, 2011)
  - SWOT (van Wijngaarden et al., 2012)
  - PDSA (plan, do, study, act) (Taylor et al., 2014)
  - Six Sigma: DMAIC (define, measure, analyze, improve, control) is employed with existing processes or projects. DMADV (define, measure, analyze, design, validate) is employed to design or create a new process or project (Antony et al., 2018).
- Offer regular check-ins with new content experts to discuss the scope of the student's project and offer support if and when difficulties arise.

PHASE 3: IMPLEMENT

Human-Centered Design Mindset: Embrace Ambiguity

The nature of capstone, as with OT practice, is fluid. Challenges and uncertainties will arise, and students should tackle them with curiosity, an open mind, and solution-based collaboration.

Key Takeaways

This phase guides students through the bulk of capstone implementation. Here students execute their plan while continually adjusting based on feedback from collaborators. Educators should consider building in structures throughout the implementation phase to gather weekly or biweekly updates from students, as needed.

Inevitably, there will be challenges. Developing clear guidelines and strategies to support students and mentors in addressing issues like misaligned expectations, scope of work changes, conflicts with colleagues, or unexpected obstacles is critical. While the experiential plan will outline expectations surrounding mentorship and supervision and encourage students to reach out if they are unsure how to address a problem. You may consider providing students with a template to document barriers and process what strategies they are using to overcome them (coordinate with AFWC for resources that can be adapted for capstone).

It is important to prompt students to begin thinking about their sustainability plan. Will the capstone work live on in some way? If so, how? Challenge students to:

- Work with their mentor to identify who will be responsible for the work once the student transitions out of the project.
- Think about how those involved will be trained to continue the work.
- Consider how work will be attributed, signing an authorship agreement form, if appropriate.
- Ensure all collaborators can provide feedback on the sustainability plan.

Teaching Tip

- Use existing program examples of flexibility to guide students so that they can navigate "gray areas" in project work, encouraging a solution-oriented mindset.
- Use social media, program websites, blogs, or public dissemination opportunities to highlight capstone student work throughout the capstone experience. Students can create these as part of their capstone development plan or for the site and mentor.
- Have students collaborate with their content expert for a plan to maintain or transition their project after their capstone is completed. Thinking about sustainability during implementation allows students to consider all aspects and contexts of their program with and without them (see Chapter 8).

PHASE 4: MEASURE

Human-Centered Design Mindset: Conscientiously Advocating

As students approach the midpoint and later stages of their capstone experience, educators can support students in reflecting on power dynamics and the impact of their project, ensuring it meets the authentic needs of the site, population, mentor, and their own learning.

Key Takeaways

In the measurement phase, students evaluate their progress, refine their objectives, and ensure that the project is viable and sustainable. Educators should, at the very least, ask content experts to complete a midterm evaluation near week 7 and a final evaluation at week 14 to assess student progress. This is also an opportunity for the student and content expert to ensure there is alignment between the student's project outcome expectations and the site goals. Some educators may request more frequent evaluations from the content expert.

As the capstone experience progresses, provide students with assignments or activity suggestions that encourage them to gather insights on their deliverables and project progress. Consider embedding prompts into weekly objectives or the activity tracking log(s) (see Appendix 9.F for an example). It may also be helpful to ask students to submit drafts of their project deliverables with evidence of feedback from their mentor. This holds students accountable for starting the work early, gathering insights from collaborators, and iterating on their ideas. Reiterate the value of collaboration, and emphasize the importance of creating space for diverse perspectives and opinions. Educators can support students by requesting that they submit drafts or prototypes of their deliverables alongside their time logs or reflections. This encourages students to embrace the iterative mindset and seek feedback from mentors and colleagues.

Teaching Tip

- Guide students in reflecting on the power dynamics of their project and impact. This could be a required reflection paper or recorded response or something smaller, like a discussion board post. Consider adapting a rubric from prior assignments that is familiar to students and demonstrates scaffolding on previous learning. Areas to focus on might include:
  - How is diversity, equity, inclusion, and justice addressed in their capstone?
  - Are the site(s) and academic institution's mission, vision, and values reflected in student work?
  - How are students considering and incorporating diverse perspectives in their work?
- Measurement can be viewed from many perspectives. Consider what your program needs to gather in terms of various student perspectives (self, site, content expert, benefits, challenges, and process), the mentor (self, student, benefits, drawbacks, and future needs), site, and others.

Table 9-6. Questions for Educators to Consider When Transitioning or Wrapping Up a Capstone

QUESTIONS TO CONSIDER WHEN TRANSITIONING OR WRAPPING UP A CAPSTONE
Site Environment, Policies, Procedures
• What does your student need to be turned into the site (e.g., badge, computer)?
• Do you need to cancel network access or change passwords?
Experience Wrap-Up
• Did you prompt your student to provide a summary of your experience to your capstone mentor and site?
• Are there student dissemination expectations beyond the program requirements?
• Did you send the mentor a certificate confirming their participation (e.g., to support CEU requirements)?
• Have you sent a thank-you message to site mentors?
• Do you need permission from the site to share materials or examples of student work?
• Do you have access to the necessary digital materials?
Mentorship Plan
• Have you gathered feedback and perceptions of the overall experience from the site mentor?
• What advice do they have for future capstone mentors?
• What feedback do they have to the OT program in terms of logistics, student preparedness, communication, and overall success of the capstone mentoring experience?
Next Steps
• Is the capstone mentor willing to collaborate again in the future? Why or why not?
• Have you provided the site and collaborators with your contact information and/or obtained their future contact information?
• Have all collaborators completed a feedback and outcome survey?

- Explore what you as an educator can discover or measure that can inform students, content experts, and future capstone program development.

PHASE 5: TRANSITION

Human-Centered Design Mindset: Iterating and Collaborative Relationships

Especially at the end, iteration and collaboration are crucial. Students should focus on collecting feedback, finalizing deliverables, and preparing for the transition of both the project and mentor relationship.

Key Takeaways

The final phase of implementation focuses on wrapping up the project and transitioning responsibilities while disseminating project outcomes to stakeholders. It might be valuable to have students submit sample deliverables as evidence of achieving their capstone objectives. These can also be used, with permission, as samples to demonstrate the value of a capstone student collaboration with future sites.

Each program will have different expectations around dissemination. As an educator, be explicit with students, content experts, and sites about how information will be disseminated. Remember to reiterate HIPPA and confidentiality expectations to students who are presenting their work publicly. Students should also be intentional about attributing work to their collaborators.

Teaching Tip

- Students can document the wrap-up process and provide recommendations to transition the mentor–student relationship, if appropriate.
- Table 9.6 offers examples of questions to consider when transitioning or wrapping up a capstone.
- Encourage mentors for one last time to reflect on the capstone's success and areas for improvement. Examples include access to self-assessments, conduct of focus groups, surveys, conduct of interviews, or invitations to collaborate on presentations at the state and national levels.

EDUCATOR CHAPTER SUMMARY

This section highlights the importance of clear communication, mutual goal setting, and adaptability in fostering successful mentorship relationships. It underscores the dynamic relationship between mentees and mentors, which drives professional growth and can enhance the overall capstone experience.

REFERENCES

Accreditation Council for Occupational Therapy Education. (2023). *2023 Accreditation Council for Occupational Therapy Education (ACOTE®) standards and interpretive guide.* https://acoteonline.org/accreditation-explained/standards/

Ahmed, N., & Stafford, C. (Hosts). (2022, November). Inclusive design mindsets [audio podcast episode]. In *Creative confidence.* IDEO U.

Antony, J., Palsuk, P., Gupta, S., Mishra, D., & Barach, P. (2018). Six Sigma in healthcare: A systematic review of the literature. *International Journal of Quality & Reliability Management, 35*(5), 1075–1092. https://doi.org/10.1108/IJQRM-02-2017-0027

Armstrong-Heimsoth, A., Hahn-Floyd, M., Williamson, H. J., & Lockmiller, C. (2020). Toward a defined role for occupational therapy in foster care transition programming. *The Open Journal of Occupational Therapy, 8*(4), 1–8. https://doi.org/10.15453/2168–6408.1726

Biwer, F., Wiradhany, W., oude Egbrink, M. G. A., & de Bruin, A. B. H. (2023). Understanding effort regulation: Comparing 'pomodoro' breaks and self-regulated breaks. *British Journal of Educational Psychology, 93*(52), 353–367. https://doi.org/10.1111/bjep.12593

Bowman, J., Mogensen, L., Marsland, E., & Lannin, N. (2015). The development, content validity and inter-rater reliability of the SMART-goal evaluation method: A standardized method for evaluating clinical goals. *Australian Occupational Therapy Journal, 62*(6), 420–427. https://doi.org/10.1111/1440–1630.12218

Cirillo, F. (2018). *The pomodoro technique: The acclaimed time management system that has transformed how we work.* Currency.

Courtney, M. E., & Dworsky, A. (2006). Early outcomes for young adults transitioning from out-of-home care in the USA. *Child & Family Social Work, 11*(3), 209–219. https://doi.org/10.1111/j.1365–2206.2006.00433.x

DeIuliis, E., & Bednarski, J. (Eds.). (2019). *The entry level occupational therapy doctorate capstone: A framework for the experience and project.* Slack.

Jacobson, D., & Mustafa, N. (2019). Social identify map: A reflexivity tool for practicing explicit positionality in critical qualitative research. *International Journal of Qualitative Methods, 18.* https://doi.org/10.1177/1609406919870075

Kemp, E. L., Domina, A., Stephenson, S., & Start, A. (2022). Perceived value & usefulness of the entry-level occupational therapy doctoral capstone. *Journal of Occupational Therapy Education, 6*(3), 11. https://doi.org/10.26681/jote.2022.060311

Landfried, M., Chen, E., Savelli, L.B, Cooper, M, Price, B. N., & Emmerling, D. (2023). MPH capstone experiences: Promising practice and lessons learned. *Frontiers in Public Health,* 1–11. https://https://doi.org/10.3389/fpubh.2023.11299330

Mezirow, J. (1997). Transformative learning: Theory to practice. *New Directions for Adult and Continuing Education,* (74), 5–12. https://doi.org/10.1002/ace.7401

Stavros, J. M., & Hinrichs, G. (2011). *The thin book of SOAR: Building strengths-based strategy.* Thin Book Publishing.

Stephenson, S., Ivy, C., Vonier, M., & Sweets, D. (2024). Building bridges: A mentor education program for occupational therapy practitioners. *Journal of Occupational Therapy Education, 8*(1), 19. https://doi.org/10.26681/jote.2024.080119

Stephenson, S., Rogers, O., Ivy, C., Barron, R., & Burke, J. (2020). Designing effective capstone experiences and projects for entry-level doctoral students in occupational therapy: One program's approaches and lessons learned. *The Open Journal of Occupational Therapy, 8*(3). https://doi.org/10.15453%2F2168–6408.1727

Taylor, M. J., McNicholas, C., Nicolay, C., Darzi, A., Bell, D., & Reed, J. E. (2014). Systematic review of the application of the plan–do–study–act method to improve quality in healthcare. *British Medical Journal Quality & Safety*, 23(4), 290–298. https://doi.org/10.1136/bmjqs-2013–001862

van Wijngaarden, J. D., Scholten, G. R., & van Wijk, K. P. (2012). Strategic analysis for health care organizations: The suitability of the SWOT-analysis. *The International Journal of Health Planning and Management*, 27(1), 34–49. https://doi.org/10.1002/hpm.1032

Wiggins, G., & McTighe, J. (2005). *Understanding by design* (2nd ed.). Association for Supervision and Curriculum Development.

APPENDICES

Appendix 9.A Capstone Flyer Assignment Template

Appendix 9.B Example Flyer

Appendix 9.C Doctoral Capstone Experience and Project Weekly Planning Guide

Appendix 9.D Communication Log

Appendix 9.E Reflection Prompt Ideas

Appendix 9.F Week-by-Week Activity Log Example

Appendix 9.A
CREATE A CAPSTONE FLYER ASSIGNMENT TEMPLATE

Instructions: Take a moment to create a **one-page** capstone flyer that explains what your capstone is, what your project entails, and what you envision for your 14 weeks. Consider the following as a structure:

1. **Who you are.**

   In this section, take a moment to introduce yourself. You may answer:
   - What personal and professional experience led you to pursue this capstone topic?
   - What excites you about your capstone?
   - How does your capstone align with your core values and long-term goals as an OT?

2. **Purpose of project.**

   Briefly summarize the rationale or need for this project.

3. **What to expect.**

   Highlight the strategies or methods you will use to engage in your experience and implement your project.

4. **Outcomes.**

   Outline your expected outcomes.

5. **Contact information.**

   Be sure to include contact information so people can get in touch with you!

6. **Email template.**

   Draft an email that accompanies your flyer to support you in reaching out to collaborators.

Appendix 9.B

EXAMPLE FLYER – CONSIDER YOUR AUDIENCE SO THAT YOU CAN CUSTOMIZE THIS TO YOUR NEEDS

STUDENT PICTURE HERE OR QUOTE

CAPSTONE

YOUR PROGRAM NAME OR LOGO

Capstone with (Your University) is a 14 week full time collaboration between a student and a site mentor. The overall goal is to (insert the preferred language of your program)

Dates for the capstone:
Addressing Sexuality in OT Rehabilitation Services

◆ CAPSTONE

14-week collaboration with student and a site mentor who has expertise in a my focus area.
Inpatient rehabilitation capstone focus on clients with spinal cord injury and best practice for OT addressing sexuality

◆ MENTOR BENEFITS

Student support on focused topic
PDU certificate for NBCOT
Presentation to state or AOTA conference
INSERT- link to a relevant article or website that supports your capstone work

◆ MY PROJECT IDEAS

- Review of current evaluation practices by OT and nursing
- Identify current sex positive and sex forward literature for SCI
- Collaborate with other health professionals to create a flow chart for addressing sexuality

◆ MY FOCUS AREAS

- Spinal Cord Injury evaluation and interventions
- Sexuality, sex positive therapeutic services, and addressing sexuality and sex topics in the rehabilitation environment

◆ MY PROJECT GOALS

- Collaborate with mentor(s) on a quality improvement project to understand staff practices of providing sexuality information.
- Create sex and sexuality resources for the unit, patients, and their families.
- Identify sex and sexuality focused evaluations and interventions that can be used by the occupational therapy staff.
- Develop education resources for sex positive and sex forward language

◆ CONTACT

Student and Capstone Coordinator Information

Program mission or social media

Appendix 9.C

DOCTORAL CAPSTONE EXPERIENCE AND PROJECT WEEKLY PLANNING GUIDE

Area of Focus:

WEEK	INDIVIDUALIZED LEARNING OBJECTIVE	WEEKLY GOALS	SPECIFIC TASKS TO MEET WEEKLY GOALS	DATE COMPLETE
1				
2				
3				
4				
5				
6				
7				
8				
9				
10				
11				
12				
13				
14				

Appendix 9.D

COMMUNICATION LOG

DATE	COMMUNICATION (MEETING, UPDATED, INTERACTION) *(SHARED DOCUMENT MAY BE USEFUL)*	NEXT STEPS AND ACTION ITEMS *(BE SPECIFIC WITH TIME AND ACTIONS)*
xx/xx	Met with content expert. Reviewed: *[list topics]* Updated on: *[list topics]* Items to discuss: *[list]* Feedback for my mentor: *[write it out]* Feedback for me: *[write it out]* *(These are topic suggestions to prompt discussions during meetings. Find what prompts work for you, and these can drive the discussions in your meetings with mentors)*	

Appendix 9.E

REFLECTION PROMPT IDEAS DURING IMPLEMENTATION PHASE

Instructions: Use the following reflection prompts to challenge the capstone student to think more deeply about their self-directed learning process, goals, and needs.

- Pre-implementation (week 1)
  - What impact do I anticipate?
  - What uncertainties do I have?
  - What resources will I need at the beginning?
  - How will I measure success?
- During implementation (week 7)
  - How is the project compared to my initial expectations?
  - What challenges have I faced? How did I manage these?
  - What additional resources did I need? What will I need in the future?
  - How am I managing my time and workload?
  - Am I meeting project expectations?
- End of implementation (weeks 13/14)
  - What are two things I knew/learned/need to explore further?
  - What did I learn?
  - What am I leaving behind?

Appendix 9.F

WEEK-BY-WEEK ACTIVITY LOG EXAMPLE

WEEK 1		
Overall summary of the week: *[This can be a narrative "snapshot" of the week.]* What went well this week? *[What are you proud of this week or feel good about?]* What continues? *[What carries over, or what are you still working on?]* What needs adaptation? *[What needs adjustment? Next week I need to . . .]*		
Focus Area (List Your Focus Areas)	**Activities List (Bullet or Narrative) – This Needs to Be Specific Enough That Your Faculty and Site Mentors Understand Your Work**	**Achieved/Ongoing/Changes**
Clinical skills	• Kinesio taping course • Completed the skill checklist required by the site • Updated the skills list for a future capstone student • Reviewed department 3 protocols (insert links here) • Reviewed shoulder anatomy (links here to resources) • Caseload of clients initiated – 25% of mentor's caseload assumed	• Completed • Completed with mentor • Under review for mentor • Under review for mentor • Created flash cards (link here) • Ongoing
Program Development	• Review of the initial needs assessment • Updated the needs assessment to include xxx • Created timeline and reviewed with community site and all partners	• Completed • Completed • Under review – will come back to this next week
Other focus area		

Chapter 10

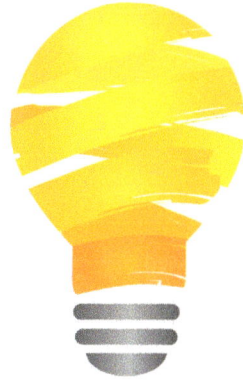

Evaluation of the Capstone Experience

Elizabeth D. Deluliis and Julie A. Bednarski

Section 1: Student Focus

Human-Centered Design Mindsets for the Doctoral Students

Human-centered design mindsets of learning from failure and iteration are important for the doctoral capstone student to continue to embrace as they near completion of the implementation phase of the doctoral capstone experience and project. Evaluating the overall experience, the student, and mentors is important in order to reflect and make adjustments for the future.

Iterate, iterate, iterate. You have been iterating throughout the implementation stage, and this is the final iteration period. Final changes are made based on outcomes, and decisions are made for future ideas based on outcomes. Evaluating your iterations and understanding how you came to the final product are important to be able to communicate how your iterations have led to the final product.

Learn from failure. Throughout the implementation phase, you have been learning from your failures, learning from things that did not go just right. Evaluating your experience and project in this, the final stage of implementation, allows you to make further changes and recommendations for the future. "When human-centered designers get it right, it's because they got it wrong first" (IDEO.org, 2015, p. 21).

INTRODUCTION FOR STUDENTS

Evaluating the learning that has occurred and your performance throughout the doctoral capstone is such an integral part of the overall doctoral capstone process. While your content expert, faculty mentor, and doctoral capstone coordinator will all most likely play a role in evaluating your completion of the doctoral capstone experience and project, you should also plan to be actively engaged within the evaluation process. Aligned with the content within Chapter 3, which helped you understand the value of being self-directed, *practice-ready*, and immersing yourself as an active participant within the mentoring relationship, there are tangible behaviors you should implement to be sufficiently prepared to engage within the evaluation process. This chapter will provide you, the capstone

DOI: 10.4324/9781003541813-13

student, a synopsis of the overall importance of evaluation within experiential learning and a snapshot of different approaches that might be used to evaluate your learning and performance during the doctoral capstone experience.

STUDENT REFLECTIVE QUESTIONS

As the implementation phase of your capstone experience nears completion, you, the capstone student, may find it helpful to reflect on the following questions:

1. How will your learning and performance be assessed during the DCE?
2. What role will you play in evaluating and providing feedback to your content expert (and other mentors/ stakeholders involved in your capstone experience)?
3. What is your understanding on how your expectations and goals on the DCE differ from level II fieldwork?
4. What are your program's policy and expectations regarding formal assessment and overall grading procedures for the doctoral capstone experience?

STUDENT OBJECTIVES

By the end of reading this chapter and completing the learning activities, the student will be able to:

1. Understand the need for evaluation of the capstone experience.
2. Compare and contrast methods for evaluation of the capstone experience.
3. Identify behaviors to be actively engaged within the evaluation process.

IMPORTANCE OF EVALUATION IN EXPERIENTIAL LEARNING

As you have learned during your studies of occupational therapy clinical practice, theories and frames of references are often used to help provide the practitioner a conceptual framework to structure understanding and guide decision-making. Just the same, educators also utilize theoretical perspectives and models, such as adult learning theory, to frame the teaching and learning process. One example which you might find applicable as a capstone student is Kolb's experiential learning cycle, which details the importance of a structured approach to learning from experience, which is essential in most progressive graduate education settings (Kolb, 1984). Kolb's cycle consists of four stages:

1. *Concrete experience.* Engaging in a new experience or encountering a new situation. In occupational therapy practice, this involves direct patient care or hands-on practice, such as formal fieldwork education or the doctoral capstone. For example, a fieldwork or

capstone student might perform an assessment or assist in the delivery of an intervention. This stage allows learners to engage actively within real-world scenarios. As you participate hands-on, expect your content expert and doctoral capstone coordinator to ask you to share your experiences.

2. *Reflective observation.* Thinking about and reflecting on the experience, noticing any discrepancies between experience and understanding. After the experience, learners reflect on what happened. In occupational therapy experiential learning, this might involve discussing cases with preceptors or mentors, reviewing patient/client outcomes, or journaling about the experience. Reflection helps identify what went well and what could be improved.

3. *Abstract conceptualization.* Formulating theories or concepts based on reflections and making sense of the experience by connecting it to existing knowledge. Based on reflections, learners develop or refine their theoretical understanding. In clinical education, this could mean integrating new knowledge about diagnostic conditions or treatment approaches and understanding how these theories apply to practice. Your content expert or doctoral capstone coordinator might guide you (or a small group of you and peers) to connect these reflections to theories or concepts learned in your curriculum.

4. *Active experimentation.* Applying the new concepts or theories in different situations to test their validity and to gain further insights. Learners then apply their new understanding to future scenarios. For example, a learner might use a new diagnostic technique or treatment approach in subsequent patient/client interactions, testing and refining their skills and knowledge. Your context expert or doctoral capstone coordinator will encourage you to apply what you have learned, as well as create opportunities for you to test this new knowledge and share outcomes with your peers.

(Kolb, 1984).

Similar to the overall doctoral capstone process, Kolb's experiential learning cycle is iterative – meaning that learning is a continuous process, where individuals keep going through these stages, refining their understanding and skills with each iteration. By cyclically engaging in these stages, you, the capstone student, can continuously develop and grow. What is going to be emphasized quite a bit in this chapter is that the experiential learning cycle spotlights the importance of reflection and application, which are crucial in developing practical skills and professional reasoning. Integrating Kolb's model helps ensure that learning is not just about acquiring knowledge but also about effectively applying and adapting that knowledge in real-world settings. This approach not only helps in understanding and refining but also reinforces a learning-oriented mindset that can be useful within the evaluation process of the doctoral capstone.

As you might assume from prior fieldwork experiences, evaluation of student performance is a necessary component in experiential learning. Not only is having a formal evaluation mechanism a requirement set by the Accreditation Council for Occupational Therapy Education (ACOTE), but evaluation also provides you, the capstone student; your content expert; and your doctoral capstone coordinator the opportunity for reflection and feedback, which promotes overall personal and professional growth. It is important to understand the perspective that evaluations are not designed by your educator or capstone coordinator to be punitive or disciplinary in nature. In fact, the evaluation process as a whole should be viewed as a wonderful opportunity to reflect, receive feedback on growth and development, and celebrate successes.

TYPES OF EVALUATION

When most people think of an evaluation or assessment, they may align it to an action or milestone that occurs at the culmination of learning. However, evaluation should be viewed as an iterative and ongoing process, and as a capstone student, you should be mindful that there are different approaches and forms that your program or content expert might use to assess your progress, learning, and performance throughout the capstone. Likewise, evaluation can be described as occurring informally or formally, or via summative or formative methods.

Informal

Informal evaluations occur on experiential learning each day. These can include more unplanned or spontaneous experiences, such as your content expert observing your performance throughout your capstone experience. Informal assessments are useful for ongoing, developmental feedback. Observation is a great informal evaluation approach to obtain objective information about performance, while also affording the opportunity for real-time feedback. For example, during a doctoral capstone experience within a residential facility for youth with mental illness, a capstone student might be responsible for participating in daily team rounds. While the capstone student is responsible for providing the occupational therapy debrief to the interprofessional team, the content expert might be in attendance to directly observe your performance. After the team meeting, your content expert might engage you in a conversation to share impressions and to provide you feedback on how you performed, including strengths as well as areas to improve for next time. Although this type of assessment might not seem as formal or significant as a written midterm or final evaluation form, all feedback received during the doctoral capstone process should be actionable and cause you, the capstone student, to think, reflect, and consider changes for the future.

Formal

Formal evaluations are usually assessment approaches that have more structure and are planned; meaning, that they can occur at specific times or intervals. These are most likely assignments listed on your course syllabi or activities prescribed by your content expert or site mentor that are scheduled and systematic to gather information and measure progress and performance. These can also be referred to as summative and formative evaluation approaches.

Formative

AOTA (2021, p. 18) defines "the purpose of formative assessment . . . to check student understanding, provide feedback, and adjust content" during the progression of learning or the experience. During the doctoral capstone, these could be activities such as discussion board questions posed by your doctoral capstone coordinator through your program's learning management system (LMS; for example, Canvas, Blackboard, Moodle, etc.) during the capstone experience, a journaling assignment requirement, or a portfolio-like assignment, which might request that you put together a comprehensive collection of artifacts or exemplars to demonstrate accomplishments and excellence. Formative evaluation approaches can be graded or ungraded and are typically used to obtain multiple points of feedback over time. Your capstone coordinator might perform a check-in (either a phone-call, web conferencing) or even a site visit with you and your content expert over the course of the 14-week DCE. In alignment with Kolb's experiential learning theory, these summative assessment approaches are usually designed to help you reflect on your learning and experience, which then prepares you well to engage in self-assessment. Your content expert or capstone coordinator might request that you engage in a self-assessment; it could be even using the same evaluation form that they will use to evaluate you.

Self-assessment is a great formative evaluation approach as it promotes self-awareness, fosters ownership and accountability, encourages reflection and critical thinking, and increases motivation and confidence. Engaging in self-assessment will also help you prepare to receive feedback more constructively and encourage dialogue when you discuss with your capstone team. Overall, engaging in a self-assessment adds depth and richness to the overall evaluation process, ultimately leading to better outcomes and personal growth.

"I completed self-assessment at my midterm and final for the DCE per my request. I felt that my DCE content expert's input was the most crucial for me to hear and utilize while moving through the implementation phase of my project. I think for me the feedback really helped me understand professional

(continued)

relationships and communication skills outside of the typical "student" environment I was used to. My conversations with my site mentor were so much more meaningful than just a grade and a sentence or two of feedback that I was used to getting on assignments in school."

– Kaitlyn Joyce, OTD, OTR/L, Duquesne University OTD class of 2023

"I engaged in self-assessment at both my midterm and final stages with my content expert. This reflective process allowed me to evaluate my strengths as well as areas for growth moving forward. This process helped me reinforce my leadership skills as I sought to have a better understanding of my own abilities. This allowed me to set realistic and relevant goals for my professional development."

– Emma Fitzgerald, OTD, OTR/L, Duquesne University OTD class of 2024

Summative

Summative approaches are typically "higher-stakes" evaluations that are used to formally measure accomplishment (or competency) of a learning goal (AOTA, 2021, p. 18). These are assessment methods, such as a mastery practical exam, final projects, or final exams. ACOTE (2023) requires doctoral programs to have "a formal evaluation mechanism for objective assessment of the student's performance during and at the completion of the doctoral capstone" (p. 44). Although there is not a formally endorsed tool at the national level to use during the doctoral capstone experience, most programs develop an evaluation tool that is used to formally objectively assess student performance during midterm (usually week 7) and at the end of the doctoral capstone experience. To be successful in passing the doctoral capstone experience, programs may create a scoring system that translates into a grading scale that is used to determine successful completion.

In summary, a 360-degree approach might be used to gather feedback and impressions from multiple sources to provide a holistic view of your strengths and areas to improve. Often, a combination of both formative and summative assessment methods provides a well-rounded evaluation, leveraging the strengths of each to support comprehensive assessment and development. Overall, these strategies can foster a culture of open communication and feedback, which in turn can enhance relationship building among your capstone team, which contributes to your personal and professional growth as an occupational therapy practitioner and professional.

While completion of that formal evaluation tool is usually dependent on your content expert or another mentor within your capstone team, there are definite expectations that are on you, the capstone student, to be actively engaged within the evaluation process. Here are some recommendations:

BEHAVIORS TO BE ACTIVELY ENGAGED WITHIN YOUR EVALUATION PROCESS

- Take responsibility for understanding how you will be evaluated. This includes actions such as critically reviewing the evaluation tool(s) *prior to* the start of the capstone experience. After reviewing the tool, what question do you have? Are you confident in all the areas that you will be assessed? Are you comfortable with the rating scales provided? If not, follow up and seek guidance.
- Be actively engaged with your own learning goals. In other words, review and take ownership of your individualized goals and objectives that you already established on the experiential learning plan.
- Actively collaborate with your context expert to develop an action plan and success criteria. When you are clearer on the learning goals and criteria for success, you will be more comfortable and prepared to take ownership of your learning.
- Maintain open communication with your context expert, and with other members of your capstone team. Take initiative and provide feedback ongoingly.
- Engage in self-assessment using your program's evaluation tool. Even if your program does not require it, self-assessment is a very beneficial activity to help instill growth and development. Identify areas you feel confident in, as well as areas that can be improved.
- Analyze all feedback you are given (formative and summative) to understand reoccurring themes or concerns. From here, use action-oriented thinking to develop recommendations for improvement or change and plan for implementation.
- Take ownership of upcoming deadlines related to activities that contribute to evaluation of your learning and performance. When are discussion board reflections or evaluations due? How will they be submitted? Are they completed by hand or electronically via a database or system such as EXXAT or CORE? Be proactive in communicating any due dates that pertain to your site mentor or context expert related to evaluations.
- Have an open mind, encourage diverse perspectives, and embrace learning. Be receptive to feedback, even if it challenges your preconceptions.

"When I initially started my DCE project, my faculty mentor really encouraged me to stay open-minded throughout the whole process, which I took to heart and implemented throughout my whole DCE year. When setting expectations for myself, my site, my team, and my research in general, it was important that I stayed flexible and open to any and all learning experiences!"

– Kaitlyn Joyce, OTD, OTR/L, Duquesne University
OTD class of 2023

By embodying these behaviors and mindsets, you will ensure that the evaluation process is thorough, effective, and responsive to the needs of all stakeholders involved within your capstone team.

STUDENT SECTION CHAPTER SUMMARY

This chapter provided you recommendations to help you be prepared to actively *experience*, *think*, *reflect*, and *act*, as these are essential steps that contribute to your overall learning and growth within the doctoral capstone experience. However, this is not the only evaluation component of your doctoral capstone. The next few and final chapters of this book will further break down evaluation approaches that can be used by your program to evaluate completion of the doctoral project.

Student Learning Activities

1. Review the course syllabi for your doctoral capstone experience course(s). What evaluation methods are listed? Would you categorize them as summative and/or formative assessment methods? Are there due dates associated with these? Put these on your calendar or in your planner, and identify a placeholder of when you get to communicate these to your content expert and mentor.

2. How is your doctoral capstone experience course graded? Letter grade or pass/fail? Review the course syllabus or your program handbook to stay informed about this.

3. Think about a time you received constructive feedback about your performance. This could be from a faculty member, fieldwork educator, or a peer student. Reflect on how you embraced the feedback. Also, how did you respond to the feedback? Can you think about how you might have changed your behaviors, actions, or attitudes to demonstrate response to the feedback?

Section 2: Educator Focus

Transformational Learning Phases and Framework for the Educator

As an occupational therapy faculty member or capstone coordinator, you aim to design student learning activities and assessment measures that make a difference to your students' lives. We want to create courses, learning activities, and assessment methods that inspire, change mindsets, and drive reflective performance during the capstone and future practice. While students are engaging in reflection throughout the entire doctoral capstone process, it really comes to a peak in these final stages of Mezirow's transformational learning theory. As students are finalizing the 14 weeks of their doctoral capstone experience (DCE) and preparing for their final evaluation, this is an opportunity to reflect on a deeper level, assess the in-depth knowledge acquired by the student, and cogitate upon the new roles and confidence they have built through the DCE. The evaluation component of the doctoral capstone experience is how you promote the initiation of Mezirow's reintegration stage (Mezirow, 1997). As you consider these evaluation components of your program's DCE, the evaluation mechanism should be about as something more than just a form or tool to "check the box" that the student was indeed evaluated. Your evaluation should promote a reflective process where areas of growth are celebrated and constructive feedback is generated. Ultimately, your evaluation of the doctoral capstone experience should help students critically examine how they have integrated new knowledge and experiences from the DCE and support students in identifying how they can continue to apply these new perspectives into their professional identity as a future occupational therapist.

INTRODUCTION FOR EDUCATOR

Not unlike the occupational therapy process, assessment (or evaluation) is an essential step in the teaching-learning process. The interrelationship between adult learning theory (andragogy) and assessment is well documented by major educational theorists, such as Bandura (1971), Cross (1981), Knowles (1970), Kolb (1984), Lave (e.g., Lave & Wenger, 1991), Revans (1980), and Rogers (1969). Although there is no single theory of adult learning that can be applied to all adults, the models represented by the aforementioned pioneers of education provide useful frameworks to conceptualize the evaluation mechanisms for experiential learning, such as the capstone. Experiential learning has influenced adult education by making educators responsible for creating, facilitating access to, and organizing experiences to facilitate higher-order learning. Experiential learning coincides closely with one of the fundamental pieces of the philosophy of occupation – learning by doing (Jackson & Caffarella, 1994). Evaluation of learning is a meaningful process for the learner and the instructor. Assessments are critical elements of instruction; they determine accomplishment of learning objectives and can provide feedback to instructors on their effectiveness. Are capstone students learning what we want them to learn throughout their capstone experience and project? Is the content expert (and other mentors involved within the capstone) providing a substantive impact on the performance of the capstone student? Did learning and growth occur within the student's chosen focus area(s)? Occupational therapy educators, specifically doctoral capstone coordinators, should be empowered to design these assessments to be more than an evaluation of what has been learned. The evaluation mechanism for the doctoral capstone can be designed to be a part of the learning process itself and a process to get data to support program evaluation measures, required by the Accreditation Council for Occupational Therapy Education (ACOTE). This chapter provides an overview of student assessment for experiential education and recommendations to guide the evaluation process during the doctoral capstone experience (DCE).

EDUCATOR REFLECTIVE QUESTIONS

During the valuation phase of the capstone, educators may find it helpful to reflect on the following questions:

1. What is your program's philosophy on student assessment?
2. What summative and formative evaluation approaches are used throughout level I and level II fieldwork to evaluate student performance in you program?
3. How would you gauge your own comfort level in developing an evaluation tool from scratch?
4. What are your institution's policies on grading during experiential learning?

EDUCATOR OBJECTIVES

By the end of reading this chapter, the educator will be able to design teaching methods to meet the stated student learning objectives:

1. Discuss theoretical approaches used to evaluate experiential learning.
2. Understand the need for evaluation of the capstone experience.

3. Compare and contrast methods for evaluation of the capstone experience.
4. Understand different strategies to design evaluation mechanisms for the DCE.

BRIEF OVERVIEW OF ADULT LEARNING THEORY

Awareness of adult learning theories is needed to develop and select evaluation systems and instruments that can measure the expected competencies and outcomes. What (to measure), how, when, and by whom are important key questions, and their answers are not always easy. Assessment should be tied to specific learning outcomes, and learners should be given whatever feedback will help them develop or consolidate their knowledge, skills, or attitudes. One principle of adult learning theory is to allow learners to determine their own learning goals. In most instructional settings, specific learning objectives must be met and are traditionally established, reinforced, and monitored by the educator. The accreditation standards surrounding the capstone require a shift in this paradigm and require that capstone student play an integral role in structuring how they show evidence of skill proficiency within their chosen focus area(s). ACOTE (2023) standard D.1.4 enforces this adult learning principle to be instituted by the creation of student-directed learning objectives as part of the experiential plan and written agreement for the capstone, discussed in Chapter 7. Knowles (1984, 1992) has contended that adults differ from younger learners in the following ways. (See Text Box 10.1.)

TEXT BOX 10.1

What Are the Basic Principles of Adult Learning?

1. They derive from adults' experiences and needs.
2. Adults need to be involved in planning their instruction and evaluating their results. (This is encompassed in the co-creation of the individualized student learning objectives within the experiential learning plan.)
3. Adults are often self-directed, and their motivation to learn is internal.
4. Adults also learn well in situations where they can experience using their new knowledge.
5. Adult learning should center on solving problems and not absorbing content.
6. Adults prefer experiential learning.

Not unlike the various lenses that practitioners use to view the occupational therapy process, assessment strategies can be developed using theoretical frameworks. For instance, Alexander Astin, a clinical and counselling psychologist, proposed the input–environment–output (I-E-O) model to develop assessment and evaluation activities in higher education. The premise of this model is that educational assessments are not complete unless the evaluation includes information on three essential elements: student inputs (I), the educational environment (E), and student outcomes (O) (Astin, 1993). Figure 10.1 shows the interrelationship among the three components of the I-E-O model.

Astin's model contends that outcomes in terms of student development are determined by both inputs (I) and learning environments (E); at the same time, inputs also influence outcomes (O). Astin's theory can be useful to occupational therapy educators as we further explore strategies to evaluate the doctoral capstone. (See Table 10.1.)

The holistic perspective of the I-E-O model and the significance of the interaction (interdependence) among the three postulates parallel many signature occupational therapy theories and models of practice, such as person--environment–occupation performance (PEOP) model (Christiansen et al., 2005), person–environment–occupation (PEO) model (Law et al., 1996), and the Canadian model of occupational performance (CMOP; Polatajko et al., 2007). Capstone students' learning and performance are a function of the students themselves, their context, and their experience. Application of the I-E-O model results in more accurate

assessment of the effects of the learning environment. Use of this model in student assessment "forces" educators to address not only outcomes but also inputs and environmental variables when evaluating student performance. Again, like the occupational therapy process, evaluation measures should be an ongoing process of establishing clear, measurable expected outcomes of student learning, ensuring that students have sufficient learning opportunities to achieve those outcomes. Assessment should include a systematic process of gathering, analyzing, and interpreting the evidence to determine how well the learner matched the stated expectations (Allen, 2004; Banta, 2002; Banta et al., 2009; Maurrasse, 2002; Suskie, 2009; see Figure 10.2). Although outcomes are important to measure, they reflect the end product of assessment, not a "complete assessment cycle" (Qualters, 2010, p. 56). As an educator, it is therefore necessary to devise unique assessment methods to measure success in both the process and the product (Moon, 2004).

Assessment strategies, consistent with Knowles's philosophy, might include case studies, role-play, simulations, and self-evaluation that enable adults to learn the process as much as the content itself. Many of these assessments are commonly used in occupational therapy education,

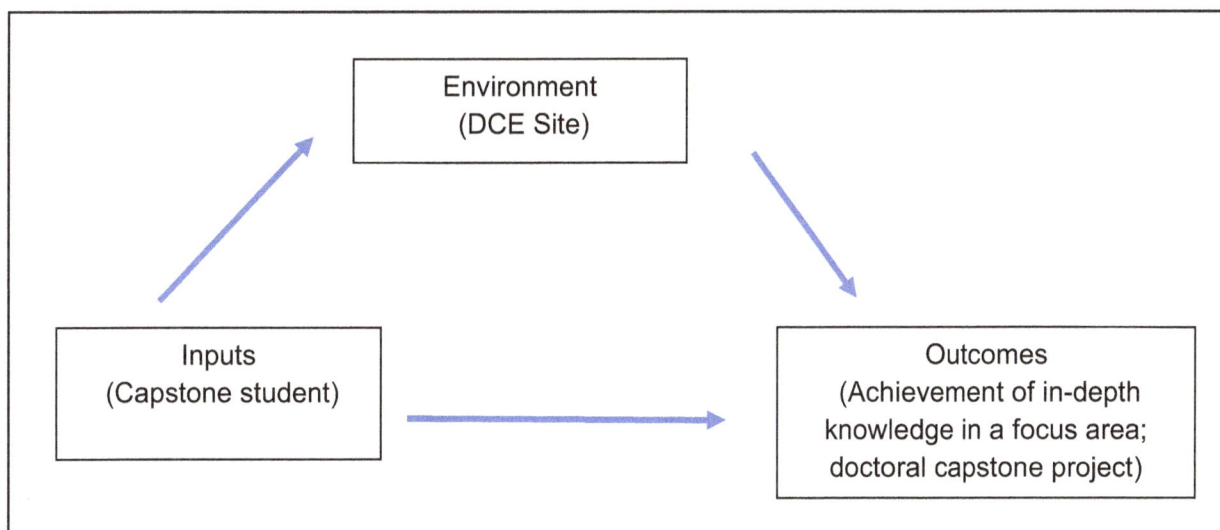

Figure 10-1. Schematic of Astin's I-E-O model.

Table 10-1. Astin's Model		
INPUT	Assess capstone students' knowledge, skills, and attitudes before a learning experience	Capstone students are required to demonstrate
ENVIRONMENT	Assess capstone students' actual experience during the capstone	Impact of content expert and site
OUTPUT	Assess the success (or talents) that we are trying to develop	In-depth skills/knowledge developed aligned with the focus area

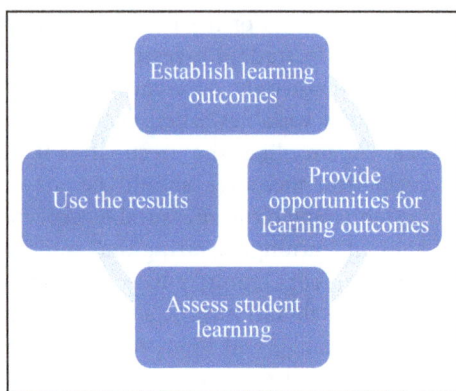

Figure 10.2. Iterative process of the evaluation of student learning.

yet do they provide a mechanism that offers holistic and ongoing feedback on the doctoral capstone student's performance during the capstone experience?

ASSESSMENT IN OCCUPATIONAL THERAPY EXPERIENTIAL EDUCATION

ACOTE (2023) provides an excellent structure for diversifying evaluation of student learning. Via the standards and the accreditation process, each occupational therapy program is required to provide evidence of student learning in the B, C, and D standards. ACOTE offers several measures for student learning assessment via their accreditation process and related documents. These include assignment, lab test, objective test, essay test, project, presentation, and demonstration. There is also an "other" selection that can be used to describe pedagogical approaches that may not be encompassed in the previous seven assessment measures. Experiential learning can be simply described as "hands-on" learning, yet it can occur via several approaches. Formal, regulated, and accredited experiential learning in occupational therapy includes fieldwork education and the doctoral capstone. Other pedagogical methods to foster "hands-on" learning can occur via community-engaged learning (Greene, 1997; Hoppes et al., 2005) and simulation (Bethea et al., 2014), which are often cited in occupational therapy literature yet not required by ACOTE. In Chapter 1 of this book, you learned that the primary objective of level I fieldwork is to "introduce students to fieldwork, to apply knowledge to practice, and to develop understanding of the needs of clients" (ACOTE, 2023, p. 38). Other accreditation standards provide additional oversight needed by the academic fieldwork coordinator in regard to having clearly documented student learning competencies expected of the level I fieldwork experience. ACOTE standards indicate that there needs to be mechanisms for formal evaluation of student performance for level I fieldwork. Previously, the American Occupational Therapy Association (AOTA) endorsed a tool, "Level I Fieldwork Competency Evaluation for OT and OTA Students" (AOTA, 2017).

While this tool was designed to complement the AOTA Fieldwork Performance Evaluation, it is no longer publicly available via online resources provided by AOTA.

Chapter 1 also discussed that the goal of level II fieldwork is to develop competent, entry-level, generalist occupational therapy practitioners (ACOTE, 2023). Standards C.1.14 and C.1.15 require that the occupational therapy education program document mechanisms for evaluating the effectiveness of supervision (e.g., student evaluation of fieldwork) and formal evaluation of student performance on level II fieldwork. Evaluation of the student performance can be completed via the AOTA FWPE or an equivalent evaluation mechanism. (See Text Box 10.2.)

TEXT BOX 10.2

Other evaluation mechanisms for fieldwork education include the FEAT and SAFECOM tools.

The **Self-Assessment Tool for Fieldwork Educator Competency** (SAFECOM) is a tool to facilitate student self-reflection and self-assessment throughout the fieldwork process. The SAFECOM can be used formally via the midterm and final evaluation time periods, or informally, to guide conversations between the student and the fieldwork educator and guide the student's growth based on site-specific learning objectives and to promote continued professional development (AOTA, 2023).

The **Fieldwork Experience Assessment Tool** (FEAT) provides a structure for the fieldwork student and the fieldwork educator to have a meaningful discussion aimed to identify strategies to facilitate the just-right challenge. This tool is meant to be used collaboratively and to help the fieldwork educator and the fieldwork student understand the unique and dynamic interaction among the environment, the fieldwork educator, and the student (Atler et al., 2001).

There are clear resources provided to occupational therapy faculty, academic fieldwork coordinators, fieldwork educators, and students provided by the AOTA regarding fieldwork education.

ACOTE D standards outline the minimum educational requirements for the doctoral capstone (ACOTE, 2023). In previous chapters, key aspects of the doctoral capstone were discussed, such as the differentiation of the capstone project vs. experience (Chapter 1), correlation with an in-depth focus area (Chapter 2), congruence with the program's curriculum design (and necessary collaboration among faculty, content expert, and the capstone student (Chapter 7). Specific to the assessment process, standard D.1.7 requires that occupational therapy doctoral (OTD) programs "document a formal evaluation mechanism for objective assessment of the student's performance during and at the completion of the DCE" (ACOTE, 2023, p. 44). As there is not a formally endorsed tool provided by AOTA or ACOTE to use for evaluation of the capstone experience, this chapter is intended to provide recommendations and resources to guide the educator regarding various methods to evaluate the evaluation of the capstone student during and at completion of the capstone experiences, as well as evaluation of the mentorship and supervision provided by the content expert.

EVALUATION OF THE CAPSTONE STUDENT'S PERFORMANCE DURING THE EXPERIENCE

The capstone student's performance and progress during the DCE should be closely monitored by the student, content expert, and capstone coordinator, and perhaps even by the faculty mentor (or faculty capstone chair). Evaluation can occur informally and formally. Informal evaluation of the capstone student can occur during feedback sessions with various members of the capstone team and during phone calls or site visits supported by the capstone coordinator. Sample forms to guide feedback sessions or for phone check-ins or site visits can be found in Appendix 10.A at the end of this chapter. These informal methods of evaluating the student's performance and providing feedback for growth can be used to satisfy evaluation mechanisms "during the capstone experience" aspect of the D.1.7 standard (ACOTE, 2023). Other strategies to evaluate student feedback during the capstone experience can be use of required student reflections. The capstone coordinator can use the academic institution's learning management system (such as Blackboard, Canvas, Design2Learn, Moodle, etc.) as means to connect, collaborate, and evaluate student performance during the capstone experience. Self-reflections and student discussion board postings can be required elements of the course listed on the syllabus and provide useful information to the capstone coordinator of the overall grading outcome of the experience. Engaging the capstone student in reflection is crucial to organize, interpret, and bring meaning and coherence to their learning experience. Similar to level II fieldwork, although the content expert or faculty mentor (or capstone chair) can provide valuable feedback on the capstone student's performance via the evaluation forms and established feedback mechanisms, as the primary faculty member responsible for the capstone, it is the doctoral capstone coordinator's responsibility to assign the overall grade for the experience. Reflections or postings can be used creatively by the doctoral capstone coordinator to exemplify congruence to curricular threads or curriculum philosophy, acknowledge the in-depth knowledge within the chosen focus area(s), and gain feedback on the capstone student's overall growth and development at specific intervals of

the 14-week experience (see Text Box 10.3). Strategies to approach the grading of the capstone are discussed later in this chapter.

TEXT BOX 10.3

Week 1

Can you believe it is the XYZ semester of your doctoral program? CONGRATULATIONS on the completion of your capstone proposal! Now it is time to put all your hard work into practice and make it a reality! Throughout the capstone journey, I would like each of you to respond to questions and also respond to your peers. I will also offer my own thoughts and suggestions. For this week. Please respond to the following questions:

1. How did your content expert respond to the final draft of your project proposal? Did they provide feedback? Share some details.
2. What updates have been made to your individual student objectives on your experiential plan through collaboration with your content expert?
3. How are things going in general? Any questions or concerns? Any questions from you or your content expert regarding the paperwork?

Week 4

Identify effective mentorship strategies that work for you, and why this type of supervision works for you. Do you feel that you are receiving the type and amount of mentorship/feedback that you need for the successful completion of your DCE? How has your content expert or mentor provided you with feedback, and how has this supported your capstone project and DCE experience thus far? Does anything need to change, and if so, how could you ask for this type of feedback?

Week 8

You are more than halfway through your capstone! How is the journey thus far?

For this week's post, please describe one aspect of interprofessional collaboration that you participated in. Who were the different professionals involved, and what role did they play? How did you participate? Why is interprofessional collaboration important at your site?

Week 12

Share with your peers how you have incorporated evidence-based practice into your role as an occupational therapist (student) at your site. Do other professionals at your site use evidence to guide their decision-making, and if so, how do they demonstrate this practice?

TEXT BOX 12-3 (continued)

Week 14

You are nearing the end of the DCE! I hope that you enjoyed the journey and grew as you experienced curves and bumps in the road along the way.

The goal of the capstone is to develop occupational therapists with in-depth knowledge. Share with your peers about an in-depth experience with the following: clinical skills, research skills, administration, program development and evaluation, policy development, advocacy, education, and/or leadership. Provide an example of how you have been exposed to two or more of the preceding focus areas that you have had a chance to develop during the DCE.

360-Degree Evaluation Approach

In addition to these informal strategies to provide feedback and evaluate capstone student performance, the use of a more formal evaluation mechanism (tool) is recommended for consideration. Similar to level II fieldwork, which uses a tool to evaluate student performance at midterm and at completion of the 12-week experience, an evaluation report can be created by the occupational therapy program to be used by the content expert, doctoral capstone coordinator, or faculty mentor (or capstone chair). This approach to evaluation is often described as a *360-degree approach* (Bracken, 2009; Cormack et al., 2018) and can be used to help maximize the functions of feedback to enhance the capstone student's learning and improve curriculum outcomes. (See examples provided in Appendices 10.B and 10.C.) This multisource feedback approach is a useful method to ensure that the evaluation process is holistic and interactive among the capstone team. (See Text Box 10.4.) The goal is to encourage reflection among the capstone team and collect feedback that will help capstone students grow and develop in their focus area. By including the content expert, faculty member (or capstone chair) in the evaluation process, the student has an opportunity to get balanced feedback and

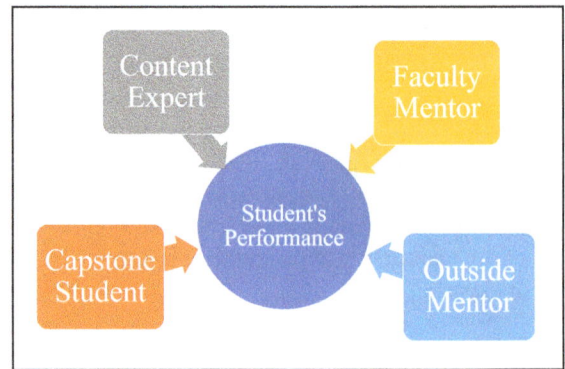

Figure 10.3. Multisource feedback approach.

encouragement for increased self-awareness (Figure 10.3). This allows students to gain a clearer picture of their progress and desired goal. It may also be beneficial to have a mechanism for the consumers (clients) who interact with the capstone student to provide feedback, if appropriate, based on the type of DCE and focus area.

TEXT BOX 10.4

Evidence indicates that the 360-degree evaluation approach can create behavior change (Goldsmith & Morgan, 2004; Goldsmith & Underhill, 2001; Smither et al., 2005), yet it is recommended that four critical design factors be taken into consideration: (1) relevant content, (2) credible data, (3) accountability, and (4) consensus (Bracken & Rose, 2011). (See Table 10.2.)

In addition to the evaluation of the capstone student being a holistic appraisal, this tool can be designed to measure progress and provide feedback at specific intervals of the DCE, such as midterm (week 7) and at completion (week 14). (See Text Box 10.5 and 10.6.)

TEXT BOX 10.5

Specific resources the capstone coordinators and OTD faculty may find useful when creating evaluation measures for the capstone can be found in the following resources:

Table 10-2. Recommended Design Features for Evaluation Tools

DESIGN FEATURE	IMPLICATIONS FOR DEVELOPMENT OF A TOOL FOR THE DOCTORAL CAPSTONE EXPERIENCE
Relevant content	Constructs being measured (hard or practice-ready skills); accessibility of tool
Credible data	Response scale; training of raters; frequency of rating
Accountability	Reviewing results among the capstone team; awareness and acceptance of feedback
Consensus	Having all members of the capstone team participate to "maximize message" (Bracken & Rose, 2011, p. 6)

Source: Adapted from Bracken, D. W., and Rose, D. S. (2011). When does 360-degree feedback create behavior change? And how would we know it when it does? *Journal of Business and Psychology, 26*(2), 183–192. https://doi.org/10.1007/s10869-011-9218-5.

- Fitzpatrick, J. L., Sanders, J. R., Worthen, B. R., & Wingate, L. A. (2022). Program evaluation: *Alternative approaches and practical guidelines* (5th ed.). Pearson.
- Presser, S., Couper, M. P., Lessler, J. T., Martin, E., Martin, J., Rothgeb, J. M., & Singer, E. (2004). *Methods for testing and evaluating survey questions*. Wiley.
- Saris, W. E., & Gallhofer, I. N. (2014). Design, evaluation, and analysis of questionnaires for survey research (2nd ed.). Wiley.

TEXT BOX 10.6

General Recommendations for Designing an Evaluation Tool

- Be concise.
- Have clear instructions for use and purpose of tool.
- Focus on measurable objectives (American Association for Public Opinion Research, 2024).
- Have a clear and understandable rating scale.
- Keep questions relevant.
- Arrange the questions used in topic areas in an organized manner (for example, you can purposefully group all the practice-ready [soft skills] together) (American Statistical Association [ASA], 1999).
- Be aware of possible limitations and biases (ASA, 2022).
- Keep the interest of the client as focus.

Designing an evaluation tool is much like writing a research paper: Before you write about your findings, you need to ask questions about and clarify your research goal and your process and break down your topic into manageable parts. Questions to ask yourself can include the following:

- "What is the purpose of this evaluation?"
- "What do I hope to learn?"
- "How will the data I collect influence my decisions?"
- "What is my target population?"

By *target population* we mean the people who you want to take your survey.

Another critical consideration when developing assessments has to do with the variability of experiential activities during the capstone experience. Because capstone students are working on different projects and in different focus area(s), they cannot all be expected to learn the exact same things, and each student may take away something different from the experience. Beyond the variability of activities, there is also variability among the students. Additional focus points to consider when creating a formal evaluation mechanism to measure the student's performance on the capstone can include rooting evaluation components in the individualized learning objectives, established in the experiential learning plan for mentorship and supervision. (See Appendices 9.B and 9.C for sample evaluation forms.) Several of these sample evaluations in the appendices offer blank space for the capstone student to specify (i.e., write in) their individualized learning objectives. Evaluation components can include a combination of technical skills (related to their chosen focus area) and practice-ready skills (elaborated on in Chapter 3). Capstone coordinators can also use Bloom's domains of learning (often referred to as KSA – knowledge, skills, and attitudes) as a guide to structure constructs of the capstone evaluation (Anderson & Krathwohl, 2001; Bloom, 1956; Table 10.3).

Table 10-3. Overview of Bloom's Domain of Learning and the Capstone

DOMAIN OF LEARNING	DESCRIPTOR	RELATIONSHIP TO THE DCE
Cognitive domain	Mental skills (knowledge)	• Adhering to the procedures of the capstone site • Problem-solving, troubleshooting an unanticipated scenario • Metacognition
Affective domain	Growth in feelings or emotional areas (attitude or self)	• Listens with respect • Culturally aware • Participation and initiation • Motivation • Self-efficacy
Psychomotor domain	Manual or physical skills (i.e., doing)	• May pertain more specifically to the focus area chosen and the type of capstone project

Source: Adapted from Bloom, B. S. (1956). *Taxonomy of educational objectives: The classification of educational goals.* Longmans, Green.

Within the 360-degree evaluation process, providing opportunities for self-reflection and self-assessment of the capstone student is crucial. Boud (2013) indicated how important self-assessment is in the learning process and the value of involving students in determining how success or achievement is defined. As part of the learning objectives for the capstone experience course, educators and doctoral capstone coordinators can specifically require that the capstone student complete and submit a self-assessment (using the same tool that their site mentor uses to evaluate their performance). Not only is this strategy an important component of adult learning that fosters self-reflection, but it can also be used to facilitate discussion among the capstone team. The use of self-assessment could occur at midterm and at completion of the DCE.

RECOMMENDATIONS FOR RATING SCALES

A Likert scale is typically a 5- or 7-point scale used to allow individuals to express how much they agree or disagree with a particular statement (McLeod, 2008). The rating scale offers a range of answer options – from one extreme to another – and includes a moderate or neutral point. In survey design, Likert scales are commonly used to measure attitudes and opinions with a greater degree of nuance than a simple "yes–no" question. The AOTA FWPE tool uses a Likert scale for the fieldwork educator to evaluate the performance of a level II fieldwork student (Table 10.4).

There are various types of response scales that can be used in a 360-degree evaluation approach:

- Effectiveness scale
- Observed frequency scale (4-point)
- Anchored observed frequency scale (typically a recommended approach where 360 is being used for behavioral development)
- Developmental rating scale

Examples of each of these types of response scales are presented in the following subsections.

Effectiveness Scale

To counter a skew of ratings when using a 5-point scale, this type of scale should be designed to have three positive response options and two negative response options (Expert Training Systems [ETS], 2024; Table 10.5).

Observed Frequency Scale (4-Point)

This scale asks raters about the frequency with which an individual displays certain behaviors (ETS, 2024. It also has an "unable to comment" response, which accounts for the fact that some of those providing feedback may not feel they have had the opportunity to observe a particular behavior. For example, if the faculty mentor (or capstone chair) is using the same tool as the content expert, there may be certain components of the evaluation that they would not be able to formally rate if they did not observe over the course of the capstone experience (Table 10.6).

Anchored Observed Frequency Scale

This scale uses percentage bandings to guide raters and ensure greater consistency in ratings (ETS, 2024. This method can reduce the likely discrepancies in ratings based

Table 10-5. Effectiveness Scale

RESPONSE OPTION CODE	DESCRIPTION
NE	Not effective (−)
SE	Somewhat effective (−)
E	Effective (+)
VE	Very effective (+)
EE	Extremely effective (+)

Table 10-4. Rating Scale of the AOTA Fieldwork Performance Evaluation

4 = EXEMPLARY PERFORMANCE	Demonstrates satisfactory competence in specific skills *consistently*
3 = PROFICIENT PERFORMANCE	Demonstrates satisfactory competence in specific skills
2 = EMERGING PERFORMANCE	Demonstrates limited competence in specific skills; inconsistencies may be evidence; displays some gaps and/or inaccuracies
1 = UNSATISFACTORY PERFORMANCE	Fails to demonstrate competence in specific skills; performs in an inappropriate manner; demonstrates significant gaps and/or inaccuracies

Source: Adapted from American Occupational Therapy Association (2020). *Fieldwork performance evaluation (FWPE) rating scoring guide (revised in 2020)*. https://www.aota.org/-/media/corporate/files/educationcareers/fieldwork/fieldwork-performance-evaluation-rating-scoring-guide.pdf.

Table 10-6. Observed Frequency Scale

VALUE	DESCRIPTION
4	Always does this
3	Does this more often than not
2	Sometimes does this and sometimes does not
1	Rarely or never does this
N/A	Unable to comment (not observed)

on individuals' different interpretation of frequencies. This scale can help bring more objectivity to the process by providing guidance on how often is "often" to enable more distinction between ratings (Table 10.7).

Developmental Rating Scale

This type of rating scale is focused on rating a person's capabilities on a particular behavior (ETS, 2024). This scale has a greater number of positive descriptors to enable more spread of ratings and to reduce a positive skew. Naturally, it is often chosen where 360-degree feedback is being used to directly inform personal or professional development plans. A developmental scale is focused on helping raters reinforce their strengths and take action to improve their development needs. It should only be used for developmental purposes and is not suitable for performance management. The "no opportunity to observe" option can be helpful for feedback providers if they are newly interacting with the capstone student or

do not work closely with the individual in certain capacities and so have not seen a particular behavior or skill being demonstrated (Table 10.8).

Some examples of terminology to consider when building a tool to evaluate the doctoral capstone can be seen in Text Boxes 10.7 and 10.8.

TEXT BOX 10.7

1 = Needs attention
2 = Not making progress
3 = Making progress
4 = Met
5 = Exceeding

TEXT BOX 10.8

NE = No evidence
S = Somewhat (incomplete/need improvement)
A = Approaching (acceptable yet developing)
G = Grasped (present)

It might also be beneficial to use qualifying words to help the evaluator further understand the rating, seen in Text Boxes 10.9 and 10.10.

TEXT BOX 10.9

- Consistently exceeds
- Often exceeds expectations
- Meets expectations
- Some improvement needed
- Major improvement needed

Table 10-7. Rating Scale of the AOTA Fieldwork Performance Evaluation

LABEL	PERCENTAGE	VALUE
Always	95% or more	6
Nearly always	75% to 94%	5
Often	50% to 74%	4
Sometimes	25% to 49%	3
Rarely	6% to 24%	2
Hardly ever	5% or less	1
No opportunity to observe	–	N/A

Table 10-8. Developmental Rating Scale

Significant development need	Slight development need	Competent	Slight strength	Definite strength	Exemplary – a role model	No opportunity to observe

TEXT BOX 10.10

- Strongly disagree
- Disagree
- Neutral/neither agree nor disagree
- Agree
- Strongly agree

An open or blank space for qualitative comments should also be provided. It should be encouraged that any scores that are rated as extremely low or high on a Likert scale should include a qualitative comment from the evaluator to help substantiate the score. An example of comments to satisfy a rating of 5 out of 5, or above expectations/exceptional, can be seen in Text Box 10.11.

TEXT BOX 10.11

"Capstone student established interprofessional team rounds with rehabilitation staff on daily basis and created a virtual communication log that led to increased care coordination."

"Capstone student completed systematic review of literature regarding rehabilitation care of the patient with traumatic brain injury and developed evidence-based protocol to be implemented on the brain injury unit."

Examples of comments to satisfy a 1 out of 5 rating, which may indicate performance that is significantly below expectations or at risk, can be seen in Text Box 10.12.

TEXT BOX 10.12

"Capstone student has difficulty initiating conversation with content expert as well as the interprofessional team members, including other occupational therapy staff, rehabilitation aides, and nurses. Interprofessional input to the capstone project has been limited due to poor communication."

"Capstone student has demonstrated poor use of evidence, citing Wikipedia and Google as primary sources used to inform the capstone project."

An important aspect of the DCE is that capstone students ultimately demonstrate in-depth skills within their focus area, through the experience and the project. One strategy to specify that the individualized learning objectives were met by the capstone student is to include a statement or attestation on the evaluation tool, such as Text Box 10.13.

TEXT BOX 10.13

Please check one:

____ All the learning objectives per the experiential plan have been accomplished, and I recommend that the student pass the DCE.

____ The student has NOT fulfilled the objectives for the DCE and is NOT recommended to pass.

The preceding information is meant to inform and inspire doctoral programs that are seeking to develop or enhance the evaluation mechanisms regarding the capstone. Regardless of the evaluation mechanisms created and chosen, the capstone coordinator should educate all members of the capstone team on the evaluation tool and related procedures and processes. One strategy to educate the capstone team, specifically the site mentor, is to develop a webinar-like training that can be used to onboard all site mentors and compare and contrast fieldwork education and the capstone.

RECOMMENDATIONS FOR GRADING SCHEMES FOR THE DOCTORAL CAPSTONE EXPERIENCE

In addition to establishing the evaluation mechanism, educational programs will need to determine the grading practice to be used in the capstone experience course. Programs could synthesize formative and summative evaluation feedback from the capstone team to assign a letter grade (using a traditional A through F letter grade scale) or have more of a benchmark measure, which may determine a final rating, such as:

- Pass with honors (H – to recognize exemplary performance of the capstone student)
- Pass (P)
- Not pass (NP)

Policies and procedures related to the doctoral capstone should include clear expectations of performance, grading process, and remediation plan. Similar to what occurs with level II fieldwork, the site mentor is able to provide input and feedback on the capstone student's performance during the experience, yet it is ultimately the responsibility of the doctoral capstone coordinator to assign the final grade or rating for the capstone student.

Requirements for successful completion of the DCE can include the following components:

- Satisfactory completion of the 14-week (560-hour) full-time experience
- Satisfactory completion and submission of all learning objectives, learning activities, and evidence via completion of the evaluation form
- Satisfactory completion of all required assignments (e.g., reflection postings and submission of other required forms)
- Completion of the "Student Evaluation of Capstone Experience" evaluation form

The doctoral capstone coordinator can synthesize information obtained from the evaluation tools as well as the capstone student's effectiveness in completing required paperwork, according to the established policy and syllabus. An example of how to use the

Table 10-9. Examples of a Pass–Fail–Honor Grading System for Doctoral Capstone Experience

GRADE	DESCRIPTOR	DATA
Honors or high pass	• Beyond exceeded score for 80% of DCE evaluation of the OTD student • Exceptional comments on DCE evaluation of the OTD student	90% to 100% on assignments (including reflections and other required tasks)
Pass	• Beyond exceeded and met for 70% of DCE evaluation of the OTD student • Above-average comments on DCE evaluation of the OTD student	80% to 89% on assignments
Fail/not pass	• Did not receive a passing score on DCE evaluation of the OTD student	Did not turn in assignments or missed assignment deadlines

pass–fail–honor grading system for the DCE is provided in Table 10.9.

The literature on pass–fail grading schemes in medical and health science education provides several advantages that should be considered by doctoral capstone coordinators and occupational therapy faculty. Pass–fail grading allows for assessment of the learner by assessing competency of an outcome rather than earning a grade. There is evidence to suggest that a significant reduction in perceived stress and potential for improvement in positive attitude is associated with pass–fail grading (Rohe et al., 2006). Dyrbye et al. (2005) stated that letter grading systems promote a competitive environment that promotes maladaptive psychosocial well-being (e.g., stress and anxiety) and increases peer competition rather than cooperative learning. A pass–fail system for experiential education has the potential to promote intrinsically self-directed learners motivated through personal growth and development (Spring et al., 2011).

The inclusion of "honors" or a "high pass" grade (as noted in Table 10.9) can be a nice way to recognize students that are above-average and consistently go above and beyond expectations set by the academic program and the site.

SUGGESTIONS FOR REMEDIATION FOR THE CAPSTONE STUDENT

Remediation of student deficiency is another essential element of the teaching-learning process and integral to adult learning andragogy. The word *remediation* can be described as a correction of maladaptive or defective performance. However, an important aspect of remediation as a teaching intervention is that it does not always have to be punitive in nature. The result of remediation can include modification of teaching strategies, giving clear, corrective feedback, and

positive reinforcement for the learner. The use of feedback and formal remediation plans (such as a learning contract or performance improvement plan) can be used to proactively identify at risk attitudes or behavior to improve the success of the student. A *learning contract* is a long-standing remedial intervention also used in fieldwork (Gutman et al., 1995; Hanson & DeIuliis, 2015; Trivinia & Johnson, 2023) and can certainly also be a useful strategy to help support the development of capstone students. (See Text Box 10.14.)

TEXT BOX 10.14

A *learning contract* is a written document developed collaboratively among the capstone team members and should:

- Identify clear, smart individualized performance goals.
- Include a time frame in which the goal should be completed.
- List action steps, resources, or strategies that the learner commits to using to be successful.
- Have responsibilities of both parties included (the site mentor should play an active role in supporting the student's success).
- Serve as formal agreement and include the signatures of all parties involved.
- Outline consequences if performance does not meet the identified goals (which could include additional counseling and advisement, extension of the capstone experience, failure of the experience, etc.).

Learning contracts can be used to improve success with hard or practice-ready skills. (See Appendix 10.D for a sample learning contract). Occupational therapy educational programs should have clear policies and procedures outlining expectations regarding remediation and specifically handling a capstone student who is not successful during the DCE. (See Text Box 10.15.) Specific aspects that should be considered in the development of remediation policies related to the doctoral capstone can include the following:

- What if the student has a history of a previous failed experiential (or fieldwork) experience?
- What if the student is on academic probation?
- Are there any ethical or legal implications?

TEXT BOX 10.15

Similar to fieldwork, content experts need to be encouraged to initiate contact with the academic program via the doctoral capstone coordinator with any signs of concern about the capstone student. Also, document, document, document! Having a paper trail that consists of things such as when concerns developed, meetings and communications that occurred, and student response to feedback and the learning contract is important data that may come in handy with the student who is not successful on the doctoral capstone.

Educational programs should have policies that outline whether students who do not earn a passing grade on the DCE are offered a second opportunity after a plan of remediation has been successfully completed or at the discretion of the doctoral capstone coordinator. If deemed eligible to continue, the capstone student would need to repeat the DCE course (experience), which may include registering again for the same course (and payment for additional credits). The capstone student should also be made aware that the dates and location of the new DCE site are dependent on the availability of placement sites, potential site mentors, and match to student's needs. Occupational therapy programs should also have policies that clearly communicate to the capstone student that he or she may be allowed to repeat only one failed DCE placement. (See Text Box 10.16.)

TEXT BOX 10.16

Doctoral capstone coordinators and occupational therapy faculty should investigate their academic institution policies of how a "fail" or "not pass" grade may affect a student's standing in the program, based on academic requirements.

EVALUATION OF THE CONTENT EXPERT, SITE, AND EXPERIENCE

Evaluation of the doctoral capstone should be a mutual experience among members of the capstone team. The capstone student plays a central role in the capstone process and should have the opportunity to have their voice heard. According to Knowles (1970, 1990), a pioneer in adult learning theory, optimal learning occurs when adults are self-directed and actively engaged in the learning process. Feedback from the student can have multifaceted purposes. It can be used to measure the student's perception of the overall experience, collaboration with the content expert and mentor, and whether the site was welcoming to the student. Feedback from the student can also be used from a program evaluation method to determine the need to develop, refine, or eliminate fieldwork and capstone sites and curriculum enhancement. Depending on the capstone focus, type of setting, or individual mentoring the capstone student, there can be great diversity among the end product of the doctoral capstone. It is important to develop assessments that measure success in both the process and the product – each area may require separate learning outcomes and criteria. One example to evaluate student performance and progress during the capstone is for the occupational therapy education program to use structured reflection prompts, which was discussed earlier in this chapter (refer back to Text Box 10.3). Obtaining feedback from capstone students about their experience at the site and their mentorship from the content expert is also important. This tool can include a combination of open- and closed-ended questions and might have a similar Likert scale that is used on the student evaluation. Other important elements of the evaluation that capstone students should complete will gauge their perception on meeting the goals and objectives on the experiential plan and achieving competence in their focus area and their perception of the supervision and mentorship received from their content expert.

Sample indicators on an evaluation tool that capstone students would use to evaluate their experience and the role of the content expert may include their perception of the:

- Orientation process at the DCE site
- Communication and feedback system with their mentor or other stakeholders at their site
- Availability of supervision from site mentor
- Content expert as a role model
- Meeting the objectives established in the experiential plan
- Achieving in-depth knowledge or competence in the chosen focus area(s)
- Content expert's contribution and impact on project

See Appendix 10.E for an example.

Students can also be prompted to consider how their new skills (in their focus area), knowledge, and experiences are transferable to other situations or environments, including those outside of a formal academic course. The evaluation tool to measure the experience from capstone students' perspective and their feedback on the mentorship received from the mentor can be gleaned in a combination of open- and closed-ended questions and the use of a Likert scale, as noted previously. Results of the evaluation completed by the capstone student can be used to develop, refine, or eliminate capstone sites.

USE OF AN EXIT SURVEY

In addition to getting subjective feedback from the capstone team using developed evaluation tools, the doctoral capstone coordinator may be interested in developing and deploying an exit survey at the completion for the entire capstone course sequence. The exit survey could also include open- and closed-ended questions and be set up to be completed anonymously by students. Exit surveys should be designed with the notion that students provide valuable insight and can help enhance curriculum and department processes and procedures. Questions can be designed to capture key data required by the academic institution or accreditors, such as ACOTE, including job placement rate and amount of student debt. (See Appendix 10.F for sample exit survey.) (See Text Box 10.17.)

TEXT BOX 10.17

To give feedback for their own professional development and growth, doctoral capstone coordinators can create and deploy student evaluation surveys specific to their role as capstone coordinator. Check with your academic institution to see if there are already surveys developed specifically for clinical, teaching, and coordinator roles that could be applicable to the DCE. (See Appendix 10.G for an example of a doctoral capstone coordinator effectiveness survey.)

EDUCATOR CHAPTER SUMMARY

This chapter has provided recommendations of how to envision and develop a holistic evaluation system, including all members of the capstone team. In addition to their own mission, vision, and curriculum philosophies at their respective academic institutions, seminal teaching and learning pillars, including Bloom's taxonomy and domains of learning, can be useful resources for doctoral capstone coordinators to use to become inspired and develop evaluation mechanisms for the capstone. Educating members of the capstone team on the evaluation tools themselves as well as the importance of their specific vantage point is an important responsibility of the doctoral capstone coordinator. Creating and maintaining clear policies (including those within a policy handbook, included on syllabi, or posted on a website) are critical aspects to ensure fair, equitable, and consistent grading practices. This chapter specifically focused on the DCE; subsequent chapters provide recommendations and strategies to design and evaluate the capstone project and final written capstone document.

LEARNING ACTIVITIES

1. Review the AOTA FWPE for the Occupational Therapy Student. For each of the 37 items, brainstorm how the skill or competency could be enhanced to measure a higher level of learning according to Bloom's taxonomy.

2. Review the evaluation process at your academic institution used to get student feedback on the level I or level II fieldwork experience. Brainstorm ideas of how it could be adapted to use on the capstone.

REFERENCES

Accreditation Council for Occupational Therapy Education. (2023). *2023 Accreditation Council for Occupational Therapy Education (ACOTE®) standards and interpretive guide.* https://acoteonline.org/accreditation-explained/standards/

Allen, M. J. (2004). *Assessing academic programs in higher education.* Anker.

American Association for Public Opinion Research. (2024). *Best practices for survey research.* https://aapor.org/standards-and-ethics/best-practices/

American Occupational Therapy Association. (2020). *Fieldwork performance evaluation (FWPE) rating scoring guide* (Revised in 2020). https://www.aota.org/-/media/corporate/files/educationcareers/fieldwork/fieldwork-performance-evaluation-rating-scoring-guide.pdf

American Occupational Therapy Association. (2017). *Level I fieldwork competency evaluation for OT and OTA students.* https://www.aota.org/~/media/Corporate/Files/EducationCareers/Educators/Fieldwork/LevelI/Level-I-Fieldwork-Competency-Evaluation-for-ot-and-ota-students.pdf

American Occupational Therapy Association. (2021). Occupational therapy curriculum design framework. *American Journal of Occupational Therapy, 75*(Suppl. 3), 7513430010. https://doi.org/10.5014/ajot.2021.75S3008

American Occupational Therapy Association. (2023). *Self-assessment tool for fieldwork educator competency revised 2023* https://www.aota.org/-/media/corporate/files/educationcareers/fieldwork/certificate/safecom.pdf

American Statistical Association. (1999). *What is a survey?* https://higherlogicdownload.s3.amazonaws.com/AMSTAT/20d2b15c-9cc4-4c39-807c-088d6a8b6228/UploadedImages/WhatIsSurvey_Lohr1999.pdf

American Statistical Association. (2022). *Ethical guideline for statistical practice.* https://www.amstat.org/your-career/ethical-guidelines-for-statistical-practice

Anderson, L. W., & Krathwohl, D. R. (2001). *A taxonomy for learning, teaching, and assessing: A revision of Bloom's taxonomy of educational objectives.* Longman.

Astin, A. W. (1993). *What matters in college: Four critical years revisited.* Jossey-Bass.

Atler, K., Brown, K., Griswold, L. A., Krupnick, W., Melendez, L. M., & Stutz-Tanenbaum, P. (2001). *Fieldwork experience assessment tool (FEAT).* https://www.aota.org/-/media/Corporate/Files/EducationCareers/Accredit/FEATCHARTMidterm.pdf

Bandura, A. (1971). *Social learning theory.* General Learning Press.

Banta, T. W. (2002). *Building a scholarship of assessment.* Jossey-Bass.

Banta, T. W., Jones, E. A., & Black, K. E. (2009). *Designing effective assessment: Principles and profiles of good practice.* Jossey-Bass.

Bethea, D. P., Castillo, D. C., & Harvison, N. (2014). Use of simulation in occupational therapy education: Way of the future? *American Journal of Occupational Therapy, 68*(Suppl. 2), S32–S39. https://doi.org/10.5014/ajot.2014.012716

Bloom, B. S. (1956). *Taxonomy of educational objectives: The classification of educational goals*. Longmans, Green.

Boud, D. (2013). *Enhancing learning through self-assessment*. Routledge Falmer.

Bracken, D. W. (2009). The art and science of 360 degree feedback (2nd ed.) [book review]. *Personnel Psychology*, 62, 652–655.

Bracken, D. W., & Rose, D. S. (2011). When does 360-degree feedback create behavior change? And how would we know it when it does? *Journal of Business and Psychology*, 26(2), 183–192. https://doi.org/10.1007/s10869-011-9218-5

Christiansen, C. H., Baum, C. M., & Bass, J. (2005). *Occupational therapy: Performance, participation and well-being* (3rd ed.). SLACK Incorporated.

Cormack, C. L., Jensen, E., Durham, C. O., Smith, G., & Dumas, B. (2018). The 360-degree evaluation model: A method for assessing competency in graduate nursing students. A pilot research study. *Nurse Education Today*, 64, 132–137. https://doi.org/10.1016/j.nedt.2018.01.027

Cross, K. P. (1981). *Adults as learners: Increasing participation and facilitating learning*. Wiley.

Dyrbye, L. N., Thomas, M. R., & Shanafelt, T. D. (2005). Medical student distress: Causes, consequences, and proposed solutions. *Mayo Clinic Proceedings*, 80, 1613–1622. https://doi.org/10.4065/80.12.1613

Expert Training Systems. (2024). *360 degree feedback rating scales: What's best practice?* https://www.etsplc.com/blog/360-degree-feedback-rating-scales-whats-best-practice

Goldsmith, M., & Morgan, H. (2004). Leadership is a contact sport: The "follow-up" factor in management development. *Strategy + Business*, 36, 71–79.

Goldsmith, M., & Underhill, B. O. (2001). Multisource feedback for executive development. In D. W. Bracken, C. W. Timmreck, & A. H. Church (Eds.), *The handbook of multisource feedback: The comprehensive resource for designing and implementing MSF processes* (pp. 275–288). Jossey-Bass.

Greene, D. (1997). The use of service learning in client environments to enhance ethical reasoning in students. *American Journal of Occupational Therapy*, 51, 844–852.

Gutman, S. A., McCreedy, P., & Heisler, P. (1995). Student level II fieldwork failure: Strategies for intervention. *American Journal of Occupational Therapy*, 52(2), 143–149. https://doi.org/10.5014/ajot.52.2.143

Hanson, D., & DeIuliis, E. (2015). The collaborative model to fieldwork education: A blueprint for group supervision of students. *Occupational Therapy in Health Care*, 29(2), 223–239. https://doi.org/10.3109/07380577.2015.1011297

Hoppes, S., Bender, D., & DeGrace, B. W. (2005). Service learning is a perfect fit for occupational and physical therapy education. *Journal of Allied Health*, 34, 47–50.

IDEO. (2015). *The field guide to human-centered design*. Ideo.org.

Jackson, L., & Caffarella, R. S. (1994). Experiential learning: A new approach. In *New directions for adult and continuing education* (vol. 62, pp. 17–28). Jossey-Bass.

Knowles, M. S. (1970). *The modern practice of adult education: Androgogy versus pedagogy*. Association Press.

Knowles, M. S. (1984). *The adult learner: A neglected species* (3rd ed.). Gulf.

Knowles, M. S. (1990). *The adult learner: A neglected species* (4th ed.). Gulf.

Knowles, M. S. (1992). Applying principles of adult learning in conference presentations. *Adult Learning*, 4(1), 11–14. https://doi.org/10.1177/104515959200400105

Kolb, D. A. (1984). *Experiential learning: Experience as the source of learning and development*. Prentice Hall.

Lave, J., & Wenger, E. (1991). *Situated learning: Legitimate peripheral participation*. Cambridge University Press.

Law, M., Cooper, B., Strong, S., Stewart, D., Rigby, P., & Letts, L. (1996). The person-environment-occupation model: A transactive approach to occupational performance. *Canadian Journal of Occupational Therapy*, 63, 9–23.

Maurrasse, D. J. (2002). Higher education-community partnerships: Assessing progress in the field. *Nonprofit and Voluntary Sector Quarterly*, 31, 131–139.

McLeod, S. (2008). *Likert scale*. https://www.simplypsychology.org/likert-scale.html

Mezirow, J. (1997). Transformative learning: Theory to practice. *New Directions for Adult and Continuing Education*, (74), 5–12. https://doi.org/10.1002/ace.7401

Moon, J. A. (2004). *A handbook of reflective and experiential learning: Theory and practice*. Routledge Falmer.

Polatajko, H. J., Townsend, E. A., & Craik, J. (2007). Canadian model of occupational performance and engagement (CMOP-E). In E. A. Townsend & H. J. Polatajko (Eds.), *Enabling occupation II: Advancing an occupational therapy vision of health, well-being, & justice through occupation* (pp. 22–36). CAOT.

Qualters, D. M. (2010). Bringing the outside in: Assessing experiential education. *New Directions for Teaching and Learning*, 124, 55–62. http://ezproxy.lib.ryerson.ca/login?url=http://search.ebscohost.com/login.aspx?direct=true&db=eric&AN=EJ912853&site=ehost-live

Revans, R. W. (1980). *Action learning: New techniques for management*. Blond & Briggs.

Rogers, C. R. (1969). *Freedom to learn*. Merrill.

Rohe, D. E., Barrier, P. A., Clark, M. M., Cook, D. A., Vickers, K. S., & Decker, P. A. (2006). The benefits of pass-fail grading on stress, mood, and group cohesion in medical students. *Mayo Clinic Proceedings*, 81, 1443–1448. https://doi.org/10.4065/81.11.1443

Smither, J. W., London, M., & Reilly, R. R. (2005). Does performance improve following multisource feedback? A theoretical model, meta-analysis, and review of empirical findings. *Personnel Psychology*, 58, 33–66.

Spring, L., Robillard, D., Gehlbach, L., & Moore Simas, T. A. (2011). Impact of pass/fail grading on medical students well-being and academic outcomes. *Medical Education*, 45, 867–877.

Suskie, L. (2009). *Assessing student learning: A common sense guide* (2nd ed.). Jossey-Bass.

Trivinia, B., & Johnson, C. R. (2023). Supporting the at risk student. In E. DeIuliis & D. Hanson (Eds.), *Fieldwork educators guide to level II fieldwork* (pp. 277–320). SLACK Inc.

APPENDICES

Appendix A
DCE Site Visit/Call/Virtual Meeting Form

Student name: _____

Site Name:_____

Content Expert: _____

Contact: ☐ Call   Zoom ☐ On-Site DCE Timeline:_____ Phone #:_____

Today's Date:_____ Setting:_____

Population(s)/Focus Area: _____

Discussion Items	Student	Site Mentor
DCE	**Orientation to Site:** ☐ Yes ☐ No **Met Staff:** **Discuss Site-Specific Objectives:** **On Track to Meet?** ☐ Yes ☐ No **Comments:**	**Orientation to Site:** ☐ Yes ☐ No **Met Staff:** **Discuss Site-Specific Objectives:** **On Track to Meet?** ☐ Yes ☐ No **Comments:**
Supervision Discrepancy noted between content expert and student	<u>**Level of Supervision:**</u> **Mentorship conducive to learning experience:** ☐ Yes ☐ No **Comments:**	<u>**Level of Supervision:**</u> **Mentorship conducive to learning experience:** ☐ Yes ☐ No **Comments:**
Mentorship Discrepancy noted between content expert and student	<u>**Level of Mentorship:**</u> **Mentorship conducive to learning experience:** ☐ Yes ☐ No **Comments:**	<u>**Level of Mentorship:**</u> **Mentorship conducive to learning experience:** ☐ Yes ☐ No **Comments:**

General Comments:		
Communication Skills Discrepancy noted between site mentor and student	**Methods of Communication/ Feedback:** Ongoing, informal communication Use of weekly communication sheets Other:_____ **Who initiates the communication?** Student Content Expert Student or Content Expert **Content mentor provides constructive feedback** Always Most of the time Sometimes Never **Communication/collaboration with other professionals:**	**Methods of Communication/ Deedback:** Ongoing, informal communication Use of weekly communication sheets Other:_____ **Who initiates the communication?** Student Content Expert Student or Content Expert **Student accepts constructive feedback** Always Most of the time Sometimes Never **Non-verbal communication:** Appropriate Inappropriate **Communication/collaboration with other professionals:**
Professional Behaviors Discrepancy noted between site mentor and student	**Problem-Solving Skills Require Guidance:** Some of the time Most of the time All of the time **Integration of Site Mentor's Feedback:** Some of the time Most of the time All of the time **Time Management:** **Professional Dress:** Yes No	**Problem-Solving Skills Require Guidance:** Some of the time Most of the time All of the time **Integration of Site Mentor's Feedback:** Some of the time Most of the time All of the time **Time Management:** **Professional Dress:** Yes No

Project Planning/ Implementation Discrepancy noted between site mentor and student	Does Student Incorporate EBP into Practice: Yes No **Utilization of EBP:** **Texts Web Journals** **Professionals Others**	Does Student Incorporate EBP into Practice: **Yes No** **Utilization of EBP:** **Texts Web** **Journals Professionals**
Preparation for DCE Need to discuss points at faculty meeting	**Was Academic Preparation Appropriate: Yes No** **Comments:**	**Was Academic Preparation Appropriate:** **Yes No** **Strengths of OTD Program:**
Strengths/Weaknesses Discrepancy noted between site mentor and student	**Strengths:** **Areas for Development:**	**Strengths:** **Areas for Development:**
Additional Learning Opportunities	**Assignments/Projects:**	**Other Activities:**

Signature acknowledges that OTD Capstone Coordinator performed on-site visit and/or virtual meeting/ phone call.

OTD Capstone Coordinator: _____

Date: _____

Content Expert Description:

Is this your first OTD capstone student? ☐ Yes ☐   No

Did the DCE placement process run smoothly? Yes ☐ No ☐

What could the OTD capstone coordinator do to facilitate success and improve communication?

Midterm Evaluation Forms:

Midterm completed and discussed: ☐ Yes   ☐ No

Goals and feedback discussed and agreed upon: ☐ Yes   ☐ No

Goals:

Overall performance:

Above expected level of competence ☐

At expected level of competence ☐

Below expected level of competence ☐

Comments:

☐ On track   ☐ Follow-up needed   ☐ Intervention required

_____

If any discrepancies were noted between content expert's and student's responses, what action was performed?

☐ Clarification only was needed from   ☐ Content Mentor   ☐ Student   ☐ Both

☐ Follow-up was performed via phone/follow-up was performed during a visit

Duquesne University Department of Occupational Therapy Doctoral Capstone Experience Evaluation of the OTD Student

Student Name: Content Expert Name:
Placement Dates: Site/Setting:
Date of Midterm Review: Date of Final Review:

Select the focus of the residency:

☐ Clinical Skills   ☐ Advocacy   ☐ Program Development/Evaluation
☐ Research Skills   ☐ Policy Development   ☐ Education
☐ Administration   ☐ Leadership   ☐ Other (please describe): _____

Instructions

The content expert will complete this evaluation form at midterm (7 weeks) and finals (14 weeks). The content expert and the OTD student will review the evaluation collectively and sign that they agree on the evaluation. The OTD student is encouraged to complete a self-assessment to guide discussion and the learning process. The self-reflection is to be completed by the student separate from and prior to meeting with the site mentor. This is used to foster self-reflection on the student's performance, including areas of growth and areas for improvement related to the learning objectives and student-specific objectives.

Learning objectives 1–11 are derived from the DU OTD Doctoral Capstone Experience Behavioral Objectives.

Note that there is space provided (potential objectives 12–14) for both the OTD student and the content expert to add three student-specific objectives, mutually decided upon by the OTD student and the content expert based on what the student wants/needs to know and what skills the student needs to develop. All objectives must be (1) relevant to the fieldwork experience setting; (2) understandable to the student, content expert, and doctoral capstone coordinator (DCC); (3) measurable; (4) behavioral/observable; and (5) achievable within the specified time frame.

Please use this scale to rate the following objectives:

5 = Exceeding, **4** = Met, **3** = Making Progress, **2** = Not Making Progress, **1** = Needs Attention
Provide comments to indicate evidence, as indicated.

DU OTD Objective #1: Student will demonstrate effective communication skills and work interprofessionally with those who receive and provide care.
Evidence of accomplishment, to be completed by student and content expert:
_____
_____

Midterm: ☐ 5 ☐ 4 ☐ 3 ☐ 2 ☐ 1
Comments: _____
_____

Final: ☐ 5 ☐ 4 ☐ 3 ☐ 2 ☐ 1
Comments: _____
_____

DU OTD Objective #2: Student will demonstrate positive interpersonal skills and insight into one's professional behaviors to accurately appraise one's professional disposition, strengths, and areas for improvement.
Evidence of accomplishment, to be completed by student and content expert:

_____

_____

Midterm: ☐ 5 ☐ 4 ☐ 3 ☐ 2 ☐ 1

Comments: _____

_____

Final: ☐ 5 ☐ 4 ☐ 3 ☐ 2 ☐ 1

Comments: _____

_____

DU OTD Objective #3: Student will demonstrate the ability to practice educative roles for clients, peers, students, interprofessionals, and others.

Evidence of accomplishment, to be completed by student and content expert:

_____

_____

Midterm: ☐ 5 ☐ 4 ☐ 3 ☐ 2 ☐ 1

Comments: _____

_____

Final: ☐ 5 ☐ 4 ☐ 3 ☐ 2 ☐ 1

Comments: _____

_____

DU OTD Objective #4: Student will develop essential knowledge and skills to contribute to the advancement of occupational therapy through scholarly activities.

Evidence of accomplishment, to be completed by student and content expert:

_____

_____

Midterm: ☐ 5 ☐ 4 ☐ 3 ☐ 2 ☐ 1

Comments: _____

_____

Final: ☐ 5 ☐ 4 ☐ 3 ☐ 2 ☐ 1

Comments: _____

_____

DU OTD Objective #5: Student will apply a critical foundation of evidence-based professional knowledge, skills, and attitudes.

Evidence of accomplishment, to be completed by student and content expert:

_____

_____

Midterm: ☐ 5 ☐ 4 ☐ 3 ☐ 2 ☐ 1

Comments: _____

_____

Final: ☐ 5 ☐ 4 ☐ 3 ☐ 2 ☐ 1

Comments: _____

_____

DU OTD Objective #6: Student will apply principles and constructs of ethics to individual, institutional, and societal issues and articulate justifiable resolutions to these issues and act in an ethical manner.

Evidence of accomplishment, to be completed by student and content expert:

_____

_____

Midterm: ☐ 5 ☐ 4 ☐ 3 ☐ 2 ☐ 1

Comments: _____

_____

Final: ☐ 5 ☐ 4 ☐ 3 ☐ 2 ☐ 1

Comments: _____

_____

DU OTD Objective #7: Student will perform tasks in a safe and ethical manner and adhere to the site's policies and procedures, including those related to human subject research, when relevant.

Evidence of accomplishment, to be completed by student and content expert:

_____

_____

Midterm: ☐ 5 ☐ 4 ☐ 3 ☐ 2 ☐ 1

Comments: _____

_____

Final: ☐ 5 ☐ 4 ☐ 3 ☐ 2 ☐ 1

Comments: _____

_____

DU OTD Objective #8: Student will demonstrate competence in following program methods, quality improvement, and/or research procedures utilized at the site.

Evidence of accomplishment, to be completed by student and content expert:

_____

_____

Midterm: ☐ 5 ☐ 4 ☐ 3 ☐ 2 ☐ 1

Comments: _____

_____

Final: ☐ 5 ☐ 4 ☐ 3 ☐ 2 ☐ 1

Comments: _____

_____

DU OTD Objective #9: Student will learn, practice, and apply knowledge from the classroom and practice settings at a higher level than prior fieldwork experiences, with simultaneous guidance from site mentor and DU OT faculty.

Evidence of accomplishment, to be completed by student and content expert:

_____

_____

Midterm: ☐ 5 ☐ 4 ☐ 3 ☐ 2 ☐ 1

Comments: _____

_____

Final: ☐ 5 ☐ 4 ☐ 3 ☐ 2 ☐ 1

Comments: _____

_____

DU OTD Objective #10: Student will relate theory to practice and demonstrate synthesis of advanced knowledge in a specialized practice area through completion of a doctoral capstone component and scholarly project.

Evidence of accomplishment, to be completed by student and content expert:

_____

_____

Midterm: ☐ 5 ☐ 4 ☐ 3 ☐ 2 ☐ 1

Comments: _____

_____

Final: ☐ 5 ☐ 4 ☐ 3 ☐ 2 ☐ 1

Comments: _____

_____

DU OTD Objective #11: Acquire in-depth experience in one or more of the following areas: clinical practice skills, research skills, administration, leadership, program and policy development, advocacy, education, and theory development.

Evidence of accomplishment, to be completed by student and content expert:

_____

_____

Midterm: ☐ 5 ☐ 4 ☐ 3 ☐ 2 ☐ 1

Comments: _____

_____

Final: ☐ 5 ☐ 4 ☐ 3 ☐ 2 ☐ 1

Comments: _____

_____

OTD Student-Selected Objective #1: _____

_____

Evidence of accomplishment, to be completed by student and content expert:

_____

_____

Midterm: ☐ 5 ☐ 4 ☐ 3 ☐ 2 ☐ 1

Comments: _____

_____

Final: ☐ 5 ☐ 4 ☐ 3 ☐ 2 ☐ 1

Comments: _____

_____

OTD Student-Selected Objective #2: _____

_____

Evidence of accomplishment, to be completed by student and content expert:

_____

_____

Midterm: ☐ 5 ☐ 4 ☐ 3 ☐ 2 ☐ 1

Comments: _____

_____

Final: ☐ 5 ☐ 4 ☐ 3 ☐ 2 ☐ 1

Comments: _____

_____

OTD Student-Selected Objective #3: _____

Evidence of accomplishment, to be completed by student and content expert:

_____

_____

Midterm: ☐ 5 ☐ 4 ☐ 3 ☐ 2 ☐ 1

Comments: _____

_____

Final: ☐ 5 ☐ 4 ☐ 3 ☐ 2 ☐ 1

Comments: _____

_____

We are interested in obtaining an accurate profile of the OTD student's capacity for the profession. We would appreciate your additional comments regarding the areas in which you rated the student on the previous pages.

Overall Strengths:

Areas for Growth:

Student's Signature _____   Date _____

Content Expert Name (Print): _____

Phone: _____

Email Address: _____

Content Expert's Signature: _____   Date _____

NOTE: *This evaluation must be completed by the student, reviewed by the site mentor, signed by both parties, and returned via EXXAT electronically to the doctoral capstone coordinator before the student will receive a grade for this capstone experience.*

Return to: *Michelle McCann, OTD, OTR/L 224 Rangos School of Health Sciences, Duquesne University, Pittsburgh, PA 15282, or email scanned copy to mccannm2@duq.edu.*

Institution:	Indiana University
Student:	
Fieldwork Educator:	
Site:	
Date:	

YOU ARE CURRENTLY IN PREVIEW MODE – THE EVALUATION CANNOT BE SUBMITTED. **Start Evaluation**

Evaluation of Student Performance: Doctoral Capstone

How to apply scoring

Please use the rating scale below in order to rate the doctoral capstone student's educational and professional outcomes at the midterm and final points of their doctoral capstone experience:

Exceeds Expectations (4)

Meets Expectations (3)

Needs Improvement (2)

Does Not Meet Expectations (1)

N/A

Section Weight: 50%

Educational Outcomes

The student is able to

		Exceeds Expectations	Meets Expectations	Needs Improvement	Does Not Meet Expectations	N/A	
Effectively identify the need or problem within the capstone setting/ population	Midpoint Required						Enter comments for midpoint
	Final Required						Enter comments for final
Demonstrate use of evidence-based practice in order to address the needs of the capstone setting population.	Midpoint Required						Enter comments for midpoint
	Final Required						Enter comments for final
Advocate for the role of occupational therapy within the capstone setting population.	Midpoint Required						Enter comments for midpoint
	Final Required						Enter comments for final
Demonstrate the value of occupational therapy within the capstone setting population	Midpoint Required						Enter comments for midpoint
	Final Required						Enter comments for final

Use knowledge to implement their student learning plan.	Midpoint Required					Enter comments for midpoint
	Final Required					Enter comments for final
Evaluate the outcomes of the capstone using evidence-based measurement practices.	Midpoint Required					Enter comments for midpoint
	Final Required					Enter comments for final
Apply theory to practice.	Midpoint Required					Enter comments for midpoint
	Final Required					Enter comments for final
Impact the health and well-being of the capstone population.	Midpoint Required					Enter comments for midpoint
	Final Required					Enter comments for final

Section Weight: 50%

Professional outcomes

The student is able to.

		Exceeds Expectations	Meets Expectations	Needs Improvement	Does Not Meet Expectations	N/A	
Collaborate and communicate with staff in professional and timely manners.	Midpoint Required						Enter Comments for Midpoint
	Final Required						Enter Comments for Final
Collaborate and communicate with clients in professional and timely manners.	Midpoint Required						Enter Comments for Midpoint
	Final Required						Enter Comments for Final
Collaborate and communicate with staff in a professional and timely manner.	Midpoint Required						Enter Comments for Midpoint
	Final Required						Enter Comments for Final
Follow the established supervision/mentorship plan.	Midpoint Required						Enter Comments for Midpoint
	Final Required						Enter Comments for Final

Be on time to all meetings and scheduled events.	Midpoint Required					Enter Comments for Midpoint
	Final Required					Enter Comments for Final
Keep site mentor aware of their schedule.	Midpoint Required					Enter Comments for Midpoint
	Final Required					Enter Comments for Final
Complete required hours each week.	Midpoint Required					Enter Comments for Midpoint
	Final Required					Enter Comments for Final
Adhere to all site policies and procedures.	Midpoint Required					Enter Comments for Midpoint
	Final Required					Enter Comments for Final
Demonstrate self-directed learnings.	Midpoint Required					Enter Comments for Midpoint
	Final Required					Enter Comments for Comments

Please provide a brief statement regarding student progress toward goals and objectives for the doctoral capstone experience and project.

Comments (Midpoint): *Comment Required   Comments (Final): *Comment Required

Enter Midponint comments	Enter Final comments

Students must score an overall average of 3.0 or higher on the FINAL EVALUATION to receive a Satisfactory score in order to pass T88.0

Evaluation Score Summary

Title: Primary Evaluation	Midpoint score	Final score 0.00	Weight 100.00%	Adj. Final Score	Required

Back to Top

Appendix D

LEARNING CONTRACT/ACTION PLAN

Performance Issue/Concern (Be Specific)	Expected Performance Goal (Behavioral Goal – SMART)	Strategies, Actions, and Resource(s) Required to Meet the Goal	Plan for Follow-Up/ Timeline (Establish Date/Time for Performance to Be Re-Evaluated)

By providing signature, both parties are acknowledging the above performance issues and agree to participate in the performance improvement plan as outlined above. It is the student's responsibility to access resources, carry out these and/or other strategies to improve their performance, and implement feedback in the identified problem areas. Failure to meet expected performance in established timeline may indicate disciplinary action and/or failed capstone experience.

Student signature:_____ Date: _____

Content Expert's signature: _____ Date: _____

Doctoral Capstone Coordinator signature: _____ Date: _____

_____

For use at follow-up meeting.
Learning Contract/Action Plan REVIEW OUTCOME

Evidence to demonstrate change in performance/outcome:

_____Review met expectations.

_____Review did not meet expectations. *Disciplinary action may be necessary.*

Student's Signature: _____ Date: _____

Content Expert's Signature:_____ Date: _____

Doctoral Capstone Coordinator's Signature: _____Date:_____

STUDENT EVALUATION OF DOCTORAL CAPSTONE EXPERIENCE

OTD Student:

Content Expert:

Doctoral Capstone Experience Site:

Dates of Doctoral Capstone Experience:

INSTRUCTIONS: The OTD student will complete this evaluation form at the completion of the 14-week experience. Both the content expert and OTD student will review the evaluation collectively and sign that they have discussed. The student will then submit the form to the doctoral capstone coordinator within three days from the last day of the experiential.

I.   Please use the scale below and rate the following:

1 = Strongly Disagree

2 = Disagree

3 = Neither Agree/Disagree (Neutral)

4 = Agree

5 = Strongly Agree

Objective	Rating					Comments
1. My content expert was accessible and available.	1	2	3	4	5	
2. My content expert communicated regularly with me.	1	2	3	4	5	
3. My content expert's behavior and attitude is an example of professionalism.	1	2	3	4	5	
4. My content expert made sure to provide ample time to ask questions and provide feedback.	1	2	3	4	5	
5. I was provided ongoing feedback in a timely manner.	1	2	3	4	5	
6. My content expert reviewed written work in a timely manner.	1	2	3	4	5	
7. My content expert made specific suggestions to me to improve my performance.	1	2	3	4	5	
8. My content expert provided clear performance expectations.	1	2	3	4	5	
9. My content expert sequenced learning experiences to grade progression.	1	2	3	4	5	
10. My content expert used a variety of instructional strategies. List those used:	1	2	3	4	5	

11. My content expert identified resources to promote student development.	1	2	3	4	5	
12. My content expert facilitated advanced clinical reasoning.	1	2	3	4	5	
13. My content expert demonstrated expertise in my chosen focus area(s).	1	2	3	4	5	
14. I learned new things about myself and how they relate to future OT practice.	1	2	3	4	5	
15. Professional growth occurred for me during this DCE experience.	1	2	3	4	5	
16. Overall, this DCE Placement experience met my expectations.	1	2	3	4	5	

II. Student Reflections

1. Before beginning a doctoral capstone experience at this site, a student should study/read/prepare by:

2. The most rewarding part of this DCE was:

3. The most challenging part of this DCE was:

Content Expert Signature: _____Date: _____
Student Signature: _____ Date: _____

NOTE: This evaluation must be completed by the student, reviewed by the content expert, signed by both parties, and returned to the doctoral capstone coordinator before the student will receive a grade for this capstone experience.

Return to: *Michelle McCann, OTD, OTR/L 224 Rangos School of Health Sciences, Duquesne University, Pittsburgh, PA 15282, or email scanned copy to: mccannm2@duq.edu.*

Appendix F

OTD EXIT SURVEY EXAMPLE

	Strongly Agree	Agree	Disagree	Strongly Disagree
Q1. The OTD curriculum prepared me to . . . [**INSERT STUDENT LEARNING OUTCOME**]. Example: **Apply evidence-based practice**. (Graduates will search, review, analyze, synthesize, and apply knowledge to inform best practice in occupational therapy and education.)				
Q2. The OTD curriculum prepared me to. . . [**INSERT STUDENT LEARNING OUTCOME**].				
Q3. The OTD curriculum prepared me to . . . [**INSERT STUDENT LEARNING OUTCOME**].				

	Strongly or Agree	Agree	Disagree	Strongly Disagree
Q4. The OTD curriculum prepared me to . . . [**INSERT STUDENT LEARNING OUTCOME**].				
Q5. The OTD curriculum prepared me to . . . [**INSERT STUDENT LEARNING OUTCOME**].				

Q6. Practice scholarship and professional development are important components of the mission and curriculum philosophy within the Department of Occupational Therapy. Please indicate from the following selections which experiences you engaged in as a doctoral student at Duquesne University (check all that apply):	
Contributed to a manuscript for publication	
Volunteered for an organization, population, or individual	
Attended annual AOTA conference	
Participated in faculty research project	
Was involved in a leadership role	
Received an academic award	
Presented at undergraduate research symposium	
Presented at national AOTA conference	
Presented for local organization/agency on a practice-related topic	
Was nominated for an academic award	
Attended a scholarly journal club	
Led or co-led a scholarly journal club	

Presented at international conference	
Attended state association conference	
Was awarded a grant	
Presented at graduate research symposium	
Participated in the application for a grant	
Presented at state OT association conference	
Presented at an international conference	
Attended district/regional association meeting	

	Strongly Agree	Agree	Disagree	Strongly Disagree
Q7. When I needed it, I received information, class schedules, etc. on a timely basis from OT faculty and staff.				
Q8. When I needed it, I received sufficient assistance in solving education-related problems from OT faculty and staff.				
Q9. Overall, I feel that the Department of Occupational Therapy provides high levels of student–faculty contact.				
	Excellent	Good	Average	Below Average
Q10. How would you rate your marketability as an OTD graduate from the OT program?				
Q11. Have you completed a professional interview for an OT-related position?			Yes	No
Q12. As of today, how many formal OT-related positions have you interviewed for?				
Q13. Did you interview or obtain a job offer based upon your doctoral capstone?				

	Accepted Job	Have Offer, No Accepted Position	Applied, But No Offer	Have Not Applied
Q14. Which of the following statements about your job search is most accurate as of today?				
Q15. If you have received a job offer or accepted a job offer, please choose the range of annual salary offered. If part-time, indicate your equivalent full-time salary. For example: If employed half-time making $30,000, check the box indicating $60,000.				

	Strongly Agree	Agree	Disagree	Strongly Disagree
Q16. I would recommend the entry-level OTD curriculum at this program to someone else.				

Q17. In what ways do you believe that your completion of the OTD program will help you meet your personal and/or professional goals? Please explain.

Q18. Faculty recognize the cost of higher education is a challenge and becoming more so. We are committed to advocating for our students with university administration to hold the line on tuition costs. Data on our students' debt load may help us develop strong, convincing arguments. Which of the following most accurately reflects your total student loan debt?

Greater than $200,000	
$180,000–$200,000	
$160,000–$180,000	
$140,000–$160,000	
$120,000–$140,000	
$100,000–$120,000	
$80,000–$100,000	
$60,000–$80,000	
$40,000–$60,000	
$20,000–$40,000	
Less than $20,000	

Appendix G

Example Doctoral Capstone Coordinator Questionnaire for Student Feedback

Rating Scale

- Strongly Agree
- Agree
- Neither Agree/Disagree
- Disagree
- Strongly Disagree

My doctoral capstone coordinator . . .

- Provided an adequate orientation and provided information about the requirements of the doctoral capstone process
- Selected (or assisted me in selecting) an appropriate setting for my doctoral capstone
- Selected (or assisted me in selecting) an appropriate content expert to serve as a site mentor
- Was available to me as a resource person via email, phone, site visits, LMS site, and/or during office hours during the doctoral capstone
- Was responsive to my questions/concerns regarding my doctoral capstone
- Provided feedback about my performance during the doctoral capstone
- Reinforced expectations for demonstrating professionalism during the doctoral capstone
- Was an effective professional role model

I felt comfortable contacting the doctoral capstone coordinator via email, phone, or during office hours regarding the doctoral capstone.

 Overall, the doctoral capstone coordinator is an effective capstone coordinator.

 [Open-ended] **What aspects of the doctoral capstone coordinator's teaching were most effective?**

 [Open-ended] **How could the doctoral capstone coordinator improve their performance within the doctoral capstone process?**

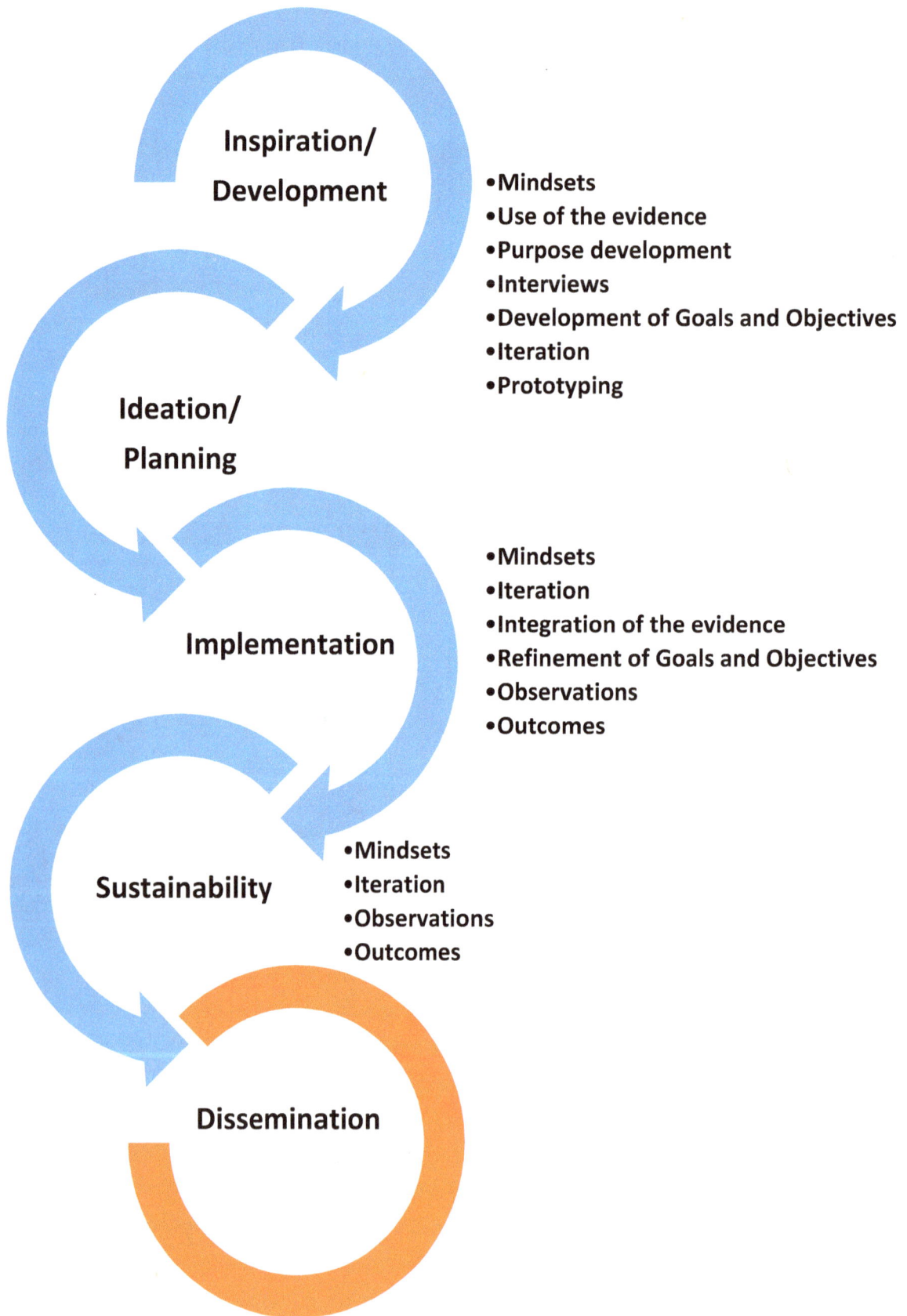

Inspiration/
Development

- Mindsets
- Use of the evidence
- Purpose development
- Interviews
- Development of Goals and Objectives
- Iteration
- Prototyping

Ideation/
Planning

Implementation

- Mindsets
- Iteration
- Integration of the evidence
- Refinement of Goals and Objectives
- Observations
- Outcomes

Sustainability

- Mindsets
- Iteration
- Observations
- Outcomes

Dissemination

PART IV DISSEMINATION

The final step in the doctoral capstone process is addressing dissemination of results. This phase allows capstone students to share the doctoral capstone experience and project with others, including the site, the client group or population involved, stakeholders, occupational therapists, and other health-care professionals. In this phase, capstone students communicate what was done, why it is important, and how the results have had an impact on the client. The dissemination allows capstone students to reflect on how taking on the mindset of a human-centered designer and the process phases of inspiration, ideation, and implementation led them to have an impact in the world. SHARE THE IMPACT!

DOI: 10.4324/9781003541813-14

CHAPTER 11

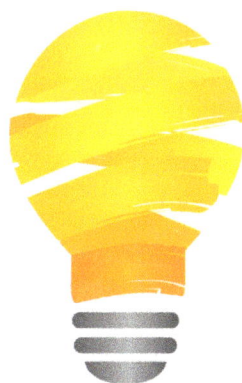

Dissemination Considerations and Impact of the Capstone

Sally Wasmuth

Section 1: Student Focus

Human-Centered Design Mindsets for Doctoral Students

The doctoral capstone experience and project are ending, and your choice to disseminate is an important one. How will you let other professionals, consumers, and stakeholders know what you have done and the outcomes of your work? You need to disseminate, and using the human-centered design mindset concepts of optimism and learning from failure will assist you in this endeavor.

Optimism. You have come so far. It is important to keep an open mind and an optimistic outlook as you think about dissemination. What is the best way to disseminate your work? Optimism will drive you forward as you think of all the potential possibilities. Keep an open mind and understand that you will find the best way to disseminate your work.

Creative confidence. Do not be limited by fear of failure as you think about how you will disseminate. Often, proposals for papers or presentations are not accepted on first attempts. Learn from feedback, and keep submitting until you are accepted. Do not give up!

INTRODUCTION FOR STUDENTS

Occupational therapy doctoral capstone experiences (DCEs) and projects have had considerable impacts on clients (improving wellness outcomes for individuals and groups), families (improving communication, caregiver support, and resource provision), society (reducing policies rooted in societal stigma that impede occupational justice), and health-care professions (illustrating the need to include occupational therapy services in specific contexts, such as mental health). The scholarly deliverables resulting from DCEs serve to deepen and extend the impact you can have in these areas. This chapter outlines several potential means for disseminating knowledge and information gained through your capstone project. It will examine factors to consider when deciding how to disseminate your work, as well as some potential challenges, and will illuminate the impact you can have through various forms of dissemination.

DOI: 10.4324/9781003541813-15

STUDENT REFLECTIVE QUESTIONS

During the dissemination phase of the capstone, you may find it helpful to reflect on the following questions:

1. Why is dissemination important? What is your plan?

2. What are the next steps after your DCE is complete? How will you or others continue the work you have begun?

3. How does your doctoral capstone project link to the vision of the American Occupational Therapy Association (AOTA) and the occupational therapy profession as a whole?

STUDENT OBJECTIVES

By the end of reading this chapter and completing the learning activities, you should be able to:

1. Compare and contrast types of project dissemination methods.

2. Understand the purpose and process of professional writing to communicate your impact in the field of occupational therapy.

3. Explain recommendations for written capstone dissemination.

4. Explain recommendations for oral capstone dissemination.

5. Identify additional formats for capstone project dissemination.

LINKING THE DOCTORAL CAPSTONE PROJECT TO AOTA VISION 2025

Vision 2025 of AOTA (2018) states, "As an inclusive profession, occupational therapy maximizes health, well-being, and quality of life for all people, populations, and communities through effective solutions that facilitate participation in everyday living" (p. 1). Three critical elements can be gleaned from this vision as pertinent when considering the impact and scholarly deliverables of your DCE and capstone project. First, the profession is focused on health, well-being, and quality of life. This basic tenet provides focus to the doctoral capstone. Regardless of the population served and whether the project focuses on individual clients, policy issues, therapists' clinical skills, organizational staff and structure, or something else altogether, the results of your efforts should enhance health, well-being, and quality of life for those affected. Second, occupational therapy practitioners strive to provide services that reach all people, emphasizing occupational justice – the notion that all people should be afforded the right to engage in and benefit from personally meaningful activities and that this should be central to occupational therapy practice (Bailliard et al., 2020). Thus, occupational therapy practitioners especially focus their efforts on people who are stigmatized, are marginalized, or for other reasons, are likely to lack opportunities for occupational participation or access to occupational therapy services. In addition to providing services to individuals, occupational therapy practitioners consider population health approaches and community-based practices (including service to organizations) as central to the profession. Third, occupational therapy practitioners promote health, well-being, and quality life by facilitating participation in everyday living. This aspect of Vision 2025 emphasizes the centrality of occupation-based intervention and the belief within the profession that meaningful participation in life is critical to human health and can reverse disease processes, improve quality of life, and enhance well-being (Steptoe & Fancourt, 2020). Taking Vision 2025 into consideration, your DCE should include an exploration of ways to **use** and **emphasize** the health-promoting power of meaningful participation in life, especially for those likely to be deprived of this universal human need.

Five guideposts define in more detail the tenets of AOTA's Vision 2025:

1. *Accessible.* Occupational therapy provides culturally responsive and customized services.

2. *Collaborative.* Occupational therapy excels in working with clients and within systems to produce effective outcomes.

3. *Effective.* Occupational therapy is evidence-based, client-centered, and cost-effective.

4. *Leaders.* Occupational therapy is influential in changing policies, environments, and complex systems.

5. *Equity, inclusion, and diversity.* We are intentionally inclusive and equitable and embrace diversity in all its forms.

(AOTA, 2018)

These guideposts can further focus your capstone project and provide structure for discussions between you and your site or faculty mentors. Table 11.1 lists some discussion questions rooted in these guideposts. Conversations steered by these questions can help pinpoint opportunities for collaborative scholarship that capitalizes on the strengths of all involved. Answers to these questions may illuminate potential avenues for scholarly deliverables.

IMPACT POTENTIAL OF THE DOCTORAL CAPSTONE PROJECT

As an occupational therapy capstone student, you have enormous impact potential on many levels. Capstone projects can impact clients, families, societies, and health-care professions. Following is a discussion of how occupational therapy capstone students can have an impact at each of these levels.

Table 11-1. Discussion Questions to Determine Focus and Scholarly Deliverables

AOTA VISION 2025 GUIDEPOSTS	QUESTIONS TO CONSIDER WITH CONTENT EXPERT AND FACULTY MENTOR
Accessible: Occupational therapy provides culturally responsive and customized services.	• Who receives services at my site – what is the client population? • Is the primary population racially, ethnically, or otherwise diverse? • Are most clients from a group that has been harmed by stigma? • Is the population inherently diverse? • Are current assessments at the site able to capture nuanced differences between clients?
Collaborative: Occupational therapy excels in working with clients and within systems to produce effective outcomes.	• What are considered effective outcomes at this site according to personnel? • What would clients consider to be effective outcomes of services? • What systemic factors impact client care within the site? • What type of outcomes need attention at the site?
Effective: Occupational therapy is evidence-based, client-centered, and cost-effective.	• Does the site provide services supported by current evidence? • How does the site determine client needs and wants? • To what extent or in what way are client needs and wants addressed by current services? • Are occupational therapy services currently provided at the site? • Are other professionals providing services that fall in the scope of occupational therapy practice? • Would service changes related to occupational therapy impact cost at the site? How?
Leaders: Occupational therapy is influential in changing policies, environments, and complex systems.	• In what ways can occupational therapy benefit clients within the capstone site? • What barriers currently prevent beneficial occupational therapy services within the site? • How does/can change occur within the site?
Equity, inclusion, and diversity: We are intentionally inclusive and equitable and embrace diversity in all its forms.	• How do inequities and health disparities impact clients within the capstone site? Do I have sufficient training in cultural humility to recognize and acknowledge my own biases? • What steps could be taken within the site to promote equity, inclusion, and diversity? • Are all client forms and practices sufficiently updated to promote inclusive and equitable care to diverse groups?

Source: Adapted from American Occupational Therapy Association (2018). *Vision 2025.* https://www.aota.org/Publications-News/AOTANews/2018/AOTA-Board-Expands-Vision–2025.aspx.

Clients

Capstone projects focused on impacting individual lives can demonstrate their impact in several ways, including, but not limited to, client surveys, evaluation of individual changes documented in electronic health records, and surveys completed by those who work with the individual clients and may observe changes.

Client surveys. A capstone student conducting a community-based leisure group for clients with substance use disorders may administer a survey to participants to determine how the leisure group impacted individuals. Questions should stem from literature documenting key wellness outcomes for this population, such as social participation (Vigdal et al., 2022), mood and emotion regulation (Stellern et al., 2023), and culturally sensitive measures of substance use (Jordan et al., 2022).

Electronic health records. A capstone student implementing a wellness group in a hospital setting may demonstrate impact by recording functional assessments documented in occupational therapy evaluations and treatment sessions before and after the group was implemented to examine the possibility that the group impacted occupational therapy treatment progress.

Surveys completed by someone who works with clients. A capstone student in a school-based setting implementing an interoceptive awareness program for students may demonstrate impact through a survey in which teachers can report observed changes in classroom dynamics and/or the ability of students to self-regulate.

Families

You can impact families by including them when developing new programming or delivering client services. Literature supports the inclusion of family members in occupational therapy and rehabilitation efforts across populations. For example, the importance of caregiver education and support to prevent burnout is well-documented (Koller et al., 2022; Kwon et al., 2021; Ricou et al., 2020). For conditions such as substance use disorders, family dynamics can have a considerable impact on recovery outcomes; as such, family-based interventions can be more effective than individual interventions (Hogue et al., 2022). You may want to consider how to engage families when developing new programs in clinical or community settings. Engaging families may also become the focus of your DCE and/or capstone project. For instance, in a hospital setting, you may develop a protocol for how to increase family engagement.

Societies

You can impact societies through doctoral capstones that focus on systemic issues, such as racism, ableism, heterosexism, transphobia, and other forms of stigma that limit occupational participation, performance, and justice. Measures such as the Acceptance and Action Questionnaire-Stigma (AAQ-S; Levin et al., 2014) have been used to demonstrate the impact of occupational therapy stigma reduction tools (Wasmuth et al., 2021, 2023).

If your capstone site is in the community or if you work directly with research faculty, you can develop projects that address societal needs. For instance, you may focus on developing community collaborative efforts to promote safe social participation in society or convening experts to address a societal problem, such as food desserts, limited resources, and/or unsafe living conditions. Advocacy is central to the profession of occupational therapy and can therefore serve as an innovative but important focal point if you are seeking to impact societies through your doctoral capstone.

Health-Care Professions

Some doctoral capstones can impact how health-care professions operate, which can have a cascade of positive impacts. For example, you may demonstrate the need for occupational therapy services within a sector that does not typically include occupational therapy services. In a Midwest hospital setting, a DCE resulted in the development of an occupational therapy program within a neonatal intensive care unit (Gibbons, 2024). Another capstone project demonstrated the need for occupational therapy within an outpatient gender wellness program in a public hospital, resulting in the creation of a part-time occupational therapy position within that setting (Schrader, 2024). One capstone project used narratives to educate health-care professional students about the presence and impact of lead exposure in a large Midwestern site (Belkiewitz, 2023; Belkiewitz & Wasmuth, 2025). The impact of this capstone project on health-care professions was that more providers knew to advise families to get tested for lead exposure, and health-care practitioners were equipped to recognize and treat symptoms of lead exposure in youth. Additionally, literature suggests doctoral capstone projects can significantly impact capstone students themselves, thereby influencing the future occupational therapy practitioner workforce. For example, Bekmuratova et al. (2022) found international capstone projects increased cultural humility of capstone students, preparing them to provide more inclusive and equitable occupational therapy services in the future.

PURPOSE AND IMPORTANCE OF DISSEMINATION OF PROJECT

At the culmination of the DCE, you have performed a needs assessment, fine-tuned the focus for your capstone project, and documented the process and findings that resulted from your work. After completing the final papers and receiving a passing grade for the DCE and project, it may be tempting to avoid or indefinitely postpone dissemination of scholarly works. At this stage, it is important for you to recognize the expertise you have gained by undergoing a unique experience in the field of occupational therapy. Your DCE results in you gaining unique insight into the workings of an organization, understanding the needs of a specific population of clients, and recognizing issues pertaining to occupational justice, evidence-based practice, and effective policy. You identify gaps in health care that occupational therapy practitioners can address. Without dissemination of scholarly works, other clinicians cannot learn from this expertise. Clients outside of an individual capstone site cannot benefit from the treatment planning and service models you have created. Organizations cannot acquire knowledge about the widespread roles of occupational therapy practitioners and the impact they can have. Upon completion of the capstone experience, you are equipped with insights and new knowledge that others can benefit from. It is an ideal time to disseminate your scholarly work.

DISSEMINATION PLANNING

The main goal of dissemination is to share with others the knowledge, information, or results that you have gathered or produced with your project. It is important first to understand knowledge translation as a paradigm to close the gaps that exist between your findings and the implementation of those findings to change practice. The World Health Organization and Pan-American Health Organization define *knowledge translation* as "the synthesis, exchange, and application of knowledge by relevant stakeholders to accelerate the benefits of global and local innovation in strengthening health systems and improving people's health" (Pan American Health Organization, 2024, n.p.). There are many knowledge translation models or frameworks that one can adopt when initially preparing for a dissemination plan to ensure application of the project results into practice. When developing a dissemination plan, it is important to be strategic with the overall approach to ensure that your project results will be utilized. For the capstone project dissemination plan, you will want to write several objectives outlining the following information:

- The information or message that will be disseminated
- The audience or to whom the message will be delivered
- The methods that will be used to disseminate the information
- The resources that will be used and who will deliver or disseminate the information
- Timing (timeline) of dissemination

When starting to develop a plan and writing objectives, it is helpful to consider overall steps in developing a dissemination strategy. See Table 11.2 for steps in developing a dissemination strategy.

Table 11-2. Steps in Developing a Dissemination Strategy

- Devise dissemination objectives.
- Determine audience.
- Develop messages.
- Decide on dissemination approaches and methods.
- Review available resources.
- Consider timing and window of opportunities.
- Evaluate efforts.

Step 1: Devise Dissemination Objectives

When considering objectives, it is helpful to identify what you hope to achieve by delivering the results of the doctoral capstone project. When writing objectives, consider why you wish to communicate findings to particular stakeholders. Additionally, it is important to consider purpose. Is the purpose of dissemination to increase awareness, understanding, or action? Keep in mind that your project will have multiple stakeholders that will require different ways for disseminating findings and results.

- *Dissemination for awareness* refers to delivering and receiving of a message and is often used for those target audiences that do not need detailed knowledge of your work but it is still important for them to be aware of the outcomes of the project (Harmsworth et al., 2000).
- *Dissemination for understanding* refers to engaging an individual into a process or allowing for those target audiences to build a deeper understanding of your project and results (Harmsworth et al., 2000).
- *Dissemination for action* is the transfer or changing of a process, product, or practice due to the results of the project (Harmsworth et al., 2000). Dissemination for action targets audiences that can influence and bring about change. Clear and easy-to-understand language should be used to articulate your objectives for dissemination. Objectives should identify the message(s) targeted for delivery, to what audience(s) they are intended, who will deliver the messages, and in what time frame.

Step 2: Determine the Audience(s)

Understanding the various stakeholders of the project and, more broadly, the target audience(s) is pertinent in developing your project's dissemination strategy. A *stakeholder* is a group or an individual that is affected or who can affect the achievement of the capstone project, and a *target audience* are the different groups of stakeholders connected to the project (Harmsworth et al., 2000).

Therefore, the need to identify stakeholders as well as target audiences is essential. Keep in mind the various target audiences will perhaps require a different message and delivery (dissemination approach).

Step 3: Develop the Message

In this step, you identify what message(s) you want to disseminate that relate(s) to your findings and tie each to the previously identified targeted audiences. Messages should be clear, with easy-to-understand language (avoid professional jargon) if any of the target audiences are beyond the occupational therapy profession. For example, if your project used an assessment tool that is familiar to the occupational therapy profession to capture individual change, you will want to ensure that audiences beyond occupational therapy can understand the tool's purpose, as well as why it is appropriate to demonstrate change for the project. Therefore, messages should be written solely for one audience, with an identification of a dissemination approach that caters to their needs.

Step 4: Decide on Dissemination Approaches and Methods

Many doctoral capstone projects have multiple stakeholders and target audiences involved within the process of collaboration, development, designing, and implementation. As such, the dissemination of project results and findings can and should be distributed to various communities, stakeholders, and appropriate wider audiences affected by the outcomes of the project. Although there is a plethora of dissemination methods or approaches, it is of utmost importance to select the correct one(s) to get the message to target audience(s) clearly and efficiently and achieve your purpose. Therefore, thinking of the purpose of the dissemination will better assist with identification of appropriate methods. Targeting methods of dissemination is essential because it will guide requirements, tools, and resources needed for dissemination, writing style, and inclusion of pertinent information for the designated stakeholder.

Step 5: Review Available Resources

It is important to consider what resources you have access to for dissemination either from the university level or from the capstone site and who might help assist with dissemination efforts. Resources can include copies of materials or handouts for newsletters, reports, workshops, conference presentations, and support for poster printing or publication fees for journal submission. Additionally, you will want to consider who will assist with dissemination efforts. The capstone team can include the content expert, faculty mentor (or capstone chair), doctoral capstone coordinator, or any other content and site experts who assisted with supervision, mentorship, and feedback of the capstone experience and project. Often, those who are on the team will have varied resources to pull together

to assist with dissemination efforts, so knowing what each person brings to the table will be important in driving the method(s) of dissemination. When writing the dissemination objectives, you will want to include who will be a part of disseminating each objective. Often, this entails discussion of authorship, inclusion and order for publications, and professional conference opportunities. Refer to Chapter 7 for discussion of the importance of an initial authorship agreement determination when developing the experiential plan.

Step 6: Consider Timing and Window of Opportunities

A timeline for disseminating your results to each of the specified targeted audiences should be included in the dissemination plan. Each objective should clearly state the anticipated due date of dissemination. Keep in mind that some dissemination efforts might happen after graduation. When writing the dissemination objectives, include who will assist with each objective and the timeline.

Step 7: Evaluate Efforts

An effective dissemination strategy embodies a constantly developing process. Therefore, it will be critical to review project progress toward the dissemination objectives continuously to ensure success. Keep in mind that during implementation of your doctoral capstone project, adjustments may need to be made to the dissemination plan objectives.

As you contemplate these aforementioned seven steps, Appendix 11.A provides an example framework to formally document a dissemination plan in collaboration with your faculty mentor and context expert.

IMPLEMENTING THE DISSEMINATION PLAN

While implementing the dissemination plan, you need to keep in mind that each stakeholder or target audience might have various expectations that will guide method(s) of delivery. Some of the stakeholders that you will want to build within the dissemination plan are the university, the capstone site, the community, and the occupational therapy profession. Expectations of each of these stakeholders should be understood and verified. Given each stakeholder's expectations or culture, the preferred method of delivery for the capstone results could range from presentation(s), papers or journal articles, briefings, or engagement in community events, each of which requires sound communication and professional preparation.

COMMUNICATION PRINCIPLES

Regardless of the method of delivery chosen, it is critical to ensure that your message is carefully designed to enhance the audience's understanding of the capstone results. The following are recommended principles from the Agency for Healthcare Research and Quality (2014) to enhance communication with various target audiences:

- *Have a clear and factual message.* The message should be clear, be easy to understand, and use language suitable for the target population. For example, if you are disseminating results to a community partner that does not have occupational therapy services, you would want to avoid using professional language that the stakeholder might not fully understand. Additionally, you will want to ensure that the message is correct and realistic.
- *Tailor the message to the receiver.* The message should be targeted to each audience and should deliver what it should know about the results of your doctoral capstone project.
- *The message should invoke action and may be repeated.* The message should create an understanding of action among the audience members and how they can produce that action. For example, if you are disseminating results to a community site to which you brought occupational therapy services, stakeholders at the site should understand how they can act with the presented results in the future. Additionally, you may repeat key messages to the audience to reinforce them.

DETERMINING AND NEGOTIATING AUTHORSHIP

Authorship is a primary means of recognizing your contributions to the project process as well as the collaborators involved. Order of authorship should be discussed from the beginning with the site mentor and university faculty mentor, and the discussion should be ongoing throughout the course of the project, if necessary, as dissemination can be a dynamic process. Once authorship order and responsibilities have been agreed on by all parties, a statement should be placed into the capstone experiential plan delineating the agreed-on terms. Beginning this process early on will ensure that all contributors' expectations are considered. It is important that everyone in the process understand that the order of authorship can change throughout the project to best reflect all collaborators' contributions. Often, authorship order changes are situation-dependent but should be decided on by considering all collaborators' perspectives and their contributions. Revisions to the experiential plan should be updated throughout the process to continuously reflect changes in authorship terms. Keep in mind that order of authorship might vary depending on which method of dissemination is chosen (presentation at a conference vs. a peer-reviewed journal article). Some of your mentors might have more guidance and expertise in a selected method of delivery; therefore, their contributions might increase and warrant authorship order changes. Ongoing and open communication while navigating the authorship process is key to ensuring the dissemination of your capstone project is professional, respectful, and above all, successful.

PRESENTATIONS

Presentations can be a way to promote your doctoral project and its outcomes to various stakeholders. Keep in mind that multiple presentations might be a possibility to ensure that outcomes have been disseminated to the proper stakeholders, such as the academic institution, community and site partners, state associations, and national associations. If you are considering preparing a presentation for a professional conference, whether state, national, or international, it is critical to align the writing of the proposal to the purpose of the conference. You will also want to carefully consider what type of presentation will effectively disseminate results, whether it be poster sessions, short courses, platform presentations, workshops, or another format. When responding to a call for submissions to a particular conference, it is important that you follow the designated criteria set forth by the organization, such as length requirements, number of adequate references, objectives, and abstract materials. Allow for plenty of time before submission for the entire capstone team to review and proofread multiple times to provide feedback for change.

The audience of your presentation(s) will vary, so changing the delivery of content and language depending on the knowledge base of the listener is important. For example, if you are disseminating results to a community board of directors at a collaborating community site, you may need to describe what occupational therapy is before talking about the project outcomes and limit professional language to reduce confusion among the audience. However, you would not need to describe occupational therapy if you were presenting at the AOTA conference because one assumes that those attending the presentation understand the professional language being used.

In preparing for any presentation, practicing is of utmost importance to reinforce that the delivery is robust and the time frame requirements are met. Ensuring that the presentation falls within allotted time constraints and allowing time for questions from the audience are imperative. Planning and preparing answers to questions that may be asked from audience members might reduce anxiety and allow for the best preparation for professional discussion. Portraying a professional image by dressing appropriately in professional attire is critical as you are representing yourself, the dissemination team, the collaborating organization, and the university.

PUBLICATIONS

A comprehensive, well-developed, well-written, and correctly referenced report of the capstone project might be an expectation of your academic program to show that you have met the educational standards of the capstone project. Many students and their collaborators agree that it is well worth the extra time and effort to submit their capstone projects to various journals (either non-peer-reviewed or peer-reviewed, given the nature of the project). Non-peer-reviewed journals often do not have a process in place to ensure accuracy, quality, or rigor of the article; therefore, the publication time and acceptance to the journal might be less. Peer-reviewed or refereed journals use a blinded process of multiple expert reviews to ensure article quality and rigor. An article that has been refereed may be accepted, considered accepted upon recommended revisions, or rejected. If revisions are necessary, keep in mind that it can take significant time to revise; multiple attempts may be necessary to correct the article for acceptance. When targeting a journal, your timeline for dissemination will need to be considered for various reasons.

When considering which journal to submit work, you should keep in mind the type of articles the journal accepts (e.g., program development, research, expert opinion). Additionally, you should consider the target audience to which you would like to disseminate findings; this will help guide you to possible journals. Some journals appropriate for dissemination of your work might not be in the profession of occupational therapy, especially if the project was interdisciplinary in nature. Considering the journal's mission is extremely important, when writing, students should ensure that the project's work aligns with the journal's focus.

Once you identify a journal, you will want to search articles that might be similar in nature to your project that has already been published. Find at least one article comparable to what you intend to submit, and review carefully how the authors structured their writing to organize and configure the submission. Remember that space is limited, so concise writing is of utmost importance. Considering the audience may allow for either cutting information or suggest the need to elaborate on some concepts. For example, if a journal is within the occupational therapy profession, you would not need to define or reference information on the profession's scope of practice, because the audience will have this knowledge base.

Many journals have guidelines on writing document requirements, such as font and style, spacing and margins, headings, length, and preferred style for citations and referencing throughout the paper and for tables and figures. It is the author's responsibility to understand and use the preferred style manual of the targeted journal (e.g., the manuals of the American Psychological Association and the American Medical Association). The style of the targeted journal might be different from the expectations of the university's final paper. If authors fail to submit work within the targeted journal's specifications, they run the risk of immediate rejection.

ADDITIONAL FORMS OF DISSEMINATION

Beyond peer-reviewed publications and formal presentations at conferences, you may disseminate your work through other media. This may include magazine or newspaper articles; online media, such as blogs; or through a conversation on a podcast. Some students have created resource binders and informational booklets that remain within occupational therapy practice settings or that are available online via websites or university publishing services, such as ScholarWorks. Ultimately, the dissemination of the capstone project should be delivered in a way that reaches those who would benefit most from the findings of the doctoral capstone. The tools in this chapter are meant to be used as a guide to make informed decisions about the best dissemination strategy, as each capstone student is unique, as is each doctoral capstone experience and project.

Chapter 12 will go into a bit more detail regarding ways to actually build and structure your final dissemination, which is typically what is used to formally evaluate your capstone project.

STUDENT SECTION CHAPTER SUMMARY

Where do you go from here? How can you leave your legacy with the capstone site? Completion of a DCE and project and dissemination of key findings is an important accomplishment for both the student and the profession of occupational therapy. As discussed earlier in this chapter and in other parts of this book, capstone projects affect clients, families, societies, and health-care professions. In addition, however, capstone experiences greatly influence the doctoral students who have completed them. New, in-depth knowledge will guide the future practice of an occupational therapy student who has completed a doctoral capstone. The mentorship, advocacy, program development, client interactions, and clinical skills built through a capstone experience may guide future clinical reasoning, career choices, and interactions with other clients and professionals. Therefore, it is worth spending time at the completion of a capstone project to reflect on the knowledge that has been gained and disseminated.

- What were the critical components and key findings of the capstone experience?
- How have they influenced you as a future occupational therapy practitioner?
- What impact did they have on the capstone site?
- What are the implications of findings obtained through the capstone project?
- How can they be carried forward?

In considering answers to these questions, you may want to explore ways in which your work can be carried forward. Was a group protocol created that can be implemented by other practitioners when you leave? Were organization changes made, and if so, did you take measures to support the site's ability to maintain these changes? Did your capstone experience result in publications that will influence other practitioners' future clinical work or scholarship? Reflecting on these questions after project completion and dissemination can ensure that the efforts put forth during capstone experiences are sustained and that you take an active role in leaving behind a legacy that is the culmination of your hard work.

Section 2: Educator Focus

Transformational Learning Phases and Framework for the Educator

As this book has revealed, transformational learning theory provides a useful guide for educators to stimulate a human-centered design mindset for students, including after the doctoral capstone experience and project are complete. As students enter the dissemination component of the doctoral capstone, they lean into Mezirow's final stage of transformational learning theory, reintegration (Mezirow, 1997). Transformational learning theory is useful in this context because it has been shown to contribute to the development and implementation of educational methods, including both learning activities and assessments of learning, that are sustainable (Rodríguez et al., 2020). Lived experiences, social learning, and competencies to ensure sustainability are critical aspects of transformational learning.

Human-centered design places the student at the core of the learning process, requiring educators to become keenly aware of students' needs, experiences, strengths, and limitations to facilitate learning that solves problems and produces results that are important to the student and their DCE.

As students evaluate and disseminate their project outcomes, integration happens as the students synthesize the knowledge gained and grow in their beliefs and transform as they transition from student to practitioner.

The following sections will provide suggestions for engaging capstone students in transformational learning, capitalizing on the key aspects of these two theoretical frameworks. At the center of both frameworks is an emphasis on the people involved (students, educators, others), their connection, and their ability to solve problems and achieve goals in unique and context- and person-specific ways.

INTRODUCTION FOR EDUCATOR

As described earlier, facilitating transformational learning involves partnership between educators and learners. This section of the chapter outlines some suggestions and tools to help facilitate this partnership. As with any partnership, consideration of the strengths and limitations of all partners can serve the team in creating a plan and strategies that align with all involved. Magolda and King (2023) describe three principles to ground educators as partners in students' learning: (1) validating learners' capacity as knowledge constructors; (2) situating learning in learners' experience; and (3) defining learning as mutually constructing meaning. Occupational therapy doctoral capstone experiences provide a unique opportunity in which the profession and its future leaders can pave the way for occupational therapy practice. In order to do that, as educators, we must enable our learners to see their own potential for changing health-care knowledge and practice by recognizing and drawing out their unique skills and perspectives, and by ensuring they are active participants in the construction of meaning through their doctoral capstone experience and project engagement.

EDUCATOR REFLECTIVE QUESTIONS

During the dissemination phase of the capstone, educators may find it helpful to reflect on the following questions:

1. What are your strengths and limitations as an educator?
2. How have you disseminated your own work? What types of dissemination have you observed from others in your field? Were they effective? Why or why not?
3. What have you accomplished/achieved in your educator role that may be useful to students?
4. What resources are you familiar with or do you have access to?
5. What do you need to learn/know about this student and their doctoral capstone to facilitate attainment of student objectives?

EDUCATOR OBJECTIVES

By the end of reading this chapter, the educator will be able to apply principles of transformational learning theory to structure learning activities, assignments, and/or assessments in order to promote the capstone student's ability to:

1. Compare and contrast the types of project dissemination methods.
2. Understand the purpose and process of professional writing in the field of occupational therapy.

3. Explain recommendations for components of a written capstone dissemination.
4. Explain recommendations for the components of oral capstone dissemination.
5. Identify additional formats for capstone project dissemination.

STUDENT OBJECTIVE 1: COMPARE AND CONTRAST TYPES OF PROJECT DISSEMINATION METHODS

A multitude of dissemination methods are available for students and mentors to consider. Being intentional about selecting dissemination methods at the start of the project can fuel excitement for the project and is a necessary step in the capstone process.

Ideas for Engaging Students With Content

One way that faculty can engage students in selecting dissemination methods is by exposing them to a wide variety of dissemination products. Students may consider reading *OT Practice* magazine articles disseminating capstone projects or review local newspaper articles. Radio and online news stories featuring occupational therapists are listed on the American Occupational Therapy Association website. Students may explore podcasts created by occupational therapists and may even pitch their work to an occupational therapy podcaster as a means of disseminating their DCE.

Student Learning Activities

Capstone coursework may include creating a literature review or annotated bibliography that contains at least five different types of disseminated work. Using the aforementioned suggestions, such learning activities may spark creativity and generate new ideas about how to disseminate the capstone project. In thinking about creative dissemination outlets, some students might even develop new or innovative ideas for how to design their DCE and project.

STUDENT OBJECTIVE 2: UNDERSTAND THE PURPOSE AND PROCESS OF PROFESSIONAL WRITING IN THE FIELD OF OCCUPATIONAL THERAPY

Teaching Tips

It is critical that the faculty mentor provide opportunities for scholarly writing about the capstone project prior to selecting dissemination methods. This will give both the mentor and the student opportunities to reflect upon the student's strengths and limitations, and to identify a dissemination method that is best suited to those strengths.

Student Learning Activities

Students motivated to disseminate their work through scholarly writing may benefit from writing exercises and habitual practices. It can be helpful for students to set aside 20 minutes a day to free-write about their doctoral capstone to keep their minds close to the project and to use free writing as a creative, expressive medium to generate and clarify ideas. This free writing can prove useful when it comes time to complete more structured writing. It can also be helpful for faculty mentors and capstone course instructors to assign small writing activities to help students practice scholarly writing styles. These drafts of literature reviews and methods can give instructors an opportunity to determine the students' professional writing skills and to make suggestions that align with students' writing when it comes to devising a dissemination plan. Some students will be more skilled at creating a resource binder and generating instructive materials to support sustainment of their DCE and project; others will be skilled in explicating theoretical underpinnings of their work and may want to publish conceptual papers or practice magazine articles. Yet others will thrive when using journal manuscript templates to create scholarly articles that disseminate scientific findings. The role of the faculty mentor is to help the student align their dissemination with their personal style and strengths.

STUDENT OBJECTIVE 3: EXPLAIN RECOMMENDATIONS FOR COMPONENTS OF A WRITTEN CAPSTONE DISSEMINATION

Ideas for Engaging Students With Content

To directly engage students with learning content for components of written dissemination of their DCE, it can be helpful for them to identify dissemination products that are similar or related to their DCE. Perhaps a prior *OT Practice* article describes a similar project, or an article in a peer-reviewed journal uses the same measurement tool. By mining existing written materials and reviewing how other authors present their findings, students gain knowledge about different ways they may present their own work.

Student Learning Activities

A learning activity that is both educational and a productive use of time is for students to identify a written dissemination product or venue and create a template for themselves to work from. For example, if a student identifies an article in the *American Journal of Occupational Therapy* that describes a project similar to their own or utilizes similar methods, it may then be a good use of their time to look at author guidelines for that journal and create a word document with each component of the written product, such as subject headings and descriptors for what should be included in each section. It can also be helpful to note how many words are allowed in each section (e.g., abstract: 250 words; paper: 4,000 words). This template will help guide students when trying to write out their DCE for dissemination.

STUDENT OBJECTIVE 4: EXPLAIN RECOMMENDATIONS FOR COMPONENTS OF ORAL CAPSTONE DISSEMINATION

Ideas for Engaging Students With Content

Students may benefit from reviewing AOTA annual conference presentations to spark ideas about how to present at conferences. Listening to other oral presentations can help students determine what is effective and what causes oral presentations to disengage audiences. Students should actively take note of their observations when listening to examples of oral presentations and reflect upon the unique characteristics and styles of presentations they find engaging.

Supplemental Readings

Gray and colleagues (2022) have noted limitations to traditional oral poster presentations.

Oftentimes, presenters are eager to share their research findings in detail, leading to complex, dense posters. Audience members attend poster presentations with the intent of coming away with new ideas and information to incorporate into practice but often feel overwhelmed by the rows of text-saturated displays. These verbose posters, in addition to lengthy "elevator speeches," limit the total number of posters audience members can consume during a session (p. 625).

As an alternative, Gray et al. (2022) describe several innovations for poster designs that can facilitate audience engagement and impact how students embark upon oral poster presentations. By allowing creativity and flexibility when designing oral presentations, capstone students gain freedom in how they present information. They may find that highlighting a particular aspect of the DCE and project might be what's most important for their audience, rather than covering every detail of what was learned.

However, oral dissemination of the capstone project is not limited to conference presentations. As mentioned in a previous section, occupational therapists have shared their work on podcasts and through the creation of creative media, such as films and audio recordings. If students are considering the goals of dissemination and presenting a clear and concise message that is tailored for the intended audience, there are many options for oral dissemination of the capstone project.

STUDENT OBJECTIVE 5: IDENTIFY ADDITIONAL FORMATS FOR CAPSTONE PROJECT DISSEMINATION

One way to support a capstone student's ability to identify alternatives to traditional dissemination pathways is by encouraging them to develop collaborative networks. Sage et al. (2021) define *professional collaboration networks* as "technology-mediated, user-centered relationship constellations designed to enhance connections and professional opportunities" (p. 42). These networks are centered on a specific goal and can assist students and others in communicating information across disciplines to stay current on new scientific information and to connect with diverse others in order to expand social networks. Students may benefit from exploring innovative avenues for developing professional networks to discover opportunities for dissemination they may not have otherwise thought of.

Supplemental Readings

Following are two dissemination products that resulted from interdisciplinary collaboration and social networking. Both occupational therapy doctoral capstone students engaged in dissemination methods that resulted in nationwide interest. Since dissemination, they have received requests to speak to occupational therapy students in universities across the United States and/or have had their work shared in non-traditional venues in multiple languages. Examining these dissemination products may help students expand their thinking about their own potential DCE dissemination.

- Milton, C., & Wasmuth, S. (2021). *Occupational therapy's role in addressing the mental health of Black girls: A community-engaged program implementation project.* ScholarWorks. https://scholarworks. indianapolis.iu.edu/server/api/core/bitstreams/ e30c98be-0134–42bd-b627-b5e312605283/content

- Belkiewitz, J. (2023, March 28). *Stories of our city: Indianapolis & lead [Video].* YouTube. https://www. youtube.com/watch?v=NBtK4J9ihUc

As described earlier, there are numerous ways to disseminate capstone project findings. Students may have a dissemination plan at the start of a project that is not feasible by the end of the project due to unexpected hurdles or changes in how the project is implemented. The Consolidated Framework for Implementation Research (CFIR) website provides a wealth of information on how to describe implementation facilitators and barriers and can be a helpful way to think about dissemination when a student is unable to collect or measure variables they originally anticipated.

ASSESSING THE DISSEMINATION PLAN

Table 11.2 listed seven steps to creating a dissemination plan: (1) Devise dissemination objectives, (2) determine audience, (3) develop messages, (4) decide on dissemination approaches and methods, (5) review available resources, (6) consider timing and window of opportunities, and (7) evaluate efforts. Appendix 11.A can be used as an example assignment to draft and grade a student's dissemination plan. The following questions can assist the educator in assessing the student's dissemination plan and can be rated on a 4-point scale: 1 (not at all), 2 (somewhat), 3 (mostly), or 4 (completely). Ratings can aid in conversations between the student and educator to improve the dissemination plan along the DCE journey as needed.

1. Are the student's dissemination objectives clear? Is it evident whether they are disseminating for understanding, awareness, action, or a combination of these?

2. Is the audience appropriate, and does the capstone student have the means to access the proposed audience? Is there a need among the identified audience to receive the information the capstone student intends to disseminate?

3. Is the message evident yet? Has the student identified alternate messages to disseminate if they are unable to devise the message they initially intended? For example, a student may want to share the impact of an education-based innovation on school-age children. However, site-specific factors may limit data collection from children. In this case, the capstone student might have a backup plan to collect survey data from teachers who work directly with the children. Finally, can the message be conveyed in the language appropriate for the identified audience?

4. Does the dissemination method match the conventions of the audience? For example, some hospital settings may expect a 15-minute in-service presentation of findings of a capstone conducted at their site, whereas other settings may not have the time and capacity for such presentations. Another question to consider: Does the planned dissemination method capitalize on the capstone student's strengths, goals, and desires? Is the student a strong writer? A confident presenter? What does the student want to achieve? Does the student have a goal to become a better writer? A published author? These questions

can aid in choosing a dissemination method that is motivating to the student and will facilitate the creation of high-quality dissemination products.

5. What are the strengths of the student's mentors? Is the faculty mentor a published author? Can someone on the mentor team guide the student to successful publication? Does the university have resources to aid the student in printing a poster for presentation? Does the capstone site have a monthly in-service time during which the student could conduct a PowerPoint presentation? Considering these resources can aid in decision-making for feasible dissemination methods.

6. What are the student's plans following graduation? Is communication regarding publication of a journal article after graduation feasible? Are there steps that can be completed prior to project completion, such as editing the capstone paper to meet journal criteria? Is there a mutual desire to complete dissemination by the time of graduation?

7. Have changes occurred that are relevant to the dissemination plan? Does the dissemination plan need to be altered? To what extent are the student and mentors satisfied with and confident about the dissemination plan?

These questions can be evaluated upon completion of an initial dissemination plan and at various points throughout the capstone journey, such as when unexpected changes occur or when a student or mentor experiences doubt about the existing plan and sees a need for change.

Table 11.3 provides an exemplar rubric to assess student performance in creating a dissemination plan.

EDUCATOR CHAPTER SUMMARY

Where do you go from here? As an educator, embarking on student capstone mentorship can feel overwhelming. Some key points to remember are that knowledge is co-constructed. You are a co-collaborator and a guide for students, facilitating their journey and their knowledge dissemination by connecting them to resources and opportunities and by helping them see and develop their own strengths. The occupational therapy doctoral capstone is an opportunity to advance the discovery of knowledge and the field of occupational therapy as whole, one project at a time. It is critical to bring faculty skills and knowledge to aid students in disseminating their important work for the betterment of our profession and those we serve.

Table 11-3. Rubric for Assessing Dissemination Plan

ASSESSMENT QUESTIONS	4	3	2	1
Devise dissemination objectives.				
1. Are the student's dissemination objectives clear?				
2. Is it evident whether they are disseminating for understanding, awareness, action, or a combination of these?				
Determine audience.				
1. Is the audience appropriate, and does the capstone student have the means to access the proposed audience?				
2. Is there a need among the identified audience to receive the information the capstone student intends to disseminate?				
Develop messages.				
1. Is the message evident yet?				
2. Has the student identified alternate messages to disseminate if they are unable to devise the message they initially intended?				
3. Can the message be conveyed in the language appropriate for the identified audience?				
Decide on dissemination approaches and methods.				
1. Does the dissemination method match the conventions of the audience?				
2. Does the planned dissemination method capitalize on the capstone student's strengths, goals, and desires?				
Review available resources.				
1. Can someone on the mentor team guide the student to successful publication?				
2. Does the university have resources to aid the student in printing a poster for presentation?				
3. Does the capstone site have a monthly in-service time during which the student could conduct a PowerPoint presentation?				
Consider timing and window of opportunities.				
1. Is communication regarding publication of a journal article after graduation feasible?				
2. Are there steps that can be completed prior to project completion, such as editing the capstone paper to meet journal criteria?				
3. Is there a mutual desire to complete dissemination by the time of graduation?				
Evaluate efforts.				
1. Have changes occurred that are relevant to the dissemination plan?				
2. Does the dissemination plan need to be altered?				
3. To what extent are the student and mentors satisfied with and confident about the dissemination plan?				

REFERENCES

Agency for Healthcare Research & Quality. (2014). *Quick-start guide to dissemination for practice-based research networks.* https://pbrn.ahrq.gov/sites/default/files/AHRQ%20PBRN%Dissemination%20QuickStart%20Guide_0.pdf

American Occupational Therapy Association. (2018). *Vision 2025.* https://www.aota.org/Publications-News/AOTANews/2018/AOTA-Board-Expands-Vision–2025.aspx

Bailliard, A. L., Dallman, A. R., Carroll, A., Lee, B. D., & Szendrey, S. (2020). Doing occupational justice: A central dimension of everyday occupational therapy practice. *Canadian Journal of Occupational Therapy, 87*(2), 144–152. https://doi.org/10.1177/0008417419898930

Bekmuratova, S., Bagby, L., Domina, A., Patterson, A., & Mu, K. (2022). The impact of international doctoral capstone experience on occupational therapy clinicians' current practice. *Journal of Occupational Therapy Education, 6*(2). https://doi.org/10.26681/jote.2022.060218

Belkiewitz, J. (2023). *Knowledge, confidence, & competence: Utilizing personal narrative as a pedagogical tool for educating professional healthcare students about local lead involvement* [Doctoral dissertation, Indiana University Indianapolis]. Scholarworks.

Belkiewitz, J., & Wasmuth, S. (2025). Personal narrative as pedagogy: A model for socially responsive narrative-based education in occupational therapy. *The Open Journal of Occupational Therapy, 13*(2), 1–17. https://doi.org/10.15453/2168-6408.2302

Gibbons, M. (2024). *Exploring occupational therapy's role in optimizing positive sensory experiences in the neonatal intensive care unit (NICU).* ScholarWorks. https://scholarworks.indianapolis.iu.edu/items/ef1e6d79-4601-45d4-bc1b-0716ebd1abc7

Gray, A. L., Curtis, C. W., Young, M. R., & Bryson, K. K. (2022). Innovative poster designs: A shift toward visual representation of data. *American Journal of Health-System Pharmacy, 79*(8), 625–628. https://doi.org/10.1093/ajhp/zxac002

Harmsworth, S., Turpin, S., Rees, A., & Pell, G. (2000). *Creating an effective dissemination strategy: An expanded interactive workbook for educational development projects.* Higher Education Funding Council for England (HEFCE).

Hogue, A., Schumm, J. A., MacLean, A., & Bobek, M. (2022). Couple and family therapy for substance use disorders: Evidence-based update 2010–2019. *Journal of Marital and Family Therapy, 48*(1), 178–203. https://doi.org/10.1111/jmft.12546

Jordan, A., Quainoo, S., Nich, C., Babuscio, T. A., Funaro, M. C., & Carroll, K. M. (2022). Racial and ethnic differences in alcohol, cannabis, and illicit substance use treatment: A systematic review and narrative synthesis of studies done in the USA. *The Lancet Psychiatry, 9*(8), 660–675. https://doi.org/10.1016/S2215-0366(22)00160-2

Koller, E. C., Abel, R. A., & Milton, L. E. (2022). Caring for the caregiver: A feasibility study of an online program that addresses compassion fatigue, burnout, and secondary trauma. *The Open Journal of Occupational Therapy, 10*(1), 1–14. https://doi.org/10.15453/2168–6408.1847

Kwon, J. H., & Hong, G. R. S. (2021). Influence of self-care on burnout in primary family caregiver of person with dementia. *Journal of Korean Academy of Nursing, 51*(2), 217–231. https://doi.org/10.4040/jkan.20274

Levin, M. E., Luoma, J. B., Lillis, J., Hayes, S. C., & Vilardaga, R. (2014). The acceptance and action questionnaire–stigma (AAQ-S): Developing a measure of psychological flexibility with stigmatizing thoughts. *Journal of Contextual Behavioral Science, 3*(1), 21–26. https://doi.org/10.1016/j.jcbs.2013.11.003

Magolda, M., & King, P. (2023). *Learning partnerships: Theory and models of practice to educate for self-authorship.* Routledge.

Mezirow, J. (1997). Transformative learning: Theory to practice. *New Directions for Adult and Continuing Education,* (74), 5–12. https://doi.org/10.1002/ace.7401

Pan American Health Organization. (2024). *Knowledge translation and evidence.* https://www.paho.org/en/evidence-and-intelligence-action-health/knowledge-translation-and-evidence.

Ricou, B., Gigon, F., Durand-Steiner, E., Liesenberg, M., Chemin-Renais, C., Merlani, P., & Delaloye, S. (2020). Initiative for burnout of ICU caregivers: Feasibility and preliminary results of a psychological support. *Journal of Intensive Care Medicine, 35*(6), 562–569. https://doi.org/10.1177/0885066618768223

Rodríguez Aboytes, J. G., & Barth, M. (2020). Transformative learning in the field of sustainability: A systematic literature review (1999–2019). *International Journal of Sustainability in Higher Education, 21*(5), 993–1013. https://doi.org/10.1108/IJSHE-05-2019-0168

Sage, M., Hitchcock, L. I., Bakk, L., Young, J., Michaeli, D., Jones, A. S., & Smyth, N. J. (2021). Professional collaboration networks as a social work research practice innovation: Preparing DSW students for knowledge dissemination roles in a digital society. *Research on Social Work Practice, 31*(1), 42–52. https://doi.org/10.1177/1049731520961163

Schrader, K. (2024). *Development of an occupational therapy health promotion group protocol in a gender diverse population.* ScholarWorks. https://scholarworks.indianapolis.iu.edu/items/e188b1cd-6b86–45bb-a003–53bc440b18f8

Stellern, J., Xiao, K. B., Grennell, E., Sanches, M., Gowin, J. L., & Sloan, M. E. (2023). Emotion regulation in substance use disorders: A systematic review and meta-analysis. *Addiction, 118*(1), 30–47. https://doi.org/10.1111/add.16001

Steptoe, A., & Fancourt, D. (2020). An outcome-wide analysis of bidirectional associations between changes in meaningfulness of life and health, emotional, behavioural, and social factors. *Scientific Reports, 10*(1), 6463. https://doi.org/10.1038/s41598-020-63600-9

Vigdal, M. I., Moltu, C., Bjornestad, J., & Selseng, L. B. (2022). Social recovery in substance use disorder: A metasynthesis of qualitative studies. *Drug and Alcohol Review, 41*(4), 974–987. https://doi.org/10.1111/dar.13434

Wasmuth, S., Leonhardt, B., Pritchard, K., Li, C. Y., DeRolf, A., & Mahaffey, L. (2021). Supporting occupational justice for transgender and gender-nonconforming people through narrative-informed theater: A mixed-methods feasibility study. *The American Journal of Occupational Therapy, 75*(4). https://doi.org/10.5014/ajot.2021.045161

Wasmuth, S., Pritchard, K. T., & Belkiewitz, J. (2023). Bridging the humanities and health care with theatre: Theory and outcomes of a theatre-based model for enhancing psychiatric care via stigma reduction. *Psychiatric Rehabilitation Journal, 46*(4), 285–292. https://doi.org/10.1037/prj0000551

APPENDICES

Appendix 11.A Occupational Therapy Doctorate Capstone Dissemination Plan

OCCUPATIONAL THERAPY

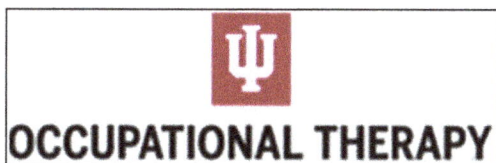

OCCUPATIONAL THERAPY DOCTORATE CAPSTONE DISSEMINATION PLAN

OTD STUDENT NAME:

_____

_____

FACULTY CAPSTONE CHAIR:

_____

_____

PRIORITY	DISSEMINATION APPROACH	INTENDED AUDIENCE	KEY MESSAGE	TIMING CONSIDERATIONS	CRITICAL PROS OR CONS
1					
2					
3					
4					
5					
Statement of Authorship: [Intentionally discuss authorship with your faculty chair. Briefly document an initial plan about authorship. A person should be recognized as an author when they have made a considerable contribution to the product.					
Statement of Ownership: [Document an initial plan about ownership. If you are creating materials (i.e., handouts, protocols, modules, manuals, etc.), consider how you are discussing this ownership with your capstone chair, site mentor, or others.]					
Self-Reflection: [Review your dissemination plan and write a brief reflection on your perceived confidence in meeting this plan.]					

CHAPTER 12

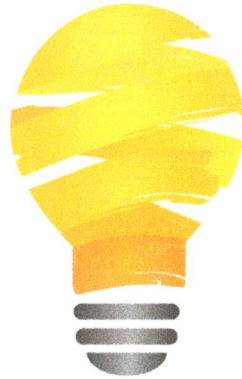

Evaluation of the Capstone Project and Dissemination Methods

Ann B. Cook and Michelle McCann

Section 1: Student Focus

Human-Centered Design Mindsets for the Doctoral Students

The mindsets of iterate, iterate, iterate and creative confidence are important as you, the capstone student, work toward your final dissemination product, whether it be a written paper, poster, webinar, or other form of dissemination. These products take on different characteristics depending on the student, the area of focus for the capstone, and your program's requirements. You will be creating some type of summative product that meets set program requirements and Accreditation Council for Occupational Therapy Education (ACOTE) standards. By being able to express your creative confidence and how multiple iterations lead to a completed project, you pave the way for other occupational therapy students and practitioners interested in taking on a human-centered design mindset.

Iterate, iterate, iterate. This will be the time to express and document how iterations of your project took shape and, ultimately, how you solved a problem and you provided a meaningful and mutually beneficial solution. You will explain how, by refining each iteration of your capstone project, learning occurred and ideas advanced. Continuous iterations may be initially frustrating, but during the creation of the final capstone dissemination product, it allows you to reflect on the iterations that ultimately led to the success of the project.

Creative confidence. You can better understand your client by being creative and documenting how this creativity led to a solution for the client. By this stage in the capstone experience and project, you will have built creative confidence within yourself; now it is time to utilize this confidence to create a superior final capstone dissemination product!

DOI: 10.4324/9781003541813-16

- 275 -

INTRODUCTION FOR STUDENTS

As learned throughout this book, the doctoral capstone is composed of a culminating experience and a comprehensive project that integrates knowledge and skills acquired within the occupational therapy doctoral curriculum. The capstone project is a high-stake learning activity that allows you to showcase critical thinking, problem-solving, and collaboration skills. This "showcase" occurs through dissemination, meaning a process of sharing your findings. As covered in Chapter 11, your "findings" may have different levels of impact, and the end result of the capstone project can take many forms, such as a final written capstone report, presentation, portfolio, or other types of publications. However, it is important to identify that a final written capstone report is not the same as a doctoral dissertation. This chapter provides an overview of suggestions on professional writing and formatting a range of dissemination products, such as capstone reports, posters, asynchronous or synchronous learning products, and formal presentations to a variety of professional and interprofessional audiences along with specific suggestions for you, the capstone student.

STUDENT REFLECTIVE QUESTIONS

When planning the dissemination of the doctoral capstone project, you may find it helpful to reflect on the following questions:

1. How do I measure my professional writing abilities and skills? How do I measure my oral presentation skills?

2. What resources are available to me through my academic institution and program to assist in my scholarly writing and/or presentation abilities?

3. What are my program's requirements for disseminating my capstone?

4. What literature in the occupational therapy profession can support scholarly writing (e.g., journal articles, position papers, evidence-based practice protocols), and how can I use them as inspirations to structure my own work?

STUDENT OBJECTIVES

By the end of reading this chapter and completing the learning activities, you will be able to:

1. Compare and contrast different types of capstone project dissemination methods.

2. Understand the purpose and process of professional writing in the field of occupational therapy.

3. Explain recommendations for components of a written capstone dissemination.

4. Describe recommendations for components of an oral capstone dissemination.

5. Identify additional formats for capstone project dissemination.

COMPARING AND CONTRASTING A DOCTORAL DISSERTATION AND A DOCTORAL CAPSTONE PROJECT

There are several differences between a doctoral dissertation and a doctoral capstone project. Both require significant scholarly effort, but they differ in their process, outcomes, and intended audiences. First, the focus of a doctoral dissertation differs from that of a capstone project. A dissertation applies action research methodology to specific situations to generate localized solutions to problems that must then be supported through a review of the literature (Herr & Anderson, 2015). The dissertation is the author's original contribution to the existing literature and theory in a particular field and is intended to fill the gap in literature while addressing a research problem (Herr & Anderson, 2015). The individual completing a dissertation is expected to create new evidence by conducting formal and rigorous research.

The dissertation process typically involves several steps. First, a problem needs to be identified, which leads the author to formulate one or more research questions. Next, a review of the existing literature should be completed to determine whether an answer to the question(s) already exists. If the review reveals a gap in the existing literature – that is, the research question cannot be answered by the existing literature – appropriate methodology should be determined to go about answering the question. From there, research should be conducted, including detailed analysis of data. Finally, the results should be disseminated, thus adding to the existing literature and filling the previous gap regarding the identified problem. Unlike a thesis or dissertation dissemination, which is focused mainly on an academic audience, a capstone dissemination may include a range of key stakeholders, such as faculty, peers, and site/organization staff.

Your doctoral capstone project is meant to have a direct impact on a real-world, practice problem that may extend or apply existing research. A capstone project involves application of best evidence, as it exists in current literature, to occupational therapy practice. In addition, a doctoral capstone project connects existing theory to practice application during the experience. Unlike a dissertation, the intended audience for a capstone is typically faculty, peers, and relevant stakeholders.

The capstone project not only expands your knowledge but also informs occupational therapy practice within your chosen focus area through scholarly inquiry and critical analysis. The capstone project can be viewed as a culminating project where you demonstrate synthesis and application of knowledge gained during the focused area

Table 12-1. Steps of Completing a Capstone Project

Step 1: Identify a real-world practice problem to address through the capstone project process. This problem can be identified through the completion of a needs assessment (ACOTE, 2023 Standard D.1.3).

Step 2: Complete an in-depth review of the current literature regarding the problem and identifying solutions to the problem evidenced in the literature. Reviewing existing literature ensures not only that the solution is evidence-based but also that the solution has proved to be successful in practice. You may find that there exists a gap in the literature regarding the particular practice problem, and therefore, the capstone project may intend to fill a gap by finding solutions to the problem identified.

Step 3: Apply evidence-based, practical strategies to find solutions to the specific problem encountered in practice and identified through the needs assessment. This is the "implementation phase" of the capstone project.

Step 4: Contribute to individual, organizational, institutional, or societal change. The capstone project should be something that not only advances your skills in a particular focus area (refer to Chapter 2 for more information on the focus areas) but also benefit the site or community and participants. The benefits of the capstone project should not end when the project is finished. ACOTE (2023) standard D.1.6 states that the dissemination of the capstone should demonstrate synthesis of knowledge in the focused area of study. In addition, the student should share any knowledge gained and pertinent information needed for the site or community to continue to carry out the project. The capstone project could be disseminated in various formats, such as a written report, a manuscript, an evidence-based practice protocol, or a handbook (see Table 12.3 for examples of various formats). In addition, products created as part of your capstone project should continue to be used at the site or in the community (e.g., patient or staff training materials, webinars, outcome measurements).

Step 5: Communicate the outcomes of your capstone project with key stakeholders and staff at the site or community organization impacted by the project, including any accompanying artifacts or deliverables. Information related to the overall process and, specifically, the results of your capstone project should be shared with the site or organization for continued benefits to be sustained after your project is complete. This could be completed through a presentation at a regularly scheduled staff meeting, or in-service through small group meetings with key stakeholders involved in or impacted by your project, or even virtually through a live webinar. It is important that the outcomes of your project are clearly communicated and that individuals at the site or organization can ask you questions to ensure the results of your project are understood. All necessary information for follow-through or continuation of your capstone project should be provided so that the site can continue to utilize this information after your project is completed. (Strategies on sustainability of the capstone were discussed in Chapter 8.)

Step 6: Disseminate the outcomes of your capstone project (ACOTE standard D.1.7). The capstone project process, including identification of the practice problem, the review of the literature, and the method of addressing the problem, data analysis, and impact, is to be disseminated and appropriate for publication or scholarly presentation (ACOTE, 2023). The requirement for dissemination ensures that you are contributing to existing information surrounding your chosen practice area as well as the knowledge of the occupational therapy community of practice. Dissemination could be completed in the form of a professional poster or platform session at the local, national, or international level and/or a written publication for a trade periodical, or maybe even a peer-reviewed journal, depending on the nature of your capstone project. Refer back to Chapter 11 for more suggestions to discuss and create a dissemination plan among your capstone team.

of study through the capstone experience (ACOTE, 2023). Similar to a dissertation, there is a process to complete a capstone project. See Table 12.1 for the suggested steps of completing a capstone project.

OVERVIEW OF PROFESSIONAL DISSEMINATION

As some level of writing is usually involved in any dissemination method, developing strong professional writing skills is essential as an occupational therapy doctoral student. The following section will provide recommendations and strategies to ensure success as you enter the dissemination phase of your doctoral capstone.

Professional Writing

Writing is an occupation that you will complete regularly as an occupational therapy practitioner. Regardless of practice setting, documentation or writing of some form must take place. The types of writing you will complete could include progress notes, evaluation reports, and other writing tasks, such as annual performance appraisals, strategic plans, or a patient education home program. As a future occupational therapist, you will need to be able to write for varying audiences and use an other-centered philosophy. Regardless of the writing task, the occupation of writing requires the development and implementation of key skills to effectively communicate. Whether your capstone dissemination takes the form of a written report, an evidence-based practice guideline, a manuscript, or some other scholarly form, you are required to communicate outcomes of your project in an organized, accurate, and concise manner with your readers in mind.

Along with other behavioral and social sciences, the occupational therapy profession uses the style of writing and formatting published by the American Psychological Association (APA). The *Publication Manual of the American Psychological Association* (7th ed.) provides guidelines for concise scientific writing with information regarding the use of punctuation and abbreviations, construction of tables, selection of headings, formatting of references, and presentation of statistics (APA, 2020). The APA manual may even be a required textbook in your program. It is highly recommended that you use APA style and the available resources through the APA when creating any written scholarly product, whether it be a manuscript for a professional journal, a conference proposal submission, or a presentation to disseminate information.

You should become familiar with the support and resources offered at your academic institution (both on campus and online). Your institution may have a writing center that assists students with APA formatting and grammar. The APA (2020) manual is a helpful resource to obtain (such as a personal copy) or use if available through the university library. There are also many online resources to assist with your writing process, as noted in Text Box 12.1. In addition, discussions regarding authorship of your final dissemination products should occur early on and then periodically throughout your capstone planning process.

TEXT BOX 12-1

Online formatting resources such as Purdue Online Writing Lab (OWL; The Purdue OWL, 2024) and reference generators such as Endnote, Zotera, and Mendeley can be resources to help you search the literature and organize the relevant literature that you find. This includes managing bibliographies, citations, and references. If you happen to be completing your doctoral capstone at a site that is not near your academic institution, you should explore whether or not your institution provides online or virtual writing support. With reference generators, be sure to explore various options and choose one that aligns with APA formatting and also helps you stay organized!

Tips for Scholarly Writing

Scientific writing is a particular style of scholarly writing with which occupational therapy students and practitioners effectively communicate information regarding practice. It is the style of writing that is recommended when writing your doctoral capstone report, a proposal submission for presentation at a conference, or a manuscript for publication. According to DeIuliis (2017), the goal of scholarly writing is to communicate information clearly, concisely, and accurately. It is not typically used to share one's opinions or beliefs but to convey facts and data. The following are tips for using scholarly writing for the final capstone product.

- *Consider the purpose of writing and your intended audience.* The purpose of your capstone product is to describe your capstone project, how it was conducted, and its results. The outcomes of your capstone project are meant to be disseminated and shared not only with the key stakeholders at the site where your project is completed but also within the profession as well. The language used to disseminate the results of your project should reflect the language of the profession, but any occupational therapy jargon should be explained, and abbreviations (e.g., ADL) should be expanded on first use.

- *Use proper grammar.* Scientific writing avoids the use of the first person (e.g., "I," "we") and is more formal than conversational grammar (Hofmann, 2017). You need to carefully choose vocabulary that reflects the specific message that you wish to communicate. Avoid the use of slang. For example, "When the client struggled, I encouraged him to hang in there." The pronoun "I" should be replaced with a noun, and the phrase "hang in there" is informal grammar, or slang. Instead, consider "When the client struggled, the capstone student encouraged the client to do their best work."

- *Write in the past tense.* Dissemination occurs after your capstone project and experience has ended; therefore, in most cases, past tense should be used throughout your report, manuscript, webinar, manual, or other form of dissemination product. Present tense is to be used for general rules and accepted facts (Hofmann, 2017). For example, when writing the results or outcomes section of your capstone report, you might write, "Following the training program, staff knowledge increased by 70%." However, in the theory section or conceptual model section of the capstone product, you may write, "The model of human occupation seeks to explain how occupation is motivated, patterned, and performed."

- *Write with active verbs* (Hofmann, 2017). Instead of using abstract nouns, use verbs to energize your writing. For example, "The client's home program was to be completed 3 days per week" uses abstract nouns. Instead, "The client was instructed to complete the home program three days per week" uses an active verb. The former is passive, whereas the latter captures the reader's attention.

- *Focus on novel ideas.* One possible outcome of the doctoral capstone is to contribute to the existing literature of the profession. Completing a thorough literature review will ensure that your project is not replicating something that has already been done or is already addressed in the literature. The outcomes of the doctoral project are intended to be useful for the site but also to provide professional clinical utility. The literature should be cited and referenced as appropriate.

- *Be concise and objective.* Scientific writing avoids the subjective, and therefore, you must avoid inserting your opinions and assumptions into your writing. Focusing on observations, facts, and data will help you write objectively and avoid bias. Scientific writing also needs to be concise and to the point. You should avoid using too many adjectives and unnecessary descriptors. For example, instead of writing, "The capstone student implemented an exciting, new program at the summer camp, and the children seemed to love it!" consider "The capstone student implemented an evidence-based sensory integration program at the summer camp across a six-week period. The children appeared to enjoy it based on their interaction level and facial expressions, and the data confirm that their quality of life improved." The latter provides a much clearer picture and includes objective data.

- *Provide evidence to support claims.* Along with being objective, you need to provide evidence regarding the outcomes of your project. Outcomes data can be qualitative and/or quantitative in nature and should clearly articulate the outcomes of the capstone project.

- *Give credit where credit is due.* It is important to give credit to any secondary authors and significant contributors to the scholarly work. The order of authorship is based on the contribution of that author (with the primary author listed first, having done the majority of the work). Additionally, individuals who have made a significant contribution to your capstone project should be recognized. This may be done by including an "Acknowledgments" section toward the beginning of the written scholarly work (before the body). (See Text Box 12.2 for an example.)

TEXT BOX 12-2

According to the APA (2020):
An author is considered anyone involved with initial research design, data collection and analysis, manuscript drafting, and final approval. . . . The primary author assumes responsibility for the publication,

---

TEXT BOX 12-2 (CONTINUED)

making sure that the data are accurate, that all deserving authors have been credited, that all authors have given their approval to the final draft; and handles responses to inquiries after the manuscript is published.
(n.p.)

Determining proper authorship is a critical step since it indicates not only who contributed to the scholarly product(s) but also who is responsible for the outcomes of the capstone project and dissemination. Disclosure of and conflicts of interest or financial affiliations associated with a project are equally connected to authorship.

Example: Sarah S. Spielson, a capstone student, created a sensory room for children in a local day care and preschool facility. She measured the outcomes of the use of the sensory room on the children's behaviors. Sarah, being the capstone student, conducted the needs assessment, did the literature review, and self-directed the project with the guidance of her content expert, Karen J. Randolph (lead teacher), and another mentor at the site, Stephen R. Carson (support staff), who often provided guidance during her time on-site. She also received support from her faculty mentor Dr. Jennifer L. Amberger and, on a couple of occasions, received advice from an expert occupational therapist in sensory integration, Lindsay T. Cooper. When completing her final capstone dissemination product, a manuscript on best practices for sensory integration using a sensory room in a childcare facility, she needed to determine authorship.

Sarah based the order of the authors of the manuscript on the overall contribution of each person to her capstone. She also discussed this order with the team, and all were in agreement. The order of authorship was as follows: Sarah S. Spielman, Karen J. Randolph, Stephen R. Carson, and Jennifer L. Amberger.

Sarah also provided an acknowledgment to Lindsay T. Cooper in a separate section to thank her for her contribution to the project. She also used the acknowledgments section to thank her peers who provided encouragement and support throughout the process.

The Role of Artificial Intelligence (AI) in Writing

With the advent of AI and the increasingly endless possibilities for integration in everyday life, including scholarly writing, comes the responsibility of using these large language models (LLMs) transparently (Bowen & Watson, 2024). Being aware of your institutional policies regarding the use of AI in the capstone project is essential. While there are many innovative and creative possibilities for integration within the capstone experience and project, AI literacy is essential to determine acceptable forms of usage from idea formation to AI-assisted writing prompts (Bowen & Watson, 2024). Harnessing the possibilities of AI comes with downsides; specifically, AI is not perfect and is prone to errors, such as biases, inaccuracies, or confabulating information from sources (Mollick & Mollick, 2023). Errors such as confabulation can be hard to detect, but these made-up "facts" are commonly known as "hallucinations" and are often seen in quotes, sources, and statistical information taken out of context (Mollick & Mollick, 2023).

In addition, if you plan to disseminate your capstone through a scholarly peer-reviewed manuscript or other publication, it is pertinent that you consult and abide by any policies enforced by the journal or publisher for incorporating AI. Many journals have author guidelines that should be referenced for this information due to bias risks, such as portraying specific viewpoints or privacy disputes related to ownership of outcomes or data loaded by a student into unrestricted AI platforms (Bowen & Watson, 2024). Prior to dabbling in the use of AI, be sure to consult your course syllabi and individual assignment guidelines, which might deter you from using AI and/or require you to disclose its use. Conference call for abstracts and/or journal publication author guidelines might also stipulate specific disclosure expectations and requirements regarding AI.

The Scholarly Writing Process

Scholarly writing is a process. You should not expect the process to be linear, in that you create the title page and continue writing until the document is finished. Writing a capstone report or other scholarly product involves ongoing steps, such as editing, rewriting, and seeking peer review. In fact, the evolution of your dissemination product might actually span across several semesters within your program. Due to the dynamic nature of a capstone project, you will be continuing to search and incorporate literature throughout the final capstone product, reflecting on feedback you've received and noting any changes made during the implementation of your project. In addition, you should continue to critically evaluate your writing as a scholarly product.

As previously mentioned, using any reputable resources, such as your academic institution's writing center, can help you at any point in the writing process. It is better to receive consultative assistance early on and frequently throughout the writing process than toward the end, as any substantial revisions may take time. Peer review is an important aspect of writing because it allows you to receive feedback from various individuals with a specific skill set and viewpoint. For example, you may have a peer reviewer who has expertise in your chosen focus area to provide feedback on content. Another peer reviewer might have strong writing skills to provide feedback on your scholarly writing. See Figure 12.1 for a schematic of the writing process.

RECOMMENDATIONS FOR THE FORMAT OF THE FINAL CAPSTONE REPORT OR MANUSCRIPT* PUBLICATION

If your program has a requirement for a written final capstone report, the next section provides some recommendations to help you develop an outline or overall

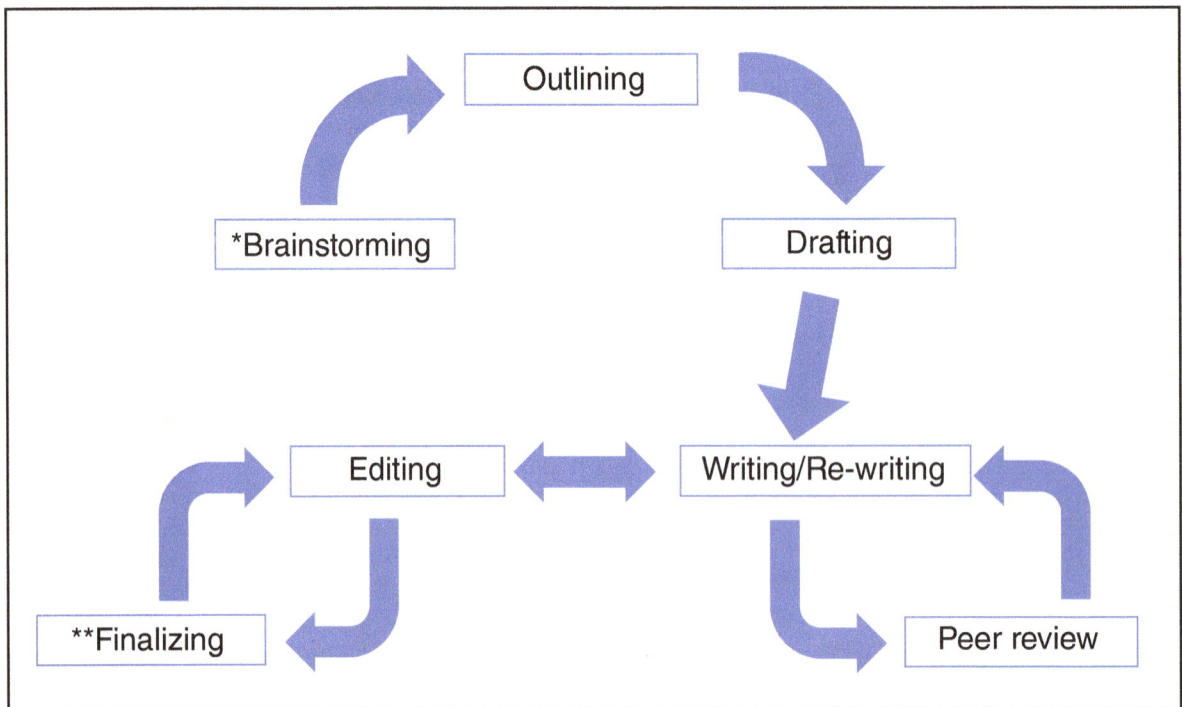

Figure 12-1. Writing as a process.

framework to showcase the process and outcomes of your capstone project. Although not every capstone report will fit neatly into the following headings, these are general suggestions for creating a well-defined, evidence-based, and comprehensive final written capstone report. To help you conceptualize how the components fit together, the headings of the capstone report can be viewed through a lens aligned with the occupational therapy process (American Occupational Therapy Association [AOTA], 2020). (See Figure 12.2.)

*Please note that when preparing a manuscript for publication, the author should consult the author guidelines for the journal to which they intend to submit their draft manuscript.

Title Page

The title of your capstone report gives the reader a clear idea of the subject matter and should be formatted according to APA (2020) guidelines. Next, your name is listed. Then list any contributing authors, such as your content expert and faculty mentor. Do not include their credentials, but do include their affiliations. A running head and page number is included in the header and will be carried throughout the capstone document. Each institution may require different information on the title page, such as the address of the university; you need to follow any guidelines provided by your institution. Refer to Appendix 12.A for an example.

Acknowledgments

The "Acknowledgments" section is unrelated to the capstone content itself but is an important place to recognize individuals who made meaningful contributions to your

capstone project. You may recognize members of your capstone team, including your content expert and any faculty who played an important role in your capstone project, as well as other key stakeholders at your capstone site who provided guidance or feedback on your project. It is also an area where you may want to thank those who supported or inspired you throughout your doctoral program, such as your family, friends, and significant others. A more formal dedication may also be included as a separate section, following the acknowledgments.

Table of Contents

The table of contents clearly outlines the contents of your capstone report with page numbers. The report may be organized by chapters, headings, and subheadings created as needed. You may also include the titles of any tables, figures, and appendices within the table of contents as well. If the list is extensive, each may be listed as a separate section or heading.

Chapter I: Introduction

The introduction captures the reader's attention and provides a context for your capstone report. Information about your capstone site itself is included. Details may include the practice setting, population served (common diagnoses, ages, or number of clients), programs offered, professionals employed, or other information that provides the reader with a mental picture of your capstone site and its operations. You will describe your chosen focus area(s) for your capstone experience and how your site provides a context for your focus area(s). The issue addressed by your capstone project is clearly defined and based in literature, addressing a larger problem of practice;

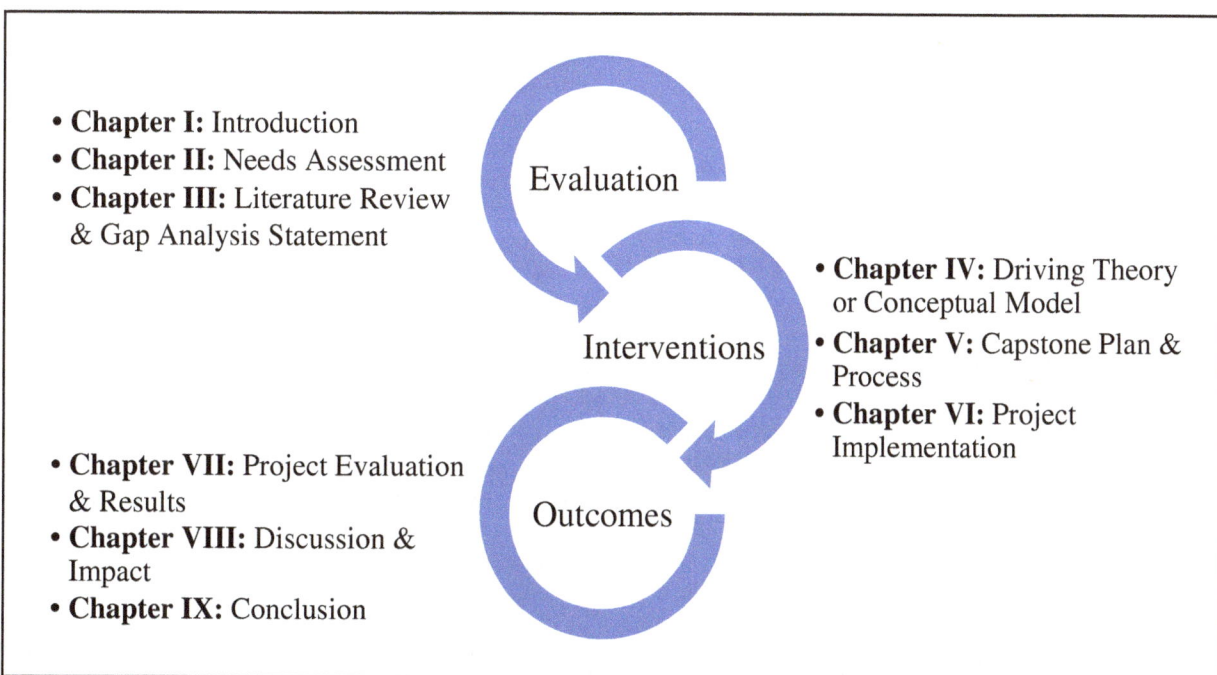

Figure 12-2. The writing process aligned with the OT process.

therefore, rudimentary information related to the issue being addressed is used as a transition to lead into your needs assessment.

Chapter II: Needs Assessment

The purpose of the needs assessment section is to identify the issue, problem at the site, or identification of a population's needs or services needed. To recap what was covered in Chapter 6, the following list provides examples of various purposes for completing a needs assessment:

- To document the existence of an ongoing/exacerbating problem.
- To prioritize the need for services or gaps of services within a community or population of interest.
- To determine whether interventions and other resources to address the identified needs exist in a community, including strengths and weaknesses.
- To determine whether existing interventions are known to or are acceptable to potential clients.
- To examine strengths and limitations of various service delivery models (e.g., medical, educational, community, social) on occupational therapy programming.
- To determine major barriers (e.g., access, environmental, policies, reimbursement) preventing clients from accessing existing services.
- To determine whether there are enough clients with a particular problem to justify creating a new program.
- To obtain information for prioritizing needs for specific targeted and mutually established outcomes for a client population.

As a quick review, see Text Box 12.3 for some prompts that will help you think about areas that you will have already explored during your needs assessment process.

TEXT BOX 12-3

Questions to Consider to Identify Issues

Who are the participants? You will need to consider various possibilities, including the clients themselves, family members or caregivers of clients, and the staff themselves.

What are the common wants and needs of the participants? Informal discussions or interviews with the participants and key stakeholders (e.g., administration at the site) will provide insight into such needs. Asking open-ended questions regarding current needs will encourage participants to freely share their thoughts and opinions. Follow-up, probing questions can then be used to target more specifics about the need. It is important to gain input from more than one participant if possible, to ensure that there is agreement that this is indeed something that is an issue that can and should be addressed. It is essential to consider both personal

---

TEXT BOX 12-3 (CONTINUED)

and cultural values, beliefs, and attitudes regarding health during these discussions.

What are the barriers to achieving these wants and needs? Once the need has been identified, determining why the need has not been addressed will uncover barriers that you will need to overcome. Common barriers include lack of time to address the need, limited resources or staff availability, and/or lack of knowledge on how to best address the need or health disparities. Discussions with participants and key stakeholders are key to determining barriers and why they have not been addressed.

Are there gaps in the service that you could fill to support these needs? There may be several areas of need identified; however, it is important that you determine which area(s) can be realistically addressed as a capstone project. Consider the structure and operations of the site, potential supports and barriers, and your own knowledge and time frame for completion. Your capstone project should address an area that is within the profession's scope of practice, as well as meet the objectives of the capstone itself.

Within a final written capstone report, you do not necessarily just want to copy and paste the "needs assessment assignment" that you completed in one of your preparatory capstone courses; rather, summarize a synopsis of the process and outcomes.

It is important to include details regarding how you conducted the needs assessment in the final capstone product. First, you should share where and when the needs assessment took place. It could have taken place over several days or weeks, and it may have been on-site or virtual. Documentation of meetings with your content expert, administration, staff, and other key stakeholders is included. Also, include the types of questions that were asked, themes that emerged during face-to-face or virtual discussion or interviews, and relevant observations made on-site. Finally, include the outcomes of your needs assessment. Although many needs may be identified, be sure to focus on the need or needs that directly influenced your capstone project and any supports or barriers presented. Include a problem statement to clearly identify the area of need to be addressed by your capstone project.

After completing the needs assessment, a written or verbal proposal should be presented to your capstone site stakeholders for approval. Information regarding this proposal process and any adjustments made to your project from the resultant feedback should be included. (See Table 12.2 for tips for writing a persuasive proposal.)

Chapter III: Literature Review and Gap Analysis Statement

Literature review. As discussed in Chapter 5, when determining whether a particular need at a site should be

Table 12-2. Tips for Writing a Persuasive Paper

MEET A NEED	When performing the needs assessment, keep in mind that the capstone project is other-centered in design and focus. The capstone proposal must meet a need identified by the site stakeholders. It is key that you collaborate with stakeholders during the needs assessment to clearly identify what is needed at the site, as well as the barriers to meeting that need. If you present a proposal for a project that is not needed, site stakeholders will likely reject your proposal. Even so, with any proposal, you should be prepared to alter the details of your proposal based on feedback from the stakeholders.
HAVE INTELLECTUAL MERIT	The capstone proposal needs to be written clearly and be intellectually sound. Robinson et al. (2008) suggest that proposals meet the "3Cs" (p. 371): • *Creativity.* Use innovative ideas to solve the problem at hand. Consider what has already been attempted in the past to solve the problem and why it did not work. • *Credibility.* Proposals should be evidence-based. Cite literature throughout your proposal to support the proposed program components. • *Competence.* You need to highlight your competence and the role of occupational therapy in meeting the need. This is especially important for role-emerging sites.
HAVE A BROADER IMPACT ON SOCIETY	Your capstone project should align with AOTA's Vision 2025, which states that "[a]s an inclusive profession, occupational therapy maximizes health, well-being, and quality of life for all people, populations, and communities through effective solutions that facilitate participation in everyday living" (AOTA, 2018, n.p.).

addressed by a capstone project, you need to complete a thorough literature review. The review of literature may occur at various points before your actual capstone project, such as before visiting your capstone site, during the formal needs assessment on-site, and after the on-site needs assessment has occurred. In addition, it is important that you continue to review the literature during your doctoral capstone experience, because you need to remain current with any new literature being published regarding your capstone topic. It is important to provide a comprehensive, current, and evidence-based review of what information is available regarding the topic and what related research has already been completed.

When reviewing the literature, consider quality sources of information, such as peer-reviewed journal articles and texts. After exhausting all possibilities for information, appraise the literature, and then select only the evidence that is relevant, recent (unless theoretical or foundational in nature), and of high quality (consider the level of evidence, from level I evidence being a randomized controlled trial, to level V evidence being expert opinion).

Within the literature review section, you should include methods used to search the literature, such as databases and search terms used, as well as how the articles were selected. Search parameters such as publication date will also be included. This data may be presented in a table.

Next, the report will contain your actual literature review findings. You should state what was found in the literature in regard to the identified need. Presenting the literature in an organized manner is important for your reader to understand your project focus and the gap found in the literature. General information on the topic should be presented first, with specifics toward the end of the literature review section. Gaps in the literature relevant to the needs assessment will lead to the question or problem statement, also known as a gap analysis statement (what was not known or had not yet been researched).

Gap analysis statement. The question or problem statement will be used to write the gap analysis statement. Once the gap in the current literature has been identified, be sure to clearly identify the lack of literature or evidence. To indicate to the reader what was missing from the literature, you can use certain key phrases. Robinson et al. (2008, p. 205) provided numerous examples of gap statements:

• "Questions remain unanswered about . . ."
• "Much has been learned about X, Y remains poorly understood . . ."
• "The next step is to apply X to . . ."
• "Additional studies are needed . . ."

Following are examples of gap analysis statements:

• "Although the literature clearly indicates that occupational therapy plays an important role in the recovery of clients who are burn-injured, the role of occupational therapy in addressing self-image of burn survivors has not been studied."
• "Occupational therapists play a key role in addressing sensory deficits in children with autism spectrum disorder; however, it is important to address the carryover of sensory interventions in the home."

Next, explain how you intend to "fill the gap." This can be done by simply stating the purpose of your capstone in one to two sentences. Some phrases that you might use to indicate how you intend to "fill the gap" are as follows:

- "The student will analyze . . ."
- "In this project, the student will investigate . . ."
- "Therefore, the purpose of this project is to . . ."
- "In this paper, the student reports . . ."

You should keep in mind that when writing your capstone report, you will eventually need to write in the past tense because the project will be complete. Following are examples of purpose statements written in the past tense:

- "The student therefore analyzed the perceived role of occupational therapy practitioners in an inpatient acute care hospital in addressing self-image with burn-injured clients."
- "Therefore, the purpose of this project was to determine if and how occupational therapy practitioners are addressing carryover of sensory interventions in the home and to address any barriers identified through the capstone project."

After providing the gap analysis statement and before discussing the project plan, the capstone student will discuss the driving theory or conceptual model used to frame the capstone project.

Chapter IV: Driving Theory or Conceptual Model

You may choose (or be required) to include a conceptual model or theory to support and frame the design of your capstone project. While the description and rationale for the theory may be written in a defined chapter of your capstone report, the theory itself will be woven throughout your report because it informs the entire process of designing and completing your doctoral capstone project.

Boniface and Seymour (2012) supported the use of theory and its role in informing evidence-based practice for occupational therapy practitioners. "Conceptual professional models not only enable therapists to connect with the theoretical foundation of their work, but they also articulate the nature of their profession" (Reagon, 2012, p. 160). Models and frameworks specific to occupational therapy often consider the person or client, the environment or context, and the task or occupation. In other words, a model helps you think conceptually about the potential participants, the identified problem or need, and any influencing factors (e.g., environmental, societal, cultural, institutional). In line with Vision 2025 (AOTA, 2018), a model helps you consider how to best address the problem through creative solutions. An occupation-based focus is key to ensuring the project is grounded in the domain of the profession.

Chapter V: Capstone Plan and Process

Plan. In this section, you will describe the goals that were identified through your literature review and needs assessment, as well as the plan and process to achieve the goals. You need to keep in mind that the occupational therapy profession is client-centered and that goals and objectives to reach the goals need to have been developed in collaboration with your site mentor to ensure that your project was meaningful to the site and benefitted key stakeholders. Consider writing SMART goals (specific, measurable, action-oriented, realistic, and timely), just as you would when working with an individual client during traditional fieldwork. Then, list short-term objectives or steps to meet the goals. The following is an example of a goal with short-term objectives:

- *Goal.* Within 4 weeks of program implementation, rehabilitation staff members will implement their knowledge of fall prevention measures, as evidenced by an average weekly decrease of one fall incident per unit.
  - *Objective:* Within 1 week of program implementation, 90% of rehabilitation staff will attend one in-service on fall prevention measures.
  - *Objective:* Within 3 weeks of program implementation, 90% of rehabilitation staff will demonstrate two strategies for fall prevention during patient handling.

Process. You would be wise to provide an action plan for carrying out your project. The plan should also include a timeline to give the audience a sense of how you planned to spend 14 weeks accomplishing your project. You may want to consider including the following:

- Time spent orienting to the site, becoming familiar with processes and procedures, and meetings with key stakeholders.
- Refinement of the project plan based on feedback from the content expert, stakeholders, and faculty mentor.
- Any meetings planned in accordance with administration, stakeholders, or site mentor for information regarding approvals, budgeting, recruitment, etc.
- Regular meetings with the content expert, faculty mentor, and/or doctoral capstone coordinator, including your own evaluation meetings (midterm and final).
- Time for updating the literature review or for any research needing to be done to set a foundation for the doctoral project.
- Creation of any products or artifacts for the project (training materials, webinars, protocols, outcome measurements, etc.).

- Marketing/recruitment period for participants (staff, patients, clients, families, etc.).
- The implementation period.
- Time for data analysis.
- Planning of final presentation.
- Final presentation date and time, in collaboration with site mentor, stakeholders, faculty mentor, and capstone coordinator.
- Time for final paperwork required by the site or your occupational therapy program.

See Appendix 12.B for an example action plan in table form and a visual timeline of events for the capstone. Other important information to include in the plan is an overall budget for materials needed and any specific resources to which you will need access to complete your capstone project.

Chapter VI: Project Implementation

Following the plan and process, you will discuss how your project was actually implemented. Although the plan gives an overview of what was intended, it is common that changes are made to the plan throughout the project's implementation phase.

Within this chapter of the final capstone report, first describe your participants. The demographics of the participants will vary based on your project focus area and the site. Participants may have been clients or patients, their families or caregivers, occupational therapy practitioners, other staff, volunteers, administration, students, or others. You may choose to provide specific inclusion and exclusion criteria for participants, depending on the type of project implemented. For example, inclusion criteria for clients might include the diagnosis, age, comprehension level, and/or occupational performance level. Inclusion criteria for staff might include occupational therapy practitioners, years of practice, and practice setting.

Next, the process to recruit participants is described. If approval from the academic institution's or capstone site's institutional review board was needed and obtained, this information should be included in the capstone report. Documents such as templates for gaining informed consent, recruitment letters, or marketing flyers might also be included as appendices. Any contact that you made with participants should be described, such as holding an in-service for therapy staff or contacting a specific group of individuals via phone or email to ask for their participation.

You should note any pertinent information regarding your participants; however, no identifying information should be included in your report. The capstone report discusses the actual number of participants and any retention issues that occurred. For example, if ten participants were originally recruited but only eight fully participated, include the reason for attrition.

Next, include your project components and the specific methods that you used to carry out each component of the plan. It is recommended that you include a timeline of events. Depending on the project itself, implementation may take several consecutive weeks or a certain day(s) each week, across several weeks. Any resources used should be listed, as well as an updated budget for the project. This information may be included as appendices in the capstone report. Your site may have offered you use of its resources, or it may have been up to you to obtain resources. If grant funding was a source of your funding, include detailed information regarding the grant.

Project components and methods may vary from one capstone project to another and will be dependent on your area of focus. For example, a report discussing a program that involved patient education on health and wellness should include information on the frequency and length of the education sessions, whether they were face-to-face or virtual, group vs. individual sessions, and any actual material discussed. A project that focused on advocacy might discuss how advocacy occurred, such as letters written to legislators, information on events attended to raise awareness, and how consumers were educated regarding the issue. It is important that all deliverables be included in your report. They may be added as appendices. Examples of deliverables that might be included for a variety of capstone projects are as follows:

- Evaluation tools or outcome measurements (e.g., surveys)
- Written treatment protocols or pathways
- Webinars or educational/learning modules
- Training materials (e.g., educational handouts or manuals)
- Curricular materials
- Community resources handbook
- Written letters or advocacy statements
- Photos of products (now owned by the site) (see Text Box 12.4)

TEXT BOX 12-4

Especially given privacy laws, you need to seek permission and comply with all policies from your academic institution and your capstone site regarding the use of **any** photographs and/or video media within any of your dissemination products.

Deviations from your original plan and the cause or reasoning for the change need to be noted. Supports and barriers during the implementation phase of your project should be clearly described.

Chapter VII: Project Evaluation and Results

Evaluation. An explanation of how the data was collected and analyzed and why you chose such methods must be included. You will need to include any relevant literature to support your process of project evaluation. The evaluation will be objective in nature, include factual information, and be free from author bias. Any individuals involved in the evaluation process, including yourself or others, such as your site mentor, need to be mentioned. If the evaluation was completed by anyone in addition to yourself, describe any collaborative processes that occurred to ensure consistency of results. Your capstone report should include any training on the measures used, if applicable. Depending on your project focus area and the methods used, this may include standardized or non-standardized outcome measures (or both), pre- and post-implementation measures, and others. Refer back to Chapter 8 for recommendations and strategies for outcome measurement and program evaluation of the doctoral capstone.

Results or outcomes. The results or outcomes section is written after you have gathered and analyzed your data. This section describes your findings in relation to your project evaluation. This may include quantitative data (e.g., statistics), qualitative data (e.g., descriptive themes from interviews), or a combination of the two. Tables, graphs, charts, or other visuals to help the reader understand the data should be included in the results. Be sure to ensure that you are displaying these figures according to APA format and style. (See Appendix 12.C for examples.)

Chapter VIII: Discussion and Impact

Discussion. The discussion helps summarize the results of your project through interpretation of the data in relation to your original problem or question. You should keep in mind the information discussed in your literature review, the gap analysis statement that you formed, and the goals and objectives set for your project. Addressing each of these areas in a concise manner based on the results of the project will make for a thorough discussion. You will also need to include any limitations of your doctoral project. Limitations could relate to barriers to participation (e.g., attrition), barriers to project implementation (e.g., restrictive site policies), a lack of resources or funding, to list a few. Here is where collaboration with your faculty mentor is key to ensure that you are comprehensively and holistically identifying and discussing limitations that arose throughout the implementation of your project.

Impact. The impact section discusses your project's impact on the site, the participants, and the occupational therapy profession. The doctoral capstone project is to be mutually beneficial, as you, the student, gain in-depth knowledge and skills, and the site has a project that will continue to make an impact long after the 14-week capstone experience has concluded. This section of the capstone report is more subjective in nature than the results section. You need to include feedback received regarding your project. Feedback may have been from participants, your content expert, or the administration at your capstone site. If the project continues after you have left the

site, information regarding any changes or refinement is to be shared. In addition, plans for carryover should be included. You may also choose to discuss your project's broader implications for society or the profession.

Chapter IX: Conclusion

Within this section, be sure to provide a concise conclusion that leaves the reader with a "take-home message." This section should be to the point and may restate the purpose of your project and a concise summary of the outcomes. It is recommended that you do not share new information in the conclusion.

References

The reference section is intended to give credit to any sources of information you cited throughout your capstone document. If information is not considered "general knowledge," it should be cited in the body of your document. A good rule of thumb is, when in doubt, to cite the source. You should use APA (2020) formatting to properly format your reference list.

Appendices

An *appendix* is information that is informative but not essential. By including appendices, you provide your readers with information that they can easily locate and refer to without cluttering the body of the paper itself. Each appendix should be lettered, titled, and included in the table of contents.

You may include various items in your appendices. Following is a list of items to consider for this purpose:

- Program marketing materials or recruitment announcements
- Letters of consent or assent for participants
- Pre- and post-assessment measures
- Budgeting spreadsheets
- Flowcharts or diagrams to illustrate data collection or analysis procedures
- Actual products or portions of products created for the project

The next section in this chapter provides examples of scholarly capstone products that relate to each of the focus areas and that you may consider for inclusion as appendices of your capstone report.

EXAMPLES OF ADDITIONAL SCHOLARLY DISSEMINATION PRODUCTS BASED ON FOCUS AREAS

Throughout the doctoral capstone, the expectations of demonstrating scholarship and dissemination may vary, and you may create a range of scholarly products to highlight your findings and likewise to meet the needs of your defined stakeholders. The type and scope of the dissemination product will vary based on site, population, and focus area. While the capstone report or manuscript formation has been previously described in detail, presentations within regional, national, or even global audiences may be an additional route of dissemination that you may elect to follow or may be required by your academic program as the formal dissemination method. Selecting a stakeholder audience or conference to disseminate scholarly outcomes of the capstone is a major decision.

You may also consider and negotiate the creation of educational programs which offer training or dissemination of generalizable outcomes to specific stakeholders or client audiences specific to your target population of interest. Examples of these scholarly products may include procedure manuals regarding a specific clinical treatment intervention or application of advancements in technology for a clinical problem or chronic condition. Other educational products may be created virtually to allow a greater span of audience members or afford individual stakeholders access to materials who may be interested in distance learning or have barriers to on-site or in-person education. Individual academic program curricular instruction may vary and offer guidance regarding type or product of dissemination. In any regard, if a capstone report is a required outcome of the experience and project, you may wish to include additional products, such as the outcomes of an evidence-based practice guideline or a critical pathway. Table 12.3 provides examples of scholarly products that can be derived from the capstone experience and included as appendices within the capstone report.

Table 12-3. Examples of Scholarly Products to Be Included as Appendices

FOCUS AREA	DESCRIPTION	EXAMPLE OF CULMINATING PRODUCT
Clinical skills	You are interested in advancing your clinical skills in an area of advanced practice, specifically, lymphedema management. You advance your skills through clinical training and via direct supervision (mentorship) of a certified lymphedema therapist. You engage in continued education and take advanced certification courses to prepare to obtain a lymphedema certification after receiving licensure.	An evidence-based, comprehensive protocol for lymphedema management for the facility. The product could be a binder that included lymphedema wrapping instruction with visuals, precautions and contraindications, resources for wrapping materials, and handouts for patient education.
Research skills	You complete a needs assessment in an elementary school and determine that several students require occupational therapy in the kindergarten class to address decreased attention and sensory needs. A literature review reveals that two sensory integration techniques have proven to be effective in addressing these issues in the classroom. After obtaining approval from key stakeholders, parents, and the university's institutional review board, you use a standardized assessment to evaluate each student for attention and sensory needs to obtain a baseline score. One intervention is provided to a group of students, and the other intervention to a second group of students. This occurs over a period of 4 weeks, with intervention occurring twice each week. Student attention and sensory needs are re-evaluated to determine progress and identify whether one treatment technique is more effective than the other.	A sensory diet protocol to be used across the school district. The protocol is based on the intervention that was found to work more effectively for the students, with suggestions for individualizing the protocol based on various needs. You provide a typed protocol, along with a link to a webinar training, teachers, classroom aides, and therapists, district-wide.

continued

Table 12-3. Examples of Scholarly Products to Be Included as Appendices (continued)

FOCUS AREA	DESCRIPTION	EXAMPLE OF CULMINATING PRODUCT
Administration	You are interested in gaining advanced skills in administration and therefore use an apprenticeship model under the owner of a pediatric outpatient clinic. You assist in preparing for re-accreditation by the Commission on Accreditation of Rehabilitation Facilities (CARF), collecting data points and preparing staff for the on-site visit by CARF.	The survey application packet, which includes detailed information about leadership, the programs and services offered at the site, and quality improvement initiatives in process. All materials needed to provide evidence of quality service are included.
Leadership	You are interested in completing advanced leadership training to create a vision for inclusion and diversity in a community organization. You complete advanced leadership training through continued education courses, readings, and webinars. After training, you create a series of leadership in-services for staff regarding respect for cultural and social diversities and steps to take for including individuals with intellectual and physical disabilities in the organization. This includes contacting speakers with expertise in these areas and creating pre- and post-assessments to measure changes in staff knowledge and awareness.	A series of webinars based on the leadership in-services provided to staff, which can be used repeatedly as new staff are hired as a part of the orientation process. At the completion of the webinar, staff are required to pass online quizzes with lifelike scenarios regarding decision-making surrounding inclusion.
Program development and evaluation	You are interested in social inclusion for children with disabilities. An elementary school offers summer camps, but they lack programs that are inclusive of children with disabilities. You create a summer program for children with disabilities, with a focus on socialization and age-appropriate play. Parents are included in parent training sessions on community resources for children with disabilities and social events for their children. Quality-of-life measurements are completed pre- and post-programming to determine parents' perceived change in their children's quality of life.	A training video for parents based on the summer camp program series, with instruction and demonstrations regarding increasing social opportunities for their children. Included are links to community resources for children with disabilities, as well as events for socialization.
Policy development	You are interested in policy development and become aware of recent issues in a community outreach program regarding staff knowledge of how to best meet the needs of clients among the lesbian, gay, bisexual, transgender, queer/questioning, intersex (LGBTQIA+) community. You administer a self-assessment to staff members regarding their own preconceptions and bias regarding individuals who are LGBTQIA+. You research best practices in addressing and meeting the needs of clients who are LGBTQIA+. You get approval of the policies and procedures from administration and complete staff education on the policy's implementation.	A policies and procedures manual regarding best practices in addressing and meeting the needs of individuals who are LGBTQIA+. The manual includes a self-assessment to measure staff member's own preconceptions and bias; resources, such as links to additional information for staff; as well as community supports that the staff can share with clients.

continued

Table 12-3. Examples of Scholarly Products to Be Included as Appendices (continued)

FOCUS AREA	DESCRIPTION	EXAMPLE OF CULMINATING PRODUCT
Advocacy	You organize a campaign to increase community and policymaker awareness of health disparities affecting individuals in the local community. You attend rallies, organize petitions, write letters, and attend meetings with various stakeholders to create change.	A website for consumer advocacy is created with information on health disparities, an online discussion forum, downloadable campaign materials (including letter templates), and links to local rallies and advocacy events.
Education	You are interested in academia as a practice setting. You attend continued education on teaching pedagogy, curricular development, educational technology, classroom management, and best practices in student assessment at an academic institution. You are mentored by an experienced faculty member. You create a series of lectures and hands-on learning activities to meet course objectives and ACOTE standards. You deliver the lectures as a guest speaker in collaboration with the primary instructor.	A lecture series with slide decks, handouts, and assignment and assessment methods related to a newly designed learning activity. Information related to course objectives and accreditation standards met by the lecture series can also be included.

DISSEMINATION THROUGH ORAL PRESENTATION: POSTERS AND PRESENTATIONS

Your occupational therapy program may require you to disseminate your capstone project orally as a poster or a platform-style presentation. This may be in addition to a written product or their sole form of dissemination. However, in addition to your program's requirements, you may choose to present your capstone project at a professional conference. It is beneficial to stay abreast of any "call for proposals," during which professional organizations announce a call for potential presenters to submit their proposal for review. This may be via email to their members or through an advertisement on their website. Regardless, it is critical that you follow the guidelines of your program or the organization's conference guidelines when preparing your dissemination product. (See Text Box 12.5 for more information.) Following are several considerations for preparing an oral dissemination.

The information presented should be as clear and accurate as it would be in a written report. Scholarly posters often include a section with brief learning objectives for the intended audience, a background and literature review, research question or problem statement, methods, data analysis and results, discussions and conclusions, and references. With posters, visual representation of the information where possible will help the viewer better understand the information, and you should supplement the written material with your own verbal explanation of the information.

Be sure to practice your "pitch." For a poster, this might be a 5-minute oral summary of your work, starting with the background or problem, leading to your research question, the methods or overall gist of your capstone project, and the outcomes. Get comfortable talking with others off-the-cuff about your project. Depending on your audience, you may be talking to a clinician, a student, or a non-OT, so tailor your pitch to that audience's interests.

You may choose to provide handouts to your audience, which could include your contact information for later communication and networking, data analysis tables, and/or references for further reading on the topic. See Appendix 12.D as an example checklist and rubric that might be helpful to guide the development of a formal poster presentation.

TEXT BOX 12-5

Be sure to follow any recommendations from your program or professional conference regarding formatting your poster or session materials. For example, sizing/poster dimension guidelines should be consulted before you begin formatting, as it can be difficult to fit information on a poster in the first place without having to resize it! Regarding oral sessions, check conference communications regarding any technology needs. Some conferences may provide all audiovisual equipment needed, while others may require you to bring a laptop or to submit your presentation ahead of time.

You should consult with conference submission guides when preparing to submit your capstone product for dissemination at a conference. Conference presentations may be time-limited, ranging from brief sessions to longer sessions of 2 to 3 hours. Consider the nature of your content and what length of time you will need to disseminate, while also keeping your audience engaged. The content of a lecture-style session is similar to that of a written manuscript or poster presentation but is obviously more verbal and can be made interactive with polls, small group discussion, and even hands-on practice, where applicable. Your program might have an approved template for you to create your poster; Appendix 12.E provides an example of this.

Finalizing the Dissemination Product, Including Capstone Report

There are various ways to disseminate the outcomes of your capstone project. Your academic institution may require you to submit your capstone report in hard copy or electronically as an assignment, as well as provide evidence of completion of your capstone project. In addition, you may choose to disseminate the results to a larger audience, such as through a poster or platform presentation at a conference or through publication in a professional magazine or peer-reviewed journal. Nonetheless, the completion of the capstone project needs to be officiated through dissemination, sharing the knowledge gained in the area of focus (ACOTE, 2023).

Regardless of how the capstone is to be disseminated, before final submission, you would be wise to receive feedback on your report. You may choose to have one or more peers in your cohort provide feedback, or you may ask your faculty mentor or other professional to review your report. It is helpful if the reviewer is familiar with your subject matter, as well as APA formatting and scholarly writing. Many professional journals require a specific review process, and you should closely follow guidelines provided by the journal.

Regarding formal submission to your academic institution, your occupational therapy program may have guidelines or requirements that you should follow. If your program requires that the capstone report be bound, determining the specifications for the bound document is important. Your program may recommend a specific binding company, color, and material for the cover or require your academic institution's crest to be displayed. Your academic institution may require an electronic copy for the library database. In this case, the academic librarians may be contacted for details regarding that process.

Other considerations which need to be continuously revisited during writing or the creation of scholarly products relate to coordination of authorship as mentioned previously, as authorship may shift according to the types or breadth of product dissemination. Product ownership is also an important topic of conversation that you need to be prepared to address with members of your capstone team or key stakeholders at your doctoral capstone site. Intellectual property development and ownership expectations may vary between institutions. Thoughtful decision-making is necessary throughout the doctoral capstone experience and project plan to ensure all parties are adequately represented.

Finally, as you wind down your doctoral capstone process and inch closer to graduating and entering clinical practice, it will be important for you to document your accomplishments related to your doctoral capstone on your résumé and include in other professional portfolio artifacts.

You might identify your doctoral capstone experience under an experiential learning header on your résumé, where you also document completed fieldwork experiences. For your DCE, you should document the time frame, capstone site name and location, and a bulleted list of specific responsibilities or skill sets that you learned. Here is an example:

Doctoral Capstone Experience
Miller's Private Pediatric Clinic, Webster, NY 5/25–8/25
- Designed and facilitated the implementation of pilot kindergarten readiness program.
- Performed developmental screenings.
- Created parent education materials related to school readiness and relevant developmental areas.
- Assisted with recruitment of families for participation in pilot program.

For your capstone project, you will want to track any formal dissemination methods. For example, if present at a state or national conference, you will want to list this as a scholarly activity on your résumé under a "Scholarship Header." An example way to identify on your résumé is:

Smith, S. (2025). *Effects of a family-centered kindergarten readiness program on parenting outcomes and parents' perceptions of their child's kindergarten readiness.* Accepted as a Poster Presentation. 2025 NY State OT Conference, Old Forge, New York. December 2025.

Student Section Chapter Summary

This chapter has provided several recommendations and guidelines to consider when approaching the dissemination phase of the doctoral capstone. Completion and dissemination of an individual capstone project are a requirement of all entry-level occupational therapy doctoral programs. Although the type and format can vary, it is essential that the capstone dissemination clearly communicate the nature of the doctoral project and the greater impact that it had and will continue to have on the site, the profession, and society.

Section 2: Educator Focus

Transformational Learning Phases and Framework for the Educator

As the entire doctoral capstone process nears completion, as educators, we can view our students within Mezirow's final stage of the transformational learning process, the reintegration phase (Mezirow, 1997). The reintegration phase occurs after learners have critically assessed their assumptions and have undergone a transformation in their perspectives. In this phase, as we guide and support our students to formally disseminate their capstone project, we are able to observe how our students have integrated new learning and perspectives. Regardless of the method, dissemination generally involves some sort of professional communication and writing. This writing requires the capstone student to integrate new insights, methods, and findings into a cohesive narrative, demonstrating how they have transformed and applied their understanding to practice. Whether your program expects a formal written capstone report, a presentation, or another product, it is the hope that the dissemination offers our students a meaningful opportunity to communicate their transformation, as well as experience a reinvigorated sense of identity and a newfound readiness for professional practice.

INTRODUCTION FOR EDUCATOR

The doctoral capstone experience affords students the opportunity to apply self-directed learning in an innovative way in order to improve upon or solve an existing problem. As reviewed in previous chapters in this book, the mentorship that each student receives throughout the capstone experience and project can significantly impact the growth trajectory throughout the entire capstone experience and project. While students participate in the mentored experience, they have the ability to "try out" skill sets which can help them to not only meet the objectives of their capstone project but, more importantly, also put into practice the skills to operationalize next steps in meeting the population demands of their targeted audience within their project. As this occurs, the capstone student may use knowledge gained from their project and experience to direct new outcomes. Through this process of integrating findings into practice, the student may have a deeper appreciation of gained knowledge which they can translate

into their dissemination product(s). It is during this time of idealized influence that true transformational learning may occur.

EDUCATOR REFLECTIVE QUESTIONS

When planning the dissemination of the doctoral capstone project, the educator may find it helpful to reflect on the following questions:

1. What form(s) of dissemination align with the program's mission, vision, and curricular design?
2. How can I guide students to disseminate their project with a product that makes sense for their focus area and project outcomes?
3. What resources should I provide to my students to enhance their written and oral presentation skills?
4. What guidelines should I provide to my students to contribute to the development of their final dissemination product?

EDUCATOR OBJECTIVES

By the end of reading this chapter, the educator will be able to apply principles of transformational learning design theory to structure learning activities, assignments, and/or assessments to promote the capstone student's ability to:

1. Compare and contrast types of project dissemination methods.
2. Understand the purpose and process of professional writing in the field of occupational therapy.
3. Explain recommendations for components of a written capstone dissemination.
4. Support recommendations for components of oral capstone dissemination.
5. Identify additional formats for capstone project dissemination.

HISTORY OF DOCTORAL CAPSTONE PROJECTS

While the focus of the student's section of this chapter is to explore various types of dissemination products for the doctoral capstone, as an educator, it is beneficial to understand the history and purpose of the capstone in healthcare education programs. Although relatively newer to the occupational therapy education requirements, the idea of a capstone project is not new to health science education. Both nursing and audiology doctoral degree programs have used capstone projects to meet accreditation standards within their curricula and can provide useful information regarding the structure of such projects. In 2004, the American Association of Colleges of Nursing (AACN) voted to endorse a position statement that required the field of nursing to transition from a master's level of preparation to a doctoral level for advanced practice by 2015 (AACN, 2017). Due to changes in health care and to improve patient outcomes, advanced scientific knowledge and practice skills would be met through the academic curriculum for the practice doctorate in nursing (DNP).

The DNP degree requires a final DNP project, often referred to as a capstone project. Similarly to the occupational therapy doctoral capstone project, it is not a dissertation but requires mastery of an advanced specialty area in nursing (AACN, 2006). It is not the creation of original research (such as with a dissertation) but requires the application of existing research and literature into practical application in clinical practice. Regarding accreditation standards, it provides evidence that the DNP program has more advanced outcomes than the master's level of preparation (Berkowitz, 2015). Like occupational therapy doctoral students, DNP students are required to disseminate the results of their capstone projects. The DNP project is to produce an academic product that results from the student being immersed in practice experience. It is reviewed by a committee, which serves as an evaluation of their growth in knowledge and expertise (AACN, 2006).

The text *DNP Capstone Projects: Exemplars of Excellence in Practice* (Anderson et al., 2015) provides detailed examples of actual nursing capstone projects, including the written capstone document. Table 12.4 provides topic areas for the capstone projects.

The DNP capstone projects in Table 12.4 highlight the importance of applying evidence to practice. Although each capstone project was very different in focus and structure, each identified an area of need and addressed

it in practice. This differs from a dissertation, in which the expectation is to produce new evidence. Similar to the DNP capstone, application is key to the occupational therapy doctorate capstone.

Many programs that offer the doctor of audiology (AuD) degree require a capstone project to meet accreditation standards set by the Accreditation Commission for Audiology Education (ACAE, 2016). Standard 25, which outlines student research and scholarly activity, states that students must demonstrate knowledge of research design, be critical consumers of professional literature, and evaluate research to apply this knowledge related to evidence-based practice (ACAE, 2016). The guidelines also suggest the completion of a "mentored experiment" to meet this standard. Many audiology programs opt to require a project that demonstrates students' abilities to evaluate research and apply evidence-based practice in the form of a clinical project.

While the capstone is required for the degrees just discussed, it is not necessarily required for all practice doctorates. The physical therapy profession made the transition to the entry-level doctor of physical therapy degree (DPT) to meet the Commission on Accreditation in Physical Therapy Education (2017) time frame. During the time of the transition to the entry-level doctorate, the physical therapy profession envisioned a degree that would glean greater respect from health-care professionals, the potential for autonomous practice with increased skills, and preparation for clinical scholarship (Plack & Wong, 2002; Rothstein, 1998; Woods, 2001). Although the transition to a doctoral degree meant that programs needed to change their curriculum, it did not require the completion of a capstone. (See Text Box 12.6.)

Table 12-4. Examples of DNP Capstone Projects

Burnout as a Barrier to Practice Among Nurse-Midwives: Examining the Evidence

A replica of the 1986 national nurse–midwife study conducted by Beaver et al. (as cited in Barroso, 2015), this project re-examined the prevalence of burnout among members of the American College of Nurse–Midwives (ACNM) currently in clinical practice in Pennsylvania. Various factors associated with burnout were evaluated. This capstone project compared findings with the original study (Barroso, 2015, p. 47).

Changing the Paradigm: Diabetic Group Visits in a Primary Care Setting

The purpose was to assess the impact of introducing one component of the chronic care model (CCM), group visits, on the delivery of health care to diabetic patients in a family medicine clinic and residency training program. The group visit is one strategy to attempt improvements in redesigning the delivery of health-care delivery services. The scope of this project was to measure patient perceptions of their health care and changes in specific diabetes clinical indicators as a result of attendance at the group visits (Short, 2015, pp. 55–56).

Promoting Compassion Fatigue Resiliency Among Emergency Department Nurses

Emergency nurses work in an environment that is intellectually, emotionally, and physically demanding, with repeated exposure to the stressors of the emergency department. Compassion fatigue (CF) may result. This capstone focused on prevention of CF and promotion of resiliency among emergency department nurses (Flarity et al., 2015, pp. 67–68).

Data from 2018 indicates that 36% of accredited DPT programs offer a designated capstone (Barlow et al., 2018).

Similarly, the doctor of pharmacy degree (PharmD) does not require a capstone project; however, some programs choose to include it as part of their curriculum (Accreditation Council for Pharmacy Education, 2015).

Although the doctoral capstone project is not a new concept in health science curricula, it is a relatively evolving requirement for entry-level occupational therapy doctoral curricula. It is important for all key stakeholders (faculty, capstone students, occupational therapy practitioners, and site mentors) to understand the differences between a dissertation and a doctoral capstone project, as well as to understand the expectations of the occupational therapy capstone student throughout the completion of the capstone project and culminating capstone report.

CONSIDERATIONS FOR MEETING THE ACOTE STANDARDS FOR THE CAPSTONE PROJECT

The capstone experience and project are significant pieces of the ACOTE requirements for the occupational therapy doctorate. It is important for faculty in entry-level doctoral programs to ensure that the standards are met within their curricula. Standard D.1.6, which refers specifically to the doctoral capstone project, states: "Ensure completion and dissemination of an individual doctoral capstone project that relates to the doctoral capstone experience and demonstrates synthesis of in-depth knowledge in the focused area of study" (ACOTE, 2023, p. 44).

Educators may want to work backward when considering their curricular design to ensure it prepares students for the doctoral capstone experience and project. ACOTE standard D.1.3 states that the doctoral capstone is to be an integral part of the curriculum design (ACOTE, 2023). It benefits students to be familiar with components of the capstone even before engaging in the experience. For example, understanding the purpose of a needs assessment and how to conduct one, perhaps through a community-engaged learning course earlier in the curriculum, would be beneficial. Skills utilized in research and scholarship, such as performing a literature review, creating a research question, designing a methodology, conducting data analysis, and interpreting the results, should not be new concepts to students engaging in the capstone. Consider what you want your graduate students to "look like" when they finish their capstones – what key skills, knowledge, and characteristics do you

expect them to possess? From there, work backward through your curriculum to determine where those areas are taught, or where they can be infused. You might even consider making these curricular threads, woven throughout the progression of the curriculum. Other strategies to integrate the doctoral capstone within your curricular design were provided in the educator section of Chapter 1.

VARIATION IN DISSEMINATION METHODS OF THE CAPSTONE PROJECT

To demonstrate synthesis of in-depth knowledge in the focused area of study, your program may meet this standard by requiring the capstone student to complete a written capstone report or other form of a scholarly product that was mentioned previously in this chapter. This product should fit with the nature of the capstone project, as well as the student's focus area. For example, one form is a written manuscript to be bound and made available through hard copy in the academic institution's library or electronically through the library's virtual databases. Appendix 12.F provides a rubric for a written manuscript that is outlined in the student section of this chapter. Another form of capstone product is a written practice guideline or evidence-based protocol. Examples of content to be included in forms of culminating documents are provided in Table 12.3 in the student section of this chapter.

In addition, an oral presentation or "defense" of the doctoral capstone project may be required. Key stakeholders from the capstone site, faculty, students, and perhaps family and other supporters of the capstone student could be invited to the presentation. This provides an opportunity for your students to share the overall process and outcomes of their work while also informing key stakeholders of the program structure and how this meets a need. An oral presentation also allows the student to provide important insights into gaps in practice or the need for current evidence to be put into practice and be clarified.

Depending on the focus area, doctoral capstone experience, and project, you may require or encourage your students to prepare a manuscript of sufficient quality to be submitted to a peer-reviewed publication or a professional trade periodical (such as the American Occupational Therapy Association's [AOTA] *OT Practice* publication). Or you might encourage them to submit a proposal to present their capstone as a poster or oral presentation at a local, state, or national professional conference. Refer to Appendix 12.D for an example of a poster presentation checklist and rubric. Prepare the capstone student to seek advice from their capstone team to determine the most appropriate audience for dissemination.

STRATEGIES FOR FOSTERING PROFESSIONAL WRITING BEHAVIORS OF STUDENTS

As an educator, you're likely aware that students have varying degrees of skill when it comes to writing. It is imperative that the dissemination of their doctoral capstone be a scholarly product and be appropriately written to reach the appropriate audience. For formal dissemination, this means utilizing APA 7th edition formatting and proper grammar. For any capstone courses, you might consider requiring students to purchase the APA 7th edition manual, whether hard copy or digitally, and to refer to it often as they format their final capstone report, poster, or other dissemination product. In addition, ensure that students are aware of the support offered through the institution – such as a university writing center.

You might also craft a department policy in your program that is designed to model and stipulate professional writing expectations for your students early in your program. (See Text Box 12.7.)

Example syllabus statement:

Complete assignments using the APA 7th edition style of professional writing. Student(s) who have three or more separate, major APA errors will incur a 5% (professional year I), 7% (professional year II), and 10% (professional year III) deduction on the final grade for the assignment.

TEXT BOX 12-7

Teaching Tip: If your institution offers writing support to students, invite a staff member or consultant from your writing class to introduce themselves and share what types of writing support is offered. It is important that students know how to access the services, whether in person or virtual, the hours that services are available, and how to set up an appointment. Students should also understand the expectations for their consultation; that is, whether the staff will review grammar and APA, provide feedback on whole drafts or only sections of reports, or whether they only answer specific questions.

The conversation regarding positive professional writing behaviors requires a discussion regarding artificial intelligence (AI) and the role learning language models (LLMs) now play in many facets of our professional practice, including scholarship. The access and advancement of LLMs such as ChatGPT and platforms like the first well-known LLM continue to accelerate and become more accessible. Educators like yourself must evolve in your iteration and reflection on how AI can be utilized. As an educator, you may consider mechanisms to help your

student understand the "guidance" AI can afford as a tool to enhance their capstone ideas or creativity.

Promoting structure and transparency of any academic integrity expectations is important to establish in the forefront of the capstone process to ensure AI is used as a tool to complement traditional pedagogies in the scholarship of learning. In the past, while educators and near peers have been surrogates in reflective learning, AI is quickly becoming a component of exploring new ideas and collaborative interaction. It is essential in today's learning environment to help students learn about AI, and the inherent risks and benefits.

It is best practice as an educator to consider AI policies at both the course and the assignment levels.

PROFESSIONAL WRITING BENEFITS INCORPORATING AI

Feedback is an essential element of professional writing. Providing feedback throughout the capstone helps a student comprehend the gaps in their current understanding in order to achieve the desired learning outcomes within the capstone. However, the time to provide tailored and meaningful feedback can be intensive and tedious. With the proper infrastructure within course assignments, AI can be integrated into specific learning checkpoints to enable students to incorporate AI to receive immediate supplemental feedback in addition to your own or that of a near peer. Educators can steward the way their students utilize AI for reflective feedback, which can help improve their feedback due to the immediacy and flexibility that AI offers (McCrea, 2023). To support your student receiving useful AI-generated feedback, you can help your student critically consider the prompts they use when eliciting AI feedback to promote trustworthiness of the feedback they receive. Examples of prompt generation to enhance student writing using AI may include:

- What are some additional ways to phrase this idea to a (specific) audience?
- How can I introduce the focus area using more professional language to make the purpose of this subject clearer?
- Provide counterarguments or complementary views regarding this writing.
- Suggest ways to change the design of this program to make it clear to an audience of [specific group of individuals].
- List any complications or risks for this program idea which are not clear in the program   outline.
- Create a list of positive and critical points of feedback about this writing.

While these are just a few prompting ideas, it is important to keep in mind that while AI can generate fast and efficient feedback, the more specificity the writer can provide in each prompt, the more relevant the AI feedback may be. AI-generated feedback may enable some of your students to receive more varied feedback (Bowen & Watson, 2024). Having both feedback from yourself and AI may challenge student thinking, afford new perspectives that are outside of your own considerations, and provide access to students who may have lack of access to in-the-moment feedback due to time constraints or accessibility to specific resources. Students who may struggle with asking for help or clarification from an instructor may find AI helps them seek additional feedback in a non-threatening way (McCrea, 2023). In this way, AI may be used as a "tutor" to help explain concepts in writing that a student may be struggling with in a beneficial and timely way.

PROFESSIONAL WRITING RISKS INCORPORATING AI

Using LLMs can benefit students in their professional writing; however, LLMs are still evolving, and their potential is still unfolding. Educators must be mindful that there are general risks outside of the ethical considerations for AI use in idea formation and professional writing. For instance, LLMs can produce outputs that are not factually accurate or based on confabulation (Augenstein et al., 2023). Since AI is generating text from many sources, including those with "faulty" human input, bias may be a potential threat introduced from the multiple viewpoints of information which AI directly compiles feedback to the user.

Privacy is also a consideration that educators should inform students about when inputting their own intellectual property into generative AI platforms, which may then store and utilize their intellectual writing for other purposes (Bowen & Watson, 2024). Just like personal information needs to be safeguarded in social media platforms, information such as student identifiers, site-specific or client-specific protected information, or academic intellectual property, which is not intended for view, should not be entered into databases, which may then draw this content for future purposes. Anything which is inputted into an AI platform may become part of the data set stored for future searches. As an educator, it is also important to be informed and educate your students on any institutional policies which are specific to the academic setting or partnering organization.

In addition, while generative AI innovation is creating exciting pathways for promoting efficiency, promoting access to knowledge, and accessibility in finding key evidence and supports for effective writing, the ethical considerations of incorporating AI cannot be overlooked. There are varying views and acceptance of AI use for writing in higher education. As AI tools change the landscape of day-to-day life, educators need to consider the applicability, ethical responsibilities, and potential conflicts of interests and risk factors which may accompany using these tools. Just as the level of sophistication of AI data storage, integration of new resources, and knowledge interpretation is increasing, detection of misuse or over-reliance on AI to generate "original ideas is becoming equally difficult to detect" (Bowen & Watson, 2024). In a study concerning student attitudes and motives for using AI by Wiley (2023), while the students reported that using AI without disclosing their use of AI was wrong, 75% of the students admitted to continuing to use AI without proper acknowledgment since they felt as though their instructors were not able to detect it. Rather than ignoring the reality of AI incorporation and our student's temptation to use it in misguided ways, as educators, we must provide transparency in how our professional ethics must guide our behaviors and actions, and this includes AI. AI can be a promising source of writing feedback. We need to set mutual expectations on the incorporation of AI to allow students to make an informed decision of how they may utilize AI in their capstone within the structure of established policies and procedures for use within the capstone. An example learning activity–integrated AI can be found in Text Box 12.8.

> **TEXT BOX 12-8**
>
> **Teaching Tip:** As a learning activity, doctoral capstone coordinators can divide capstone students into various groups and have each group read one section of an occupational therapy journal article (the introduction, methods, discussion, etc.). Ask each group to highlight any words, phrases, or abbreviations that are specific to occupational therapy. Have students reflect on the amount of occupational therapy–specific language that is used and whether someone outside the field would understand the article. Consider asking the groups to edit their assigned journal sections to be more descriptive for a non–occupational therapist audience. In a "next" iteration, an educator may also provide examples of how the student can elicit feedback from AI. Students can then compare the language suggestions provided by their "human near peers" versus the AI-generated language.

RECOMMENDATIONS FOR ORAL CAPSTONE DISSEMINATION

The doctoral capstone affords a range of opportunities for capstone students to use a wide range of dissemination strategies to apply what they have learned throughout their experience and project. This range includes opportunities via multiple venues, such as the student's site, state, national, or even international presentations.

These opportunities may incorporate in-person presentations or distance learning via virtual applications. Some oral dissemination presentations may be in real time versus pre-recorded formats. This allows for innovation and creativity within these oral dissemination products as well.

Preparing students for professional oral presentations is essential. In addition to the structural components of a dissemination presentation, such as the development of learning objectives, materials being shown or demonstrated during an oral presentation, the student must also consider the delivery of a professional presentation. Considerations such as how to engage the audience and "hook" their interest through not only the written construction of the presentation but also the visual components of their presentation are paramount. Their professionalism during the presentation must reflect a balance between enthusiasm for the topic while balancing objectivity.

- *Providing a clear agenda for the oral presentation.* Establishing an outline of the presentation early in the dissemination planning process may be helpful as you help guide your student toward dissemination possibilities. Again, depending on the type of oral presentation or conference the student elects for their dissemination, the "tone" of the oral presentation may change.
- *Consider the formatting of the presentation.* Depending on the audience and type of oral dissemination setting or conference, the student will need to develop their presentation with the context of the audience and setting in mind (Stephenson et al., 2020). As an educator, helping your student reflect on the most appropriate audience for their dissemination is a good first step. In addition, determining the length of the presentation and the level of expertise of the topic will help the student focus on what type of presentation will be most effective for sharing their information and outcomes from their capstone.
- *Developing the "story" your student wants to tell.* Instead of conveying ideas on "paper," your student needs to understand the balance of telling their "story" in technical language versus layman's terminology, which may vary depending on the type of audience who is receiving their oral dissemination (Stephenson et al., 2020). This could be compared to writing a lay summary or impact statement for a research article, which is intended to provide an outline of the article content to non-specialists in the field (Tancock, 2018). The lay summary is an efficient way of conveying the essence of the project briefly and clearly. Important information to include in the lay summary are the justification, the background/context to the project, and the impact of the work, in chronological order (Tancock, 2018). In addition,

specific conferences may have guidance on the formatting of the presentation or stylistic recommendations which help set the "tone" for the conference. Tailoring the message to the core interest(s) of the participants and ensuring that there is a balance of data, examples, and anecdotal support can help the student convey the appropriate amount of information or visual information also.

Another example learning activity can be found in Text Box 12.9

> ## TEXT BOX 12-9
>
> **Teaching Tip:** Provide your students with an in-class activity or video assignment that requires them to provide a brief oral overview of their capstone project and outcomes to various audiences. For an in-class activity, students can role-play in small groups and provide feedback to each student presenter on their body language, presentation content, vocabulary (jargon), and overall presentation skills. The students who are not presenting can act as the audience and role-play their level of understanding and interest in the topic. For a video assignment, students can be assigned one or more audiences to present to and post their videos to the program's online learning platform for peer feedback. Consider assigning audiences such as the capstone site staff members, occupational therapy practitioners, laypeople, and others.

- *Audience engagement.* Coaching your student on how to engage their audience is an essential next step. Using instructional technology applications such as a poll embedded in their presentation may be a great way for them to engage the audience and solicit feedback from their audience participants. Several studies have found that polling technology increases learner satisfaction and participation (Castillo et al., 2020; Phelps & Moro, 2022; Sedghi et al., 2021). No matter if the oral presentation is in person or virtual, a poll may be a good strategy to gauge audience interest and understanding (Phelps & Moro, 2022). In addition, encouraging your student to use reflective questions or interactive activities, such as trivia, may help them engage their audience within their dissemination (Research Guide for Students, 2014). Consider instructional technologies, such as Mentimeter (n.d.) or Poll Everywhere (n.d.), which allow for polling, question-and-answer, word clouds, and more. These technologies can help create an environment of active learning and make the oral presentation less pressure for the student.

ADDITIONAL PRODUCTS RELATED TO THE CAPSTONE PROJECT DISSEMINATION

While a poster and oral presentation may be the most common forms of dissemination for capstone projects, they are not the only forms that will adequately meet the ACOTE requirement. Depending on your program, as well as the student's capstone focus, you might encourage students to "think outside the box." For example, a student who completes a project focused on applying evidence-based practice in a particular setting might create a written protocol for the occupational therapists at the site that guides them through the rationale and process of this clinical practice. Refer your students to the AOTA (2024) practice guidelines for clinical practice guideline exemplars.

Another example is a webinar or series of webinars. A capstone student might disseminate their project and results through a recorded voice-over slideshow. This is a creative way to reach audiences that may not be local to the program or capstone site or for those who may not be able to join for a synchronous session.

It may behoove you to provide examples of various forms of dissemination to your students early in the capstone planning process. Whether you create your own examples or ask permission from former capstone students whose dissemination products were excellent, it is helpful for students to visualize what various forms of dissemination might look like. Consider posting these online or having them available via hard copy somewhere in the program's offices.

A suggestion for your program to repurpose capstone dissemination products can be found in Text Box 12.10.

TEXT BOX 12-10

Teaching Tip: Consider re-packaging capstone dissemination products as a way to offer continued education and professional development to your alumni, fieldwork educator community, content experts, or local occupational therapy practitioners. Inviting them to attend the capstone disseminations (or view asynchronous presentations) is a fantastic way to celebrate student accomplishments with a robust audience while reconnecting and networking with practitioners who not only benefit from continued education but also may be able to serve as capstone mentors in the future! Check with your state regulations to see if you are able to offer continuing education contact hours or professional development units for these sorts of events.

EDUCATOR CHAPTER SUMMARY

This chapter has provided several recommendations and guidelines for you, the educator, to consider when guiding your students through the preparation and execution of a written and/or oral dissemination of the doctoral capstone project. Ensuring that the capstone aligns with the program's curricular design and communicates the impact of the capstone project with the intended audience(s) are keys to an impactful dissemination. As the capstone product may take on various forms, it is essential that the educator clearly communicates institutional requirements and provides the student with resources for additional dissemination at the local, national, or international levels as appropriate.

LEARNING ACTIVITIES

1. Require students to make an appointment with the writing center within your academic institution for review/discussion of at least one section of their written dissemination product to gain feedback.

2. Have students access the Purdue OWL (2024) website, and bookmark it in their search browser. Have them review the APA Manual (2020) and tab important/frequently utilized sections. Ask them to share the most helpful portions that they found with the class.

REFERENCES

Accreditation Commission for Audiology Education. (2016). *Accreditation standards for the doctor of audiology (Au.D.) program.* https://acaeaccred.org/standards/

Accreditation Council for Occupational Therapy Education. (2023). *2023 Accreditation Council for Occupational Therapy Education (ACOTE®) standards and interpretive guide.* https://acoteonline.org/accreditation-explained/standards/

Accreditation Council for Pharmacy Education. (2015). *Accreditation standards and key elements for the professional program in pharmacy leading to the doctor of pharmacy degree.* https://www.acpe-accredit.org/pdf/Standards2016FINAL.pdf

American Association of Colleges of Nursing. (2006). *The essentials of doctoral education for advanced nursing practice.* http://www.aacnnursing.org/DNP/DNP-Essentials

American Association of Colleges of Nursing. (2017). *DNP fact sheet.* http://www.aacnnursing.org/News-Information/Fact-Sheets/DNP-Fact-Sheet

American Occupational Therapy Association. (2018). *Vision 2025.* https://www.aota.org/Publications-News/AOTANews/2018/AOTA-Board-Expands-Vision–2025.aspx

American Occupational Therapy Association. (2020). Occupational therapy practice framework: Domain and process (4th ed.). *American Journal of Occupational Therapy*, 74(Suppl. 2), 7412410010p1–7412410010p87. https://doi.org/10.5014/ajot.2020.74S2001

American Occupational Therapy Association. (2024). *Evidence-based practice: Practice guidelines and evidence-based clinical resources.* https://www.aota.org/practice/practice-essentials/evidencebased-practiceknowledge-translation/practice-guidelines

American Psychological Association. (2020). *Publication manual of the American Psychological Association* (7th ed.). https://doi.org/10.1037/0000165–000

Anderson, B. A., Knestrick, J. M., & Barroso, R. (Eds.). (2015). *DNP capstone projects: Exemplars of excellence in practice.* Springer.

Augenstein, I., Baldwin, T., Cha, M., Chakraborty, T., Ciampaglia, G. L., Corney, D., DiResta, R., Ferrara, E., Hale, S., Halevy, A., Hovy, E., Ji, H., Menczer, F., Miguez, R., Nakov, P., Scheufele, D., Sharma, S., & Zagni, G. (2023). Factuality challenges in the era of large language models. *ArXiv.* https://doi.org/10.48550/arXiv.2310.05189

Barlow, S. J., Hanks, J., & Tate, J. J. (2018). A study of capstone courses utilized in United States Doctor of Physical Therapy program curricula. *Journal of Allied Health, 47,* 147–151.

Barroso, R. (2015). Burnout as a barrier to practice among nurse-midwives: Examining the evidence. In B. A. Anderson, J. M. Knestrick, & R. Barroso (Eds.), *DNP capstone projects: Exemplars of excellence in practice* (pp. 45–53). Springer.

Berkowitz, B. (2015). The emergence and impact of the DNP degree on clinical practice. In B. A. Anderson, J. M. Knestrick, & R. Barroso (Eds.), *DNP capstone projects: Exemplars of excellence in practice* (pp. 3–16). Springer.

Boniface, G., & Seymour, A. (Eds.). (2012). *Using occupational therapy theory in practice.* Wiley.

Bowen, J. A., & Watson, C. E. (Eds.). (2024). *Teaching with AI.* Johns Hopkins University Press.

Castillo, S., Thomas, L., Yarlagadda, S., Ahmed, Y., & Newman, J. R. (2020). Poll Everywhere to encourage learner satisfaction and participation in internal medicine fellowship didactics. *Cureus, 12*(2), e7078. https://doi.org/10.7759/cureus.7078

Commission on Accreditation in Physical Therapy Education. (2017). *Standards and required elements for accreditation of physical therapist education programs.* http://www.calstate.edu/app/dpt/documents/CAPTE-criteria–2009.pdf

DeIuliis, E. D. (2017). *Professionalism across occupational therapy clinical practice.* SLACK Incorporated.

Flarity, K., Holcomb, E., & Gentry, J. E. (2015). Promoting compassion fatigue resiliency among emergency department nurses. In B. A. Anderson, J. M. Knestrick, & R. Barroso (Eds.), *DNP capstone projects: Exemplars of excellence in practice* (pp. 67–78). Springer.

Herr, K., & Anderson, G. L. (2015). *The action research dissertation: A guide for students and faculty* (2nd ed.). Sage.

Hofmann, A. H. (2017). *Scientific writing and communication: Papers, proposals, and presentations* (3rd. ed.). Oxford University Press.

McCrea, P. (2023). *Developing expert teaching: A practical guide to designing effective professional development.* Routledge.

Mentimeter. (n.d.). https://www.mentimeter.com/

Mezirow, J. (1997). Transformative learning: Theory to practice. *New Directions for Adult and Continuing Education,* (74), 5–12. https://doi.org/10.1002/ace.7401

Mollick, E. R., & Mollick, L. (2023). *Using AI to implement effective teaching strategies in classrooms: Five strategies, including prompts.* The Wharton School Research Paper. SSRN. https://doi.org/10.2139/ssrn.4391243

Phelps, C., & Moro, C. (2022). Using live interactive polling to enable hands-on learning for both face-to-face and online students within hybrid-delivered courses. *Journal of University Teaching and Learning Practices, 19*(3). https://doi.org/10.53761/1.19.3.08.

Plack, M. M., & Wong, C. K. (2002). The evolution of the doctorate of physical therapy: Moving beyond the controversy. *Journal of Physical Therapy, 16,* 48–58.

Poll Everywhere. (n.d.). https://www.polleverywhere.com/

The Purdue Online Writing Lab. (2024). https://owl.english.purdue.edu/owl/resource/551/01

Reagon, C. (2012). Using occupational therapy theory within evidence-based practice. In G. Boniface & A. Seymour (Eds.), *Using occupational therapy theory in practice* (pp. 155–164). Wiley.

A Research Guide for Students. (2014). *Chapter 3: Presentation tips for public speaking.* http://www.aresearchguide.com/3tips.html

Robinson, M., Stroller, F., Costanza-Robinson, M., & Jones, J. K. (2008). *Write like a chemist: A guide and resource.* Oxford University Press.

Rothstein, J. (1998). Education at the crossroads: For today's practice, the DPT. *Physical Therapy, 78,* 358–360.

Sedghi, N., Limniou, M., Al-Nuiamy, W., Sandall, I., Al-Ataby, A., & Duret, D. (2021). Enhancing the engagement of large cohorts using live interactive polling and feedback. *Developing Academic Practice,* 31–50. https://doi.org/10.3828/dap.2021.6

Short, P. (2015). Changing the paradigm: Diabetic group visits in a primary care setting. In B. A. Anderson, J. M. Knestrick, & R. Barroso (Eds.), *DNP capstone projects: Exemplars of excellence in practice* (pp. 55–65). Springer.

Stephenson, S., Rogers, O., Ivy, C., Barron, R., & Burke, J. (2020). Designing effective capstone experiences and projects for entry-level doctoral students in occupational therapy: One program's approaches and lessons learned. *The Open Journal of Occupational Therapy, 8*(3), 1–12. https://doi.org/10.15453/2168–6408.1727

Tancock, C. (2018). *In a nutshell: How to write a lay summary.* Elsevier. https://www.elsevier.com/connect/in-a-nutshell-how-to-write-a-lay-summary

Wiley. (2023). *Higher ed's next chapter, 2023–2024: Four trends reshaping the learning landscape.* http://www.wiley.com/en-us/network/trending-stories/trends-in-higher-education-2023-2024-shaping-the-learning-landscape

Woods, E. N. (2001). The DPT: What it means for the profession. *PT Magazine, 9*(5), 36–43.

APPENDICES

Appendix 12-A
EXAMPLE TITLE PAGE

Title of Capstone Report   1

Title of Capstone Report

First M. Last, Contributing Author Name(s)

Author's Affiliations or Academic Institution Name

School/College/Division

Appendix 12-B

Doctoral Capstone Experience (DCE) Action Plan to Achieve In-Depth Skills

This form is to be used after the experiential plan is complete. In collaboration with your site mentor, outline how you, the OTD student, will achieve your self-authored individualized learning objectives indicating activities or action steps to take and proposed evidence of achievement of your learning objectives (add rows to the table as needed). Remember that this should align with your focus areas, and that you have 14 weeks.

Individualized Learning Objectives or Learning Targets	Activities, Strategies, and/or Actions to Achieve Objectives	Proposed Timeline for Each Objective	The Skills You Possess and the Resources You Can Access to Enable You	Proposed Evidence of Achievement of Learning Objective (Success Criteria)

Signatures below signify acceptance of the above proposal and approval to move forward with implementation. It is the student's responsibility to access resources, carry out these and/or other strategies to increase their knowledge and skill, aligned with their chosen focus area.

Student signature: _____   Date: _____

Content expert signature: _____   Date: _____

Proposed Timeline for the 14-Week Doctoral Capstone Experience
(*Please include doctoral capstone project components as well.*)

Please complete the following schedule as a tentative plan of how you foresee your time spent during the 14-week doctoral experience. This plan may be general at this point and subject to change. This is a tool to help you consider how you will spend time to meet your learning objectives as well as complete your culminating capstone project. Experiences, actions, and steps that you will take should align with your chosen focus area(s). Please share this with your entire capstone team.

DCE Week	Experiences, Actions, Steps	Notes/Miscellaneous
Week 1		
Week 2		
Week 3		
Week 4		
Week 5		
Week 6		
Week 7 MIDTERM EVALUATION DUE		
Week 8		
Week 9		
Week 10		
Week 11		
Week 12		
Week 13		
Week 14 FINAL EVALUATION DUE		

TITLE OF CAPSTONE PROJECT

Timeline of Program Development

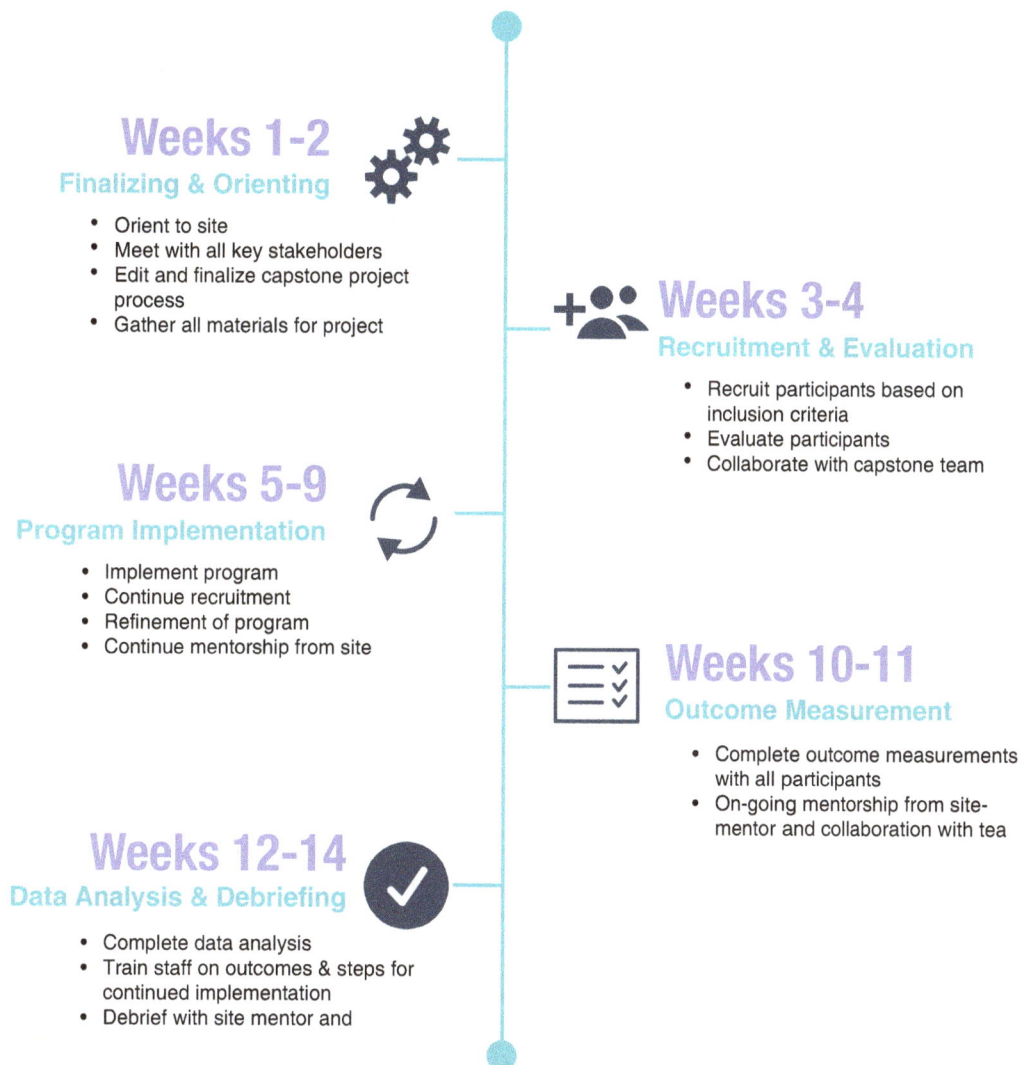

Weeks 1-2
Finalizing & Orienting

- Orient to site
- Meet with all key stakeholders
- Edit and finalize capstone project process
- Gather all materials for project

Weeks 3-4
Recruitment & Evaluation

- Recruit participants based on inclusion criteria
- Evaluate participants
- Collaborate with capstone team

Weeks 5-9
Program Implementation

- Implement program
- Continue recruitment
- Refinement of program
- Continue mentorship from site

Weeks 10-11
Outcome Measurement

- Complete outcome measurements with all participants
- On-going mentorship from site-mentor and collaboration with tea

Weeks 12-14
Data Analysis & Debriefing

- Complete data analysis
- Train staff on outcomes & steps for continued implementation
- Debrief with site mentor and

Appendix 12-C

EXAMPLE OF HOW TO DISPLAY RESULTS

Quantitative

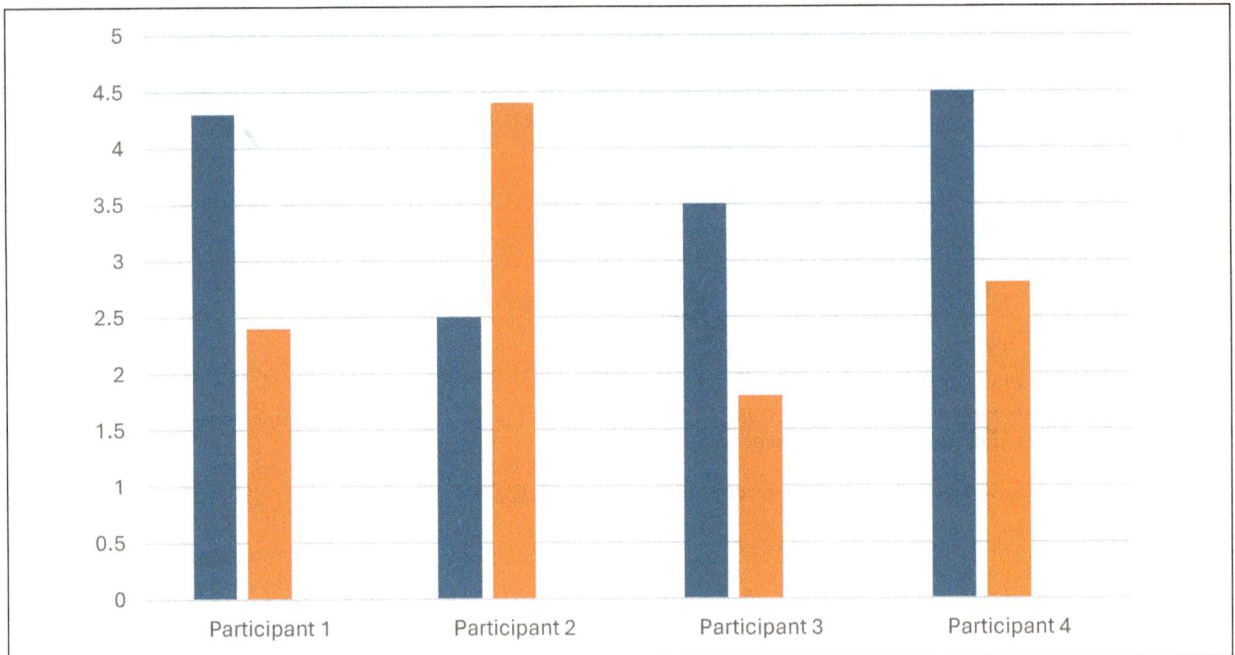

Qualitative

Participants were asked to describe their experience participating in the program. All participants noted positive experiences, and two shared that they hoped to continue utilizing the information shared even after the program had concluded. Participant 1 stated, "I really enjoyed the social nature of group therapy. It was beneficial to hear from other patients who were going through something very similar to what I'm going through, and how they are adjusting."

Example of Quantitative Data Analysis from a Capstone on Pressure Injury Education

Quantitative Data Analysis

Differences in Total Scores on Confidence in Interprofessional Pressure Injury Prevention and Management Questionnaire

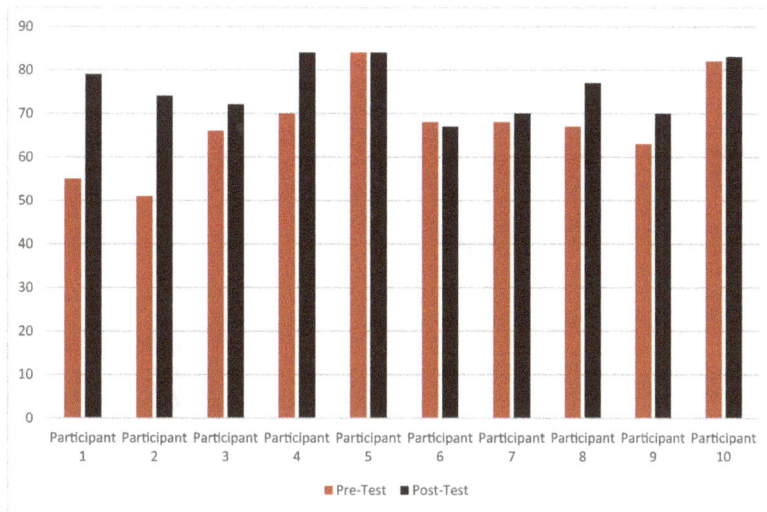

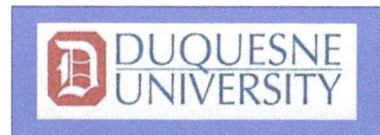

Quantitative Data Analysis Cont.

Table 1
Descriptive Statistics of Select Questions from Pre-Test/Post-Test
Collaboration Questionnaire (n = 10)

Selected Question	Mdn (IQR)	
Pre-Test Post-Test		
1. All interprofessional team members on the unit are committed to collaborative practice.	4 (5-2.75)	4 (5.25-3.75)
2. Each member's specific areas of expertise are always used for patient wound care.	3.5 (5-2.75)	4 (5-3.5)
3. Patient concerns regarding wound care are addressed effectively through regular team meetings and discussion.	2.5 (5-2)	4.5 (5-3)
4. Our interprofessional team has developed effective communication strategies to share concerns for patients at risk for developing pressure injuries.	3.5 (5-1.75)	4.5 (5-3.75)
5.Team members encourage patients to be active in their own pressure injury prevention.	5 (5-4)	5.5 (6-4.75)
6. The patient is considered a valued member of their health care team.	5 (6-4)	6 (6-4.75)

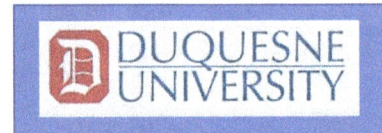

DUQUESNE UNIVERSITY

Example of Qualitative Data Analysis from a Capstone on Pressure Injury Education

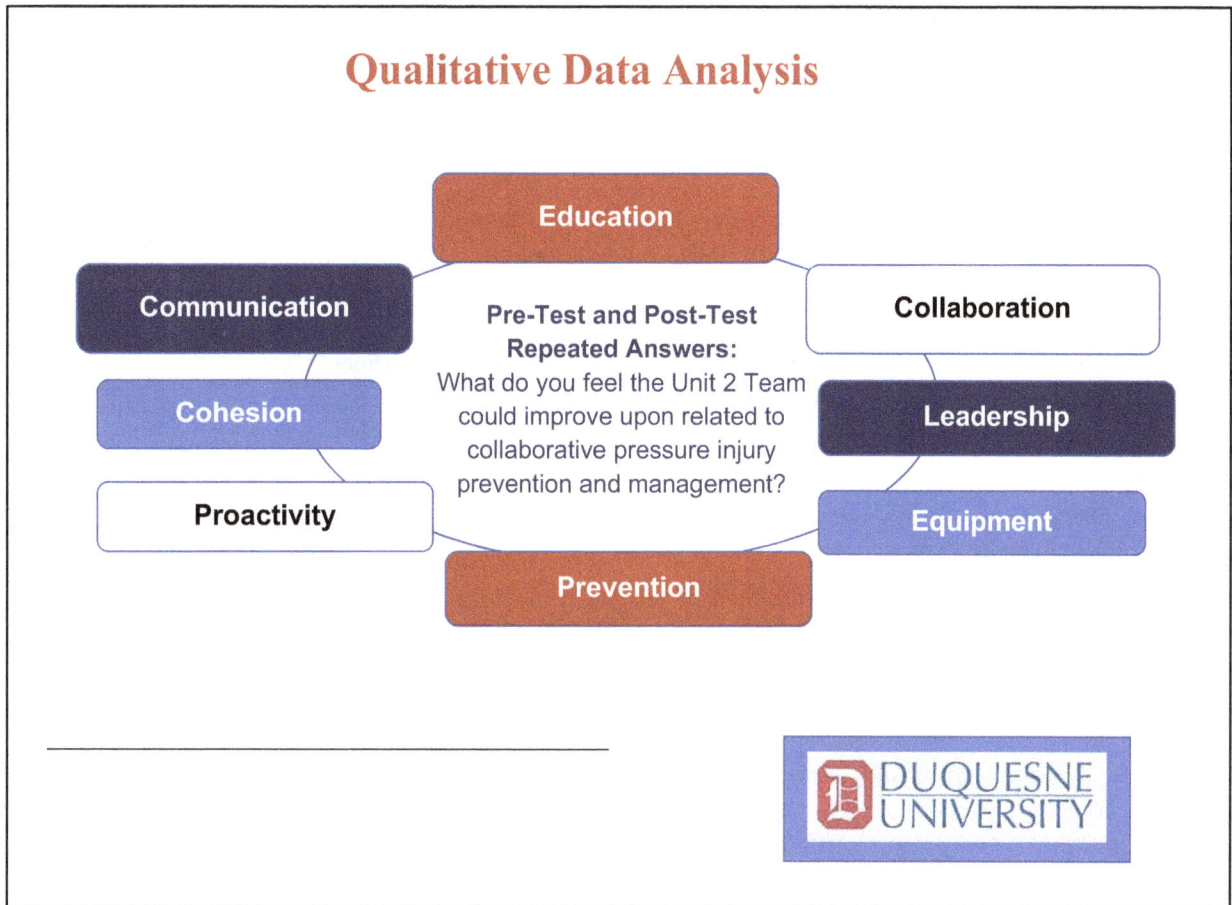

For qualitative data analysis, we analyzed open-ended responses on the questionnaires and searched for themes and repeated responses. Due to the lengthiness of responses, we felt the most impactful way to present our qualitative analysis was to showcase pretest and posttest responses to a meaningful question. The question that was selected was: What do you feel the unit 2 team could improve upon relating to collaborative pressure injury prevention and management? Responses that were repeated on both the pretest and posttest include education, collaboration, leadership, equipment, prevention, proactivity, cohesion, and communication. This shows that even after a 14-week program focused exactly on these items, the interprofessional team members still felt that they were their weakest areas. This parallels findings in literature that show prevention and collaboration are systemic barriers in health care that continuously need to be worked on and evolved to strengthen the quality of patient care provided.

– Alicia Colossi, OTD, Duquesne University, Pittsburgh, PA, class of 2024

Appendix 12-D
EXAMPLE POSTER FORMATTING AND CONTENTS CHECKLIST

_____ Poster dimensions are 36" × 38".

_____ The poster's title is in APA 7th edition formatting (e.g., Trauma-informed care for families: A doctoral capstone experience and project) – notice only the first word of the title and the first word after the colon are capitalized!

_____ The title is brief and descriptive, capturing the essence of your project.

_____ Your name, your faculty mentor's name, and the name of our institution are at the top of the poster.

- Confirm with your content expert if they would like you to include their name **and/or** site name on the poster.

_____ Any graphics used serve a purpose and enhance the verbal presentation.

_____ The font style is no less than 24 pt and permitted by APA 7th Edition guidelines.

- **Sans serif fonts**: Calibri, Arial, or Lucida Sans Unicode.
- **Serif fonts**: Times New Roman, Georgia, or Computer Modern (default font for LaTeX).

_____ The contents of the poster are written with *clarity* (apastyle.org).

- Uses language others will understand.
- Follows spelling and grammar conventions.
- Checked and edited for misplaced or missing ideas.
- Sections of the poster are easy to follow and are logically sequenced.

_____ The contents of the poster are written with *precision* (apastyle.org).

- Specific and consistent nouns and past-tense verbs.
- Provide exact numbers and statistics rather than approximations when reporting outcomes.
- Abbreviations used are consistent with APA 7th Edition abbreviations guide (see *Publication Manual* Sections 6.24–6.26).

_____ The contents of the poster are *inclusive* (apastyle.org).

- Describes communities and populations with dignity and respect.
- Calls communities and populations what they call themselves.
- Focuses on relevant characteristics.
- Uses bias-free and inclusive language.

_____ The poster's design is visually appealing and readable.

- Organized into clear sections with headings (you can use your capstone report sections as a guide).
- Graphs, charts, tables, or images illustrate your data effectively and are clearly labeled.
- The color palette provides adequate contrast and is visually appealing; it avoids use of too many colors.
- Leaves enough white/empty space to prevent clutter and improve readability.

_____ The poster includes a (summarized) Introduction section.

_____ The poster includes a (summarized) Needs Assessment section.

_____ The poster includes a (summarized) Literature Review section.

_____ The poster includes Capstone Project Plan and Process, Capstone Project Implementation, and Capstone Project Evaluation and Outcomes sections.

_____ The poster includes a *Discussion* section.

- Mentions sustainability.

_____ In-text citations are formatted using APA 7th Edition guidelines for citation style.

_____ Includes references list (e.g., QR code, printed handout, etc.).

_____ I have rehearsed/practiced the poster presentation and feel confident in my ability to present clearly, loud enough, and without a script.

Poster Presentation Scoring Rubric

STUDENT NAME	10 POINTS	8 POINTS	6 POINTS
Content, Organization, and Poster Design	The poster is clear and concise and follows a logical sequence. *You may want to use your paper sections as a loose reference for organization.*	The presentation is clear and concise and follows a logical sequence. It is, however, at times difficult to follow reasoning of the student, leading the audience to be confused.	The presentation is poorly organized and lacks logical sequencing. The audience has difficulty following the major concepts of the presentation.
Theoretical Basis	A theoretical basis for the DCE is clearly described in this presentation, and the relationship to practice is clear and well-developed.	A theoretical basis for the DCE is described in this presentation, however lacks a clear relationship to practice.	A theoretical basis for the DCE described in this presentation; however, there is minimal connection to practice and more depth of thought is needed.
Synthesis of Advanced Knowledge	The student demonstrates excellent synthesis of advanced knowledge in their focus area, and content is supported by relevant literature. ACOTE area(s) of focus are listed.	The student demonstrates good synthesis of advanced knowledge in their focus area, and content is supported by relevant literature. ACOTE area(s) of focus are not included.	A fair synthesis of advanced knowledge in their focus area is presented, and more depth is needed. ACOTE area(s) of focus are not included.
Evaluation Method and Project Outcomes	The student provides an excellent description of project evaluation and clearly states project outcomes.	The student provides a good description of project evaluation and clearly states the project outcomes.	The student does not communicate clearly a description of project evaluation and/or does not describe project outcomes.
Overall Presentation Style	The student is very well rehearsed and not just reading from a script. The student is confident in materials presented. Student speaks clearly and loud enough to be heard.	The student is rehearsed, however reads too much from a script. Student needs more rehearsal to increase confidence.	The student is just reading from a script and appears not well rehearsed. More rehearsal is needed. Student does not demonstrate confidence in materials.

Total Score = _____/50 points

Appendix 12-E

EXAMPLE CAPSTONE PROJECT POSTER PRESENTATION

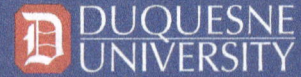

Enhancing Competence and Self-Efficacy in Direct Care Staff Through a Hybrid Dementia Education Training Program

Emma Fitzgerald, BS, OTD[1]; Elizabeth D. DeIuliis[1], OTD, OTR/L, FNAP, FAOTA; Erin McMaster[2]

[1] Duquesne University; Pittsburgh, PA; [2] Arden Courts; Pittsburgh, PA

DUQUESNE UNIVERSITY
John G. Rangos, Sr.
School of Health Sciences

BACKGROUND

- OT practitioners often provide direct services to individuals with dementia but are rarely involved in educating direct care staff (DCS) in memory care.
- Despite DCS's critical role in assisting residents, continued education is limited. From 2011 to 2021, the DCS workforce grew by 1.5 million (Gaugler et al., 2023), yet the lack of ongoing training affects job satisfaction, retention, and care quality.
- Research shows that dementia training improves staff knowledge, competence, and attitudes (Spector et al., 2016), enhancing empathetic care and job satisfaction (Rasmussen et al., 2023).
- This capstone project aimed to address this gap in education at a memory care facility.

RELEVANT LITERATURE

Relevance to Practice: Should be relevant to caregivers to ensure transfer of knowledge (Surr et al., 2016)	Non-Pharmacological Approach: Non-drug interventions are more effective than medication (Carrarini et al., 2021)
Managing Agitation & Adverse Behaviors: Agitation is common and DCS should be equipped with strategies (Carrarini et al., 2021)	Continued Education: Education is vital to maintain and enhance care quality (Rasmussen et al., 2023)

PARTICIPANT SAMPLE

- Participant sample: n=6 with a mean age of 42.17 years
- 83.3% female and 16.6% male
- All participants had a high school diploma or higher
- Years Experience with Dementia Population
  - 1-2 years: 33.3%
  - 3-5 years: 33.3%
  - 6-10 years: 16.6%
  - More than 10 years: 16.6%
- No participants have ever had additional dementia training outside of mandatory facility training

PROGRAM DESIGN

- One-group pretest/posttest design to evaluate a 10-week dementia training program for direct care staff
- 4 virtual, asynchronous training modules; two (optional) face-to-face mentoring sessions
  - *Back to Basics:* Types of Dementia and its Progression
  - *The Skill Spectrum:* Levels of Physical and Cognitive Ability
  - *Tranquility Tactics:* Addressing Agitation and Adverse Behaviors in Dementia
  - *Crafting Capabilities:* Adapting and Modifying Meaningful Activities for Residents
- Instruments:
  - Competence was measured using a 20-item multiple-choice questionnaire aligned with modules.
  - Self-efficacy was assessed via the Caring Efficacy Scale (Shrestha et al., 2023).
  - Satisfaction Survey to assess dementia training as a whole.
- Statistical significance was evaluated using the Wilcoxon Signed-Rank test.

PROGRAM OUTCOMES

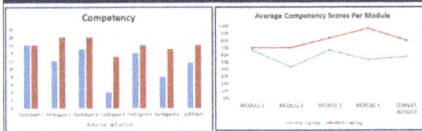

Figure 1: This shows an overall improvement in competency scores from pre-test to post-test for all participants.

Figure 2: This graph shows and increase in average competency scores across all 4 learning modules.

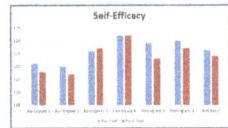

Figure 3: This bar chart compares self-efficacy pre-test and post-test scores, showing a general decline in self-efficacy following the training.

DISCUSSION

- 83.3% of participants demonstrated an increase in competency. The average & overall score increased from pre- to post-training for each module. The average overall score went from a 57.5% pre-training to an 80% post-training.
- 66.6% of participants demonstrated a decrease in self-efficacy. This suggests that while knowledge increased, new awareness of care complexities may have led to temporary doubt in their abilities. This outcome may align with the Dunning-Kruger effect, where initial overconfidence is replaced by a more realistic self-assessment post-training. However, it is also possible participants could have come to an understanding that their previous methods might not have been the most effective, thus temporarily lowering their self-efficacy score as they acknowledge their shortcomings.
- 100% of staff participants stated that they were 'very satisfied' with the training program as a whole, and also expressed its applicability and relevance to their daily responsibilities.

IMPACT STATEMENT

"I appreciate now having knowledge about the different types of dementia and how they effect residents. It helps me better understand what they are going through."

"One thing I took away from this training is that ways of engaging residents in meaningful activities can also help reduce agitation."

- These program outcomes suggest that dementia care training programs can enhance staff competence, but they may also highlight gaps in confidence due to the complexity of dementia care, requiring additional support.
- This heightened competence can translate into more effective care strategies, such as using appropriate communication techniques, recognizing early signs of agitation, and adapting activities to match residents' level of ability.
- To improve long-term outcomes, facilities should implement ongoing training, hands-on practice, and regular feedback to reinforce skills and enhance self-efficacy.

REFERENCES

Scan the QR code to view references

Appendix 12-F

EXAMPLE OF A RUBRIC FOR A FINAL WRITTEN CAPSTONE REPORT

CRITERIA	EXCELLENT (4)	GOOD (3)	SATISFACTORY (2)	NEEDS IMPROVEMENT (1)	WEIGHT
Introduction	Clear, compelling introduction; provides context, purpose, and relevance of the capstone project with thorough background information.	Clear introduction with context and purpose but may lack some depth or detail in presenting the background.	Introduction provides basic context but lacks depth, leaving gaps in understanding the project's purpose.	Weak or unclear introduction; fails to present the project's background or significance.	10%
Needs Assessment	Comprehensive assessment of the problem, including clear identification of the need, target population, and contextual factors.	Clear needs assessment but may lack detail or full consideration of contextual factors.	Needs assessment addresses the problem but is superficial or lacks clarity.	Insufficient or unclear needs assessment; does not effectively describe the issue.	10%
Literature Review	Thorough review of relevant, recent literature that critically analyzes existing research; clear synthesis of key findings.	Solid review of literature with synthesis, though may not cover all relevant studies or offer a deep analysis.	Limited review of literature; may omit key studies or fail to critically analyze sources.	Incomplete or poorly organized literature review; lacks relevance or synthesis.	15%
Driving Theory or Conceptual Model	Clearly explains and justifies the chosen theory or model; demonstrates strong connection to the project goals and objectives.	Clear explanation of the theory or model, with some connection to project objectives, though not fully explored.	Theory or model is described, but explanation is weak or only loosely connected to the project.	Theory or model is unclear, inadequately explained, or not relevant to the project.	10%
Capstone Plan and Process	Detailed, well-organized plan, with clear steps and timelines; fully addresses project goals and logistics.	Well-organized plan with clear steps, but minor gaps or lack of clarity in timeline or process.	Plan is outlined but lacks detail, or some steps are unclear or underdeveloped.	Plan is vague, is incomplete, or lacks sufficient detail to guide project implementation.	10%

continued

Project Implementation	Clear, detailed account of the implementation process; addresses challenges and describes successful strategies.	Provides a solid description of implementation, with minor gaps in explaining challenges or strategies used.	Implementation is described but lacks depth or clarity; some details are missing or unclear.	Implementation section is vague or lacks detail; does not adequately explain how the project was carried out.	15%
Project Evaluation and Outcomes	Thorough, clear evaluation of project outcomes, with clear evidence of success or areas for improvement; uses appropriate methods and analysis.	Good evaluation of outcomes with clear analysis, though some aspects may be less detailed or not fully assessed.	Evaluation is attempted but lacks depth, clarity, or appropriate methods for assessing outcomes.	Evaluation is unclear, is incomplete, or does not appropriately address the outcomes of the project.	10%
Discussion and Impact	Thoughtful, comprehensive discussion of project impact on the OT profession, community, and stakeholders; connects outcomes to broader implications.	Strong discussion of impact, though may lack depth in some areas or broader connections to the OT profession.	Impact is discussed but lacks depth or broader implications; may be overly narrow in focus.	Weak or unclear discussion of impact; fails to relate outcomes to larger context or stakeholders.	10%
Conclusion	Clear, concise, and reflective conclusion; summarizes key findings, implications, and future directions in a compelling manner.	Clear conclusion, with summary of findings and implications, but may lack a strong final reflection or future outlook.	Conclusion summarizes findings but is weak in connecting them to implications or future directions.	Weak or unclear conclusion; does not effectively summarize the report or provide future recommendations.	5%
Writing Mechanics (Grammar, Style, Clarity)	Exceptionally clear, well-organized, and professional writing; excellent grammar, spelling, and punctuation; strong sentence structure and academic tone.	Generally clear and well-organized, with few grammar, spelling, or punctuation errors; writing is professional but may lack some fluidity.	Writing is understandable but contains frequent errors in grammar, spelling, punctuation, or sentence structure; occasionally detracts from clarity.	Writing is unclear or disorganized; frequent errors in grammar, spelling, punctuation, or sentence structure significantly hinder readability and clarity.	5%

PART V. POST-PROFESSIONAL CAPSTONE

This section of the book is a comprehensive capstone project guide for the post-professional OTD student and educator. The chapter will lead the student through all the steps of the capstone project, including *inspiration*, *ideation*, *implementation*, and *dissemination*. It will equip the educator with resources to guide and coach the post-professional student through the entire process.

DOI: 10.4324/9781003541813-17

CHAPTER 13

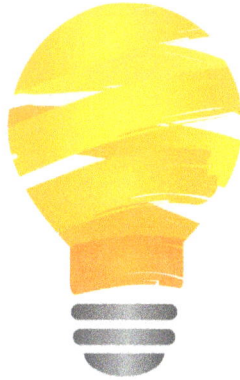

The Post-Professional Occupational Therapy Doctorate Capstone

Megan Albright and Sara Story

Section 1: Student Focus

Human-Centered Design Mindsets for the Post-Professional OT Doctoral Student

The human-centered design process of inspiration, ideation, and implementation can help guide you, the post-professional occupational therapy doctorate (PP OTD) student, through your capstone process (Asiello & Winstead, 2025). Each of these phases is evident throughout the process over the course of the specific PP OTD program. While each PP OTD program will define the phases differently, as well as the timeline for the capstone process, all are relevant as you move through your program.

Inspiration. During this phase, the mindset of **embrace ambiguity** will be important as you begin your capstone project journey. Giving yourself permission to explore and embrace not knowing the answers yet to the problem you want to solve is part of design thinking (IDEO.org, 2015). The idea for a capstone project starts even before the PP OTD student decides to pursue an advanced degree. For many, a clinical query or desire to advance clinical practice skills is the inspiration for returning to school to obtain a PP OTD, which can evolve into an idea for a capstone project. Inspiration may come from a desire to transition from clinical practice into a leadership role or shift to academia. From these ideas, the development of the project begins. During the initial semester in your PP OTD program, you will most likely be working on identifying and refining professional goals and brainstorming on how these initial conceptual ideas can be transitioned into a tangible capstone project within the time frame allowed by your program. This phase includes identifying relevant literature to support the PP OTD project. Performing a thorough literature review during this phase is helpful as it assists in identifying a gap this project will fill. Key resources and support personnel to assist in design are being defined during this phase.

Ideation. The planning phase of the project aligns with the ideation process of human-centered design. During this phase, you will focus on developing and defining the problem and purpose. Having the mindset of **creative confidence** that you have the skills to act on your big ideas and create a project is needed. "It is the belief

DOI: 10.4324/9781003541813-18

that you can and will come up with creative solutions to big problems and the confidence that all it takes is rolling up your sleeves and diving in" (IDEO.org, 2015, p. 19). During this phase, you will also **iterate, iterate, iterate**. You are problem-solving and, by continually iterating, refining and improving your project to find a successful solution to a problem (IDEO.org, 2015). Specific goals and objectives are outlined during this phase, and you will take on the task of finding solutions to assist in improving knowledge within your area of practice. Capstone team members are identified; they can include, and are not limited to, a faculty mentor, content expert, instructor of record, and other key personnel. During this time, the methods of your capstone are defined, and you will submit to the institutional review board (IRB). This section blends with the implementation phase in the sense that as it is ending, the implementation is beginning.

Implementation. The final phase of the PP OTD capstone process aligns with the implementation phase of human-centered design. This phase brings the capstone idea and planning to life; during this time, you will work on gathering data to support your capstone's purpose. The mindset of "**Optimism** is the thing that drives you forward" (IDEO.org, 2015, p. 24). You will determine how your capstone project affects the specified area of practice and what additional knowledge is provided to this area. Keep your focus on what could be, not the barriers that get in your way. Additionally, during this phase, you will focus on how the information will help with further knowledge translation and bridging gaps in the literature. Dissemination via presentation and written work is the final stage of the capstone process, which allows you to determine the sustainability of the project and how it benefits the occupational therapy profession.

INTRODUCTION FOR STUDENTS

Although this book is geared toward the entry-level occupational therapy (OTD) capstone, within this new edition, we wanted to recognize that there are limited published resources that align with the post-professional occupational therapy (PP OTD) degree. It is common for advanced graduate degrees to require a scholarly capstone-like requirement, and this chapter will take you through the capstone project. The PP OTD capstone has been described as a culminating project, with stated objectives, learning activities, and outcomes (Lampe et al., 2020).

While there are key differences between the entry-level OTD degree and the PP OTD degree, there also might be some similarities among the process of how a scholarly doctoral capstone project is developed, implemented, and disseminated. Because there are not overarching occupational therapy accreditation requirements governing how the PP OTD degree is implemented, it is common that a PP OTD curriculum and focus of a scholarly project such as a capstone is highly customizable for the working practitioner, based upon their current practice setting and/or employer. This chapter will help compare the entry-level OTD vs. the PP OTD, as well as identify, and discuss pragmatics that differ between the two-degree pathways and related capstone culminating projects. As the entry-level OTD has specific members of the capstone team, the PP OTD does as well; these members may include a faculty member within the PP OTD program who might serve as a mentor or advisor, and even a content expert that might align with your PP OTD capstone project or be within your work setting, which is probably where your project most likely will take place.

Each role is important in the design and completion of your project. The content expert will assist you with the clinical or specifics of the project, that is, what is necessary to ensure cohesion with your area of practice. Your faculty mentor is focused on the pragmatics of the project, what is realistic and attainable during the capstone time frame. This chapter will also point out how previous chapters in this book can be utilized to support the PP OTD student during completion of their capstone.

STUDENT REFLECTIVE QUESTIONS

1. What is your motivation or passion for advancing your education in occupational therapy?

2. Have you thought of some ways that you can make a practice impact on your current work setting or place of employment?

3. What considerations have you accounted for in your project, your practice, and how will these influence the capstone project?

4. What steps are you taking to ensure you can complete your project within the defined time frame?

5. How will you use feedback from your faculty, content experts, mentors, and peer cohort to refine and improve your project?

6. How will you define your relationship with your peers, your faculty, mentors, and content expert?

7. Are you aware of what your PP OTD program expectations are regarding dissemination upon completion of the capstone project?

8. How will you know your process has been effective and your project was successful?

STUDENT OBJECTIVES

By the end of reading this chapter and completing the learning activities, the student should be able to:

1. Compare and contrast doctoral dissertation vs. entry-level OTD capstone vs. post-professional (PP OTD) capstone projects.
2. Explain the roles and responsibilities of the PP OTD capstone team members.
3. Design a post-professional capstone project.
4. Evaluate outcomes of the PP OTD capstone project.
5. Compare and contrast PP OTD project dissemination methods.

HOW DOES THE PP OTD STUDENT DIFFER FROM THE ENTRY-LEVEL OTD STUDENT?

Throughout this book, you have learned that an entry-level OTD student is an individual that is pursuing their _initial degree_ in occupational therapy. Therefore, this person has obtained an undergraduate degree, is enrolled in graduate-level occupational therapy education to be eligible to sit for the national certification exam and complete licensure requirements. An entry-level OTD student that is completing their capstone has their prior fieldwork experience as clinical experience. They have not formally held an occupational therapy job or functioned as an occupational therapist in practice. An entry-level OTD student is _seeking to enter_ the occupational therapy profession.

One of the main differences between an entry-level OTD program and a post-professional OTD program is the target audience. The target audience for a post-professional OTD program are occupational therapists who already hold an entry-level occupational therapy degree (this could be a bachelor's or master's degree in OT), already are credentialed in the field (which includes national registration and/or licensure), and are seeking advanced graduate education. (See Text Box 13-1.) Post-professional programs are designed to enhance the skills and knowledge of practicing therapists. Post-professional graduate students returning for an advanced degree have determined that they are ready to take on the challenge of this type of degree program. The emphasis of each degree program can vary depending on the mission of the institution or program philosophy. Therefore, post-professional occupational therapy programs focus on furthering clinical skills knowledge, developing skills to engage in scholarly activities or leadership roles, or enhancing teaching and educational methods to impart knowledge. Students in a post-professional occupational therapy doctorate program have obtained an entry-level degree in occupational therapy (bachelor's or master's) and may work full- or part-time while completing their degree, which lends to professional growth and advancement (Lampe et al., 2020).

TEXT BOX 13-1

Bridge programs are offered at some institutions and can help individuals with a bachelor's degree earn a master's or doctorate in occupational therapy. For example, a practitioner that has a bachelor's in occupational therapy degree might be able to enroll in a PP OTD program without holding a master's degree and complete coursework that addresses gaps in knowledge and skills between a bachelor's degree and the advanced competencies required at the doctoral level. This may include competency areas such as leadership, evidence-based practice, policy, and other areas that are central to the PP OTD graduate degree. In addition to academic coursework, bridge programs often provide opportunities for clinical practice and a capstone or doctoral project.

HOW DOES A POST-PROFESSIONAL DEGREE DIFFER FROM AN ENTRY-LEVEL DEGREE?

Although this chapter is focused on the post-professional OTD degree track, there are other post-professional degrees that occupational therapists might consider to advanced their knowledge and education; these include a doctorate of health sciences (DHS), clinical sciences doctorate (CScD), doctor of philosophy or research doctorate (PhD), and doctor of education (EdD), to name a few. These degrees are generally more research-focused and prepare graduates for different career outcomes. Those practitioners who want to focus on specific knowledge areas and advanced knowledge within the field of occupational therapy align well with the scope of the PP OTD degree. While both degrees do allow for teaching in higher education, faculty tracks may be restricted as clinical doctorates may not be recognized by some academic institutions for a tenure-track position. (See Text Box 13-2.)

As discussed in Chapter 12, typically a PhD is more academically focused and research-intensive, with the expectation to establish an original line of research. The product generated to formally present the original research is called a dissertation. A clinical doctorate is more focused on applying existing research or knowledge to practical (clinical) problems and critically analyzing effective professional practices within your field of study. Practice scholarship, which involves the "discovery of knowledge in practice," is an important element within the clinical doctorate degree (Moyers & Quint, 2025, p. 1). Whereas the productivity generated from PhD and research-based degrees usually aligns with Boyer's model of scholarship, the scholarship of knowledge discovery in practice model, proposed by Moyers and Quint (2025), is a useful framework to guide the scholarly work that is generated by occupational therapy doctorate students through capstone projects.

TEXT BOX 13-2

The American Occupational Therapy Association (AOTA) defines a *terminal degree* for occupational therapists as a doctoral degree in occupational therapy or a related field (AOTA, 2022).

Although, at the national level, the occupational therapy doctorate (both entry-level and post-professional) **is** recognized as a terminal degree, note that individual academic institutions may have different parameters required for eligibility for tenure-stream or research-based faculty positions. When interested in academia as a career and going through the interview process, it is very important to clarify degree requirements and qualifications aligned with the faculty structure.

Another key difference between the entry-level OTD degree and the PP OTD degree is accreditation oversight. Currently, at the time of this book's publication, there are no current occupational therapy accreditation guidelines for post-professional occupational therapy programs. Because there is not a formal overarching accreditation governance in place, an individual interested in pursuing

advanced graduate education needs to be savvy when reviewing different program options, as there are several differences that might be observed. See Table 13-1 for a snapshot of some common differences that might be found between PP OTD programs in the United States.

Prospective PP OTD students can peruse a listing of all available PP OTD programs in the United States on the AOTA webpage, under the Education tab.

WHY DO I WANT TO RETURN TO SCHOOL FOR A PP OTD DEGREE?

Re-read the header here again. How would you answer this question? *Why do you want to return to school to pursue a PP OTD?* A helpful place to start to gather information and best practice resources is at the professional level, such as the AOTA, which outlines various reasons or motivations behind why one would obtain their PP OTD, including leadership, teaching, specialization, community impact, health-care advocacy, research, or publication (Rains & Pfaff, 2024). There are many benefits, but you need to decide why returning to school is important to you! All reasons identified to obtain a PP OTD allow you to discover and gain practice knowledge, grow in your career, and increase your engagement and contribution within the occupational therapy profession as whole. With ACOTE standards outlining the requirement of a doctoral degree for all full-time faculty in entry-level OTD

Table 13-1 PP OTD Program Variability

PROGRAM REQUIREMENT	DESCRIPTION
Admission requirements	• Varies from being able to apply as a new MS/MOT graduate to requiring a specific number of years or months working as an occupational therapist. • Some programs require an interview. • Some programs require GRE testing.
Timeline to complete program	• Around 12 months to 24 months, depending upon the level of entry OT degree (bachelor's or master's) and length of capstone project. • Part-time options may be available, which could prolong the degree completion beyond two years.
Credits to complete PP OTD	• About 30–40 credits, depending on length of program (in months/years). • Some programs offer credit for leadership or clinical experience.
Identifying a "track" or concentration	• Some programs offer a variety of specializations to pursue, such as leadership/advocacy, teaching in rehabilitation, management, and or/research. • Some programs have coursework that also contributes to the achievement of micro-credentials or certificates.
Delivery	• Many programs are 100% online, and some are taught in a hybrid model which requires synchronous courses or in-person meetings throughout the program.

programs, obtaining a PP OTD degree can be an easy decision for those that are already in academia and want to stay, but it may not be so clear for everyone (ACOTE, 2023). Understanding the benefits can be helpful in your decision-making process; growth in leadership skills, engagement in scholarly work, and increasing self-confidence as a clinician could be reasons for returning to school. Career opportunities and commitment to the occupational therapy profession may be the reason you want to return to school (Case-Smith et al., 2014). Additionally, you may want to advance your degree and background to help you climb the clinical leadership ladder where you work. If this is an area of interest to you, it does not necessarily mean you need to have one specific path to obtain a leadership position; it can also mean developing your skills to gain advanced/specialty certification, participate in company-wide committees or process-improvement projects, present to peers at continuing education events or conferences (Bitanga & Austria, 2013). These are just a few examples as to how you can improve your clinical status and professional development through an advanced degree.

Now that we have reviewed some of the contextual information that situates how a PP OTD program and student differ from the entry-level degree, this next section of the chapter will focus on the scholarly capstone component. As put forth with the rest of this textbook, the information in this chapter is to provide a generalizable resource to help guide you through the PP OTD capstone process. Each academic institution has their own specific process and expectations, so ensure that you are thoroughly reviewing your program's curriculum design and requirements.

OVERVIEW OF CAPSTONE PROCESS

Similar to the entry-level occupational therapy doctoral capstone, the post-professional doctoral capstone is process-oriented. (See Figure 13-1.) As a practicing clinician looking to advance your education and knowledge, you might consider exploring the benefits and differences between a post-professional occupational therapy degree, which is typically identified as a clinical doctorate degree, versus a research-based doctoral degree (PhD or EdD).

This book has clearly articulated that the entry-level OTD capstone project must be clearly aligned to the ACOTE D standards, with the focus on specific areas of experiential learning, including clinical practice skills, research skills, administration, leadership, program development and evaluation, advocacy, education (ACOTE, 2023). The entry-level capstone differs from the PP OTD capstone in many ways; one significant difference is the need to root the entry-level doctoral capstone to specific focus areas prescribed by ACOTE, as discussed in Chapter 2, as well as the need to have two distinct components of a 14-week experience and an individual capstone project. Although the focus areas do not specifically apply to the PP OTD capstone project, they can certainly be used to inspire brainstorming regarding potential project ideas.

PP OTD students are not confined by ACOTE standards; though the specific institution and program will have guidelines for student projects, the timeline will vary based on the program duration, which varies from university to university. Many PP OTD programs outline the capstone implementation process to range from 6 to 16 weeks, with completion required by commencement of the program.

The next following sections will move you through the six stages described in Figure 13-1 to design, implement, and evaluate a post-professional OTD capstone project.

Phase 1 Inspiration

Developing professional writing skills. Although as clinicians, we engage in various writing activities aligned with the occupational therapy progress (e.g., assessment write-ups, progress notes, transition plans, discharge summaries, individualized education programs [IEP] plans, etc.), professional or academic writing might not be something that you have engaged in for many years. Therefore, returning to school as a PP OTD student and the scholarly writing expectations associated with the coursework, and specifically the capstone project, can be daunting.

Resources and assignments to help encourage professional writing can be helpful and supportive for you as you take on the task of writing and developing your PP OTD capstone paper. Some textbooks your instructors may recommend are *A Writer's Toolkit for Occupational Therapy and Health Care Professionals*, which is designed to help writers develop confidence, tools, and skills to support their journey to becoming a writer (Whitney & Davis, 2013). This text can guide you, a novice writer, through

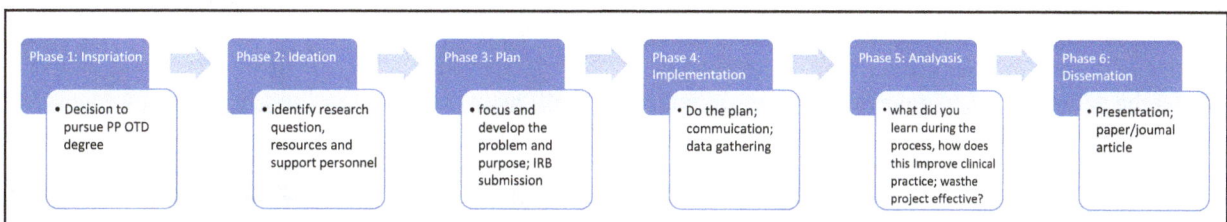

Phase 1: Inspiration	Phase 2: Ideation	Phase 3: Plan	Phase 4: Implementation	Phase 5: Analysis	Phase 6: Dissemation
• Decision to pursue PP OTD degree	• identify research question, resources and support personnel	• focus and develop the problem and purpose; IRB submission	• Do the plan; commuication; data gathering	• what did you learn during the process, how does this Improve clinical practice; wasthe project effective?	• Presentation; paper/joumal article

Figure 13-1. Overview of the capstone process.

the process of gaining confidence in writing skills, various writing styles, and types of publications. *Journal Article Writing and Publication: Your Guide to Mastering Clinical Health Care Reporting Standards* by Gutman (2017) is another resource which can help you with finalizing your writing and assist you in the process of writing a journal article. It outlines specifics necessary for each type of project being completed. Other areas of Gutman (2017) that may be helpful for you as you embark upon your first journey in scholarly writing is Chapter 13, on ethical considerations in publication. This chapter outlines the dos and don'ts during the submission process; many of these are a surprise to students upon reading this chapter (Gutman, 2017). You may benefit from the no-nonsense writing style presented in Gutman (2017), as well as providing you valuable insight into the journal submission and publication process. The American Psychological Association (APA, 2020) manual is another essential resource that will be helpful to ensure proper citations, format tables and figures, reduce language bias, and guide you much of the stylistic and formatting aspects of the scholarly writing process. Throughout the capstone process, each of the aforementioned texts can help you find your writing style and, as for many, make the transition from clinical writing to academic writing easier.

Developing evidence-based practice skills. Evidence-based practice is defined as clinical decision-making framework encouraging clinicians to integrate information from qualitative and quantitative research to assist in making decisions for clients and interventions (Sackett et al., 1996). Evidence-based practice is a key part of your clinical thinking and work as an occupational therapist. Developing skills for understanding and implementing evidence-based practice is an essential component of your capstone project. During your time as a student, you will utilize evidence-based practice skills to determine relevance for your capstone project. The following steps can help guide you in the process: Identify clinical questions relevant to your needs; search literature to identify relevance to your clinical question; review the research to determine if it is valid and, if results are clinically important, how the information can be applied in the clinical setting or with your capstone project; and review and evaluate your process each time you find relevant literature (University of Queensland, n.d.). Continued development of your evidence-based practice skills will be an area of focus throughout your capstone process. Initiating the literature search and review process early in your development will help you identify relevant literature and help identify a direction for your project. Evidence-based practice can be daunting at first, but as a clinician, you utilize evidence every day within your intervention planning processes; this takes it from the hands-on clinic view to how it will impact your capstone. As a PP OTD student, you should be working closely with your program's library and utilizing the support services provided to develop your evidence-based practice skills.

Brainstorming a direction for your PP OTD capstone. How do you decide the focus of your capstone project? This is an important question as you embark on your PP OTD journey. You might be inspired through an area of your practice or population that you work with that you have empathized with; here is where that human-centered design mindset of empathy is tapped into. Or you might have identified something within your own place of employment or area of practice that has sparked your interest, and you enjoy researching and learning more about. There are a variety of practice model groups where a PP OTD student can engage in the discovery of knowledge (Moyers & Quint, 2025). Moyers and Quint (2025) propose ten areas of scholarship of discovery in practice, which include "advocacy/policy development, practice reasoning/decision making, consumer issues, evidence-based practice, implementation science, innovation, leadership/administration, program development and evaluation, quality improvement and teaching/learning" (p. 3).

Review these areas of scholarship of discovery in practice (Moyers & Quint, 2025), and begin to think about potential ideas for your capstone project based on your career path/goals. The following ten areas of scholarship of discovery in practice have been adapted from Moyers and Quint (2025).

Advocacy/policy development. Is there a policy that you feel you may want to analyze, develop, and evaluate through advocacy? How might you empower a community in which you are involved to engage in advocacy? How can advocacy impact health and well-being within the context of your capstone?

Practice reasoning/decision-making. Do you want to explore shared decision-making in your practice area? What problem are you having in your clinical site in which decision-making and clinical reasoning may impact a solution?

Consumer issues. Do you want to focus on client satisfaction and experiences within your practice setting? Are there issues of health literacy that could be addressed to improve the experience of your clients and/or the populations you serve?

Evidence-based practice. How can you use evidence to answer a practice question? Would you be interested in developing practice guidelines or policies based on best available evidence?

Implementation science. Is there a particular intervention strategy that you would like to appraise evidence for ethical use?

Innovation. Are you interested in technology innovation and creating evidence to support the innovation? Maybe you are utilizing smart home technology with older adults or virtual reality and you would like to gain evidence to support your interventions?

Leadership/administration. What administrative changes do you want to see within your clinical setting, and how can you lead the initiative of change?

Program development and evaluation. This tends to be where many PP OTD students start their thought process. What program do I want to develop that may impact the health and well-being of those I serve, and how can I evaluate outcomes? Is there a program in place that I need to assess through program evaluation?

Quality improvement. What is the CQI process at my site? Is there a process that I feel could be improved? And if so, how can I apply the process to improve the quality of care within my clinical setting?

Teaching/learning. What do I know about teaching and learning theory, and how can I apply this to patient education, working with fieldwork students, and/or educating new practitioners?

When exploring potential capstone ideas, you should discuss this with your supervisor, professional mentor, or employer; they can provide support and assistance when developing a plan. Most likely, you are planning for your capstone project to be implemented within your clinic or workplace, and having their support will make this process easier. Program development and continuous quality improvement are two areas which can help improve overall workflow and productivity within the workplace or clinic setting. Do some research to investigate current program offerings inside and outside of your department at work. Or maybe there has been a wish list of future programming needs established by a process-improvement team. What specialty accreditations or compliance organizations does your work setting affiliate with? Think about organizations such as the Joint Commission, Commission of Accreditation for Rehabilitation Facilities, etc. Do these provide an opportunity and business rationale to support the development of your capstone project and line up well with institutional needs to collect data, track outcomes, enhance the visibility of your employer, etc.?

Clinical practice is another area in which continuous evaluation is necessary to ensure safety practices are met, hospital accreditation standards are followed, and overall client satisfaction is achieved. Completion of a capstone project with these specific areas in mind can assist you in providing valuable information to your organization and improve evidence-based practice applications. Program development may be an area in which you have had an idea for a new program to benefit your clinic and improve client outcomes; this can be a topic for your capstone. These are all examples that can mutually benefit your clinic and patient populations and also support your own personal and professional development as you embark on the PP OTD degree pathway.

Finding the right project is a combination of identifying an area you enjoy, finding a group of individuals who can support you, add knowledge and value to your project, and increase the distinct value of occupational therapy. (See Text Box 13-3.)

TEXT BOX 13-3

As a PP OTD student, think about the context of your project. Typically, students develop projects in the context of their work environment. So how might you explore your workplace environment through a needs assessment? The needs assessment, just like when you evaluate a client, allows you to evaluate the current process or state of the situation and develop a targeted plan. It is important that you develop an understanding of the needs and challenges of the individuals you are designing for. The needs assessment process allows your capstone project to be grounded in a lived experience of those it seeks to support.

There are various examples of needs assessments – many are performed based on the specific type of capstone project you are completing. Refer to Chapter 6 to get further insight into different frameworks to guide the needs assessment process.

Phase 2: Ideation (Developing and Defining Problem and Purpose, Goals, and Objectives)

Once you have solidified your idea from gathering insights from your targeted population or stakeholders, the next step in the process is defining the problem and developing a purpose. The purpose will guide you through the capstone project and assist in outlining what you will be doing over the course of the entire timeline. This process assists you in framing your clinical question into searchable or discoverable question, which is one of the initial steps in defining your problem, project purpose, and related goals and objectives. This stage encourages the creative mindset. Spend time brainstorming and coming up with a wide range of ideas. Remember the process is iterative. Refer to Chapter 7 for more information on developing a capstone purpose. The main difference between the entry-level OTD student and the PP OTD purpose development is you have a work context that you will draw upon when determining the purpose. Most likely your capstone purpose will be very personal and reflect a need within your clinical site.

PICO format. The PICO format – population, intervention, comparison, outcome – outlines the specific areas you are focusing your research on. This format works best to frame your clinical question. Each element is specifically defined and will guide you as you identify your clinical question.

P	What are the characteristics/condition of the group? This can include diagnosis, age, gender.
I	What is the assessment, treatment, or type of service you are studying or exposing the client to?
C	Is there an alternative to the assessment, treatment, or approach? There may not be a specific comparison in some situations.
O	What do you want to measure, improve, or accomplish?

Source: National Library of Medicine (n.d.).

There are a variety of resources available to help guide you through this process. Be sure to look into and utilize all the resources available to you as a student; this could be through your university library, writing center, etc., as well as other web-based resources, which can all be helpful. Refer to Chapter 5 for additional insight and examples of framing a PICO question.

Literature search/review. Once the PICO question has been framed and fully developed, performing an extensive literature search is next. Through this search, you will determine how beneficial your chosen study will be and how it will help improve practice knowledge. Identifying search terms to help guide you through this process is one of the most relevant components, but also the most challenging. Taking terms from your PICO question is a good starting point, and expanding from there is the next step. Finding the right combination of terms will provide an exhaustive list of literature – many students use search engines, such as PubMed, OTseeker, Google Scholar, and Cochrane Library. During the search, using terms which are relevant to your topic will help you in finding literature to review and synthesize to identify an existing gap in the knowledge that can be further explored. If there is a lack of literature available, then what you are proposing is how your capstone project can fill that gap. For example, if you are interested in a capstone project within rehabilitation of elbow injuries in young throwing athletes, your search terms will include variations of throwing (baseball, football, softball), elbow injuries (ligament injuries, bone, fracture, osteochondrosis dissecans). Finding literature to support a topic is one of the most difficult pieces of this process; if the search terms being used are not yielding the expected results, expanding the search, reflecting with peers to find additional terms, or taking the opportunity to do a reverse search of references within found literature can assist in identifying additional terms or resources. Performing a thorough literature search is the best way to determine if the project is timely and relevant, based on what is found or what is not found. After you have searched the literature, your next step is to synthesize and summarize the findings to guide the development of your project. This can result in the creation of a problem statement, leading to the development of your project goals and objectives.

Proposing project goals and objective. Developing the project goals and objectives is necessary to guide your methods/methodology. The goals and objectives will go through multiple iterations, just like your project itself. Taking the time to understand this process and your expectations is important; utilizing your mentors to assist you will also help define your project. You can refer to Chapter 7 for further information on how to develop project goals and objectives. Defining goals for the entry-level capstone does not differ from the post-professional capstone project. Text Box 13-4 gives examples of project aims from recent PP OTD students which guided them in the development of their project goals and objectives:

TEXT BOX 13-4

This capstone project aims to advance understanding of how modern children with disabilities play. The purpose of this project is to analyze the ways in which the availability of different toy types, specifically open-ended toys versus digital-based toys, presented in the same environment affects the play characteristics of children between the ages of 3 and 5 with a diagnosis of developmental delay (Nicole Plutino, OTD, OTR/L, BCP, Indiana University PP OTD class of 2024).

This project aims to provide a comprehensive program employing a multimodal therapy program to patients that will include a thorough evaluation of hand function and self-perceived pain levels, a custom hand-based thumb spica orthotic, manual treatment in the form of passive range of motion (PROM), education on activity modification, strengthening of first dorsal interossei and opponens pollicis, strengthening of extrinsic muscles with orthotic on, paraffin wax, and ultrasound therapy (Tor Ulla OTD, OTR/L, CHT, Indiana University PP OTD class of 2024).

Once you have developed the background, relevance, goals, and objectives of your project, you can move to the next phase, developing your methodology. The methodology will be based upon the type of capstone project you plan on implementing.

Phase 3: Planning

Methods/methodology. Thoroughly analyzing the literature, project goals and objectives, and the intended population will assist in selecting the method for data collection and analysis. As the primary lead on your capstone project, you, the student, must explain the rationale and identify how they will complete the project (Bouchrika, 2024). Note that you might initially come up with a variety of options and solutions here. Lean into your capstone team and get feedback from your intended stakeholders to see if your project meets their needs or if adjustments are necessary. Remember . . . this process is iterative and will transform and improve based upon reflection, collaboration, and feedback received.

Once more well-defined and finalized, the student can move forward with the next steps in the processes and outline their data collection plan. As you are designing your methods, you will be ensuring ethical compliance and careful consideration of the requirements related to the institutional review board (IRB) or comparable approval entity at your worksite. The IRB is a committee that reviews research involving human subjects to ensure the rights, safety, and welfare of the participants are protected (Office for Human Research Protections, 2021). Once the research methods are defined and your protocol is finalized, you will need to review the IRB requirements for the type of study you are completing. The level of review provided by the IRB will depend on your project; there are three categories: exempt, expedited, or full-board. Each type poses different levels of risk to the participants involved. *Exempt* is defined as "no risk," *expedited* is "minimal risk," and *full-board* reviews are needed if there is high risk to the participants, or if a vulnerable population is being studied (IU Human Research Protection Program, n.d.). Additionally, the level of review depends upon components of your project, which will look at the level of risk to subjects, type of research being conducted, sensitivity of the questions, complexity of the research design, and the population involved in the research. Due to the general nature of the PP OTD degree and capstone requirement, most projects will fall under the exempt or expedited categories, which pose little or no risk to the subjects involved. These types of projects include scoping/systematic reviews, program development, quality improvement, retrospective studies, clinical skill reviews, pre- and post-interviews, surveys, or how an intervention may impact a healthy participant. Full-board review is required if a study is deemed to be involving vulnerable populations; a full IRB submission must be completed (IU Human Research Protection Program, n.d.). Chapter 7 outlines the IRB process in more detail. If a capstone project aligns with continuous quality improvement activities, your worksite might have a quality improvement review process, and you might need to seek approval prior to implementation. (See Text Box 13-5 for a student testimony regarding the IRB process for a PP OTD capstone project.)

TEXT BOX 13-5

"I would need to complete a full review by the university's internal review board due to the nature of my research with a vulnerable population and the methods of my data collection utilizing videotaping. The full-review application was lengthy in nature and required a detailed protocol submission regarding how I planned to recruit children with developmental delays as participants obtain informed consent from legal guardians,

---

TEXT BOX 13-5 (continued)

the dialogue I planned to use with the participants during the data collection, and the level of security needed to store the video recording, including those obtained during data collection, in order to protect the privacy and identity of the participants. Though lengthy in nature, I was able to provide the necessary documentation and receive approval from the full-review process to begin my data collection."

– Nicole Plutino, OTD, OTR/L, BCP

Once you have developed your methods and have approval from the IRB, you might be required to develop a proposal defense, which formally presents your intended capstone project to your capstone team, or to faculty and peers within your cohort. Each program outlines this process in different ways. Overall, once you've presented your proposal and received the necessary approvals, you most likely will receive the "green light" to move forward with implementation of the project. The proposal is an important step in the process as it allows faculty and peers opportunities to address any initial concerns with the student project and outline the process moving forward. There will most likely be additional opportunities to showcase your capstone project and the related outcomes during the dissemination phase.

Phase 4: Implementation

Once your plan is finalized, and as you prepare for implementation, you will want to outline an implementation timeline. The timeline will reflect each week in the collection process and what is expected at that point in time. Timelines and expectations will vary based on the type of capstone project being completed. During this phase, to inspire reflective thinking, your faculty might expect you to engage in weekly reflections, via contributing to an online discussion board forum or maybe a journal. This practice of reflection is important and will assist in determining the next steps or if adjustments are necessary. The weekly reflective process will guide you during the semester, allowing you to determine where and when you need assistance from your faculty mentor or content expert. (See Text Box 13-6 for sample weekly reflection questions during the capstone project implementation process.) Additional strategies that can be generalized to support implementation of the PP OTD capstone can be found in Chapter 9 of this book.

TEXT BOX 13-6

Weekly Reflective Questions

- What happened that was good this week and supported your capstone project?
- What challenges did you note this week?
- Do you feel you are on track? What support do you need, or what assistance do you need?

Reflective practice assists you in critiquing your performance, evaluating and re-evaluating how your actions are shaped by values, preferences, and perspectives. Asking the questions within Text Box 13-6 each week throughout the implementation phase can guide you in determining if any additional assistance is needed.

Phase 5: Analysis

Once you have completed all components of your project, you will engage in program evaluation and analysis. Chapter 8 of this book provides many useful resources to guide this process. To evaluate your project, you should assess if it is **relevant**, **effective**, **efficient**, **impactful**, and *sustainable* (Kaldenberg & Delbert, 2024). Your project is *relevant* if the outcomes address the problem it aims to solve; it is *effective* if it has achieved the intended outcomes and objectives, the resources are being used well to achieve the intended objectives, the project has a long-term *impact* on the OT community, and if it has the ability to maintain benefits and operations overtime (*sustain*). Reflecting on each one of the aforementioned aspects of YOUR project will help you think through the overall impact of your outcomes/results. It will also give you an understanding of your project's strengths, weaknesses, and areas to improve upon. Through review and analysis of your data, you can determine if your project is relevant to your clinical practice, uses an evidence-based approach, identifies areas for improvement, and sets up your dissemination plan. Refer back to Chapter 11 for examples of ways to design your dissemination plan and to guide discussions with your faculty mentor.

Phase 6: Dissemination

As discussed in Chapters 11 and 12 of this book, most capstone projects will require some form of dissemination. Your PP OTD program might require you formally present within your program, complete a final written capstone report, or aspire to disseminate at an outside venue, such as a conference of publication. Over the course of your last semester in your PP OTD program, you will frequently discuss and finalize your dissemination plan with your faculty mentor, to ensure a set plan is in place and all are in agreement with the designation of authorship. Please be sure to be aware of the authorship and intellectual property policies that are within your academic program and at the site where your capstone project is implemented. With capstone projects, you are most likely going to be listed as the first author; your faculty mentor(s) or content experts might also be recognized as co-authors as well. Typically, at the end of your program, you will present your final project; for many, this is when they feel relief and success. Some academic programs have a poster symposium to recognize and celebrate the implementation and completion of the capstone project. Completing the presentation in a poster format will allow you to visually represent what you've done, why it was important, the methods you used, and what results you found. Having the tangible poster product ready to go will allow you to also consider formal submission of an abstract to a state or national conference to present your findings at a larger platform. Completing a peer-reviewed presentation at a professional conference is another great indicator to support your advancement and might contribute to mobility on the clinical ladder at your worksite.

TIPS FOR SUCCESS

As most PPOTD students are working professionals, it is most likely that you are now juggling several roles and needing to modify your usual habits and routines to ensure success as well as ensuring you are engaging in occupational balance.

Success in your capstone project is about balancing planning, reflection, collaboration, and flexibility throughout the process. By focusing on these tips in what follows, you'll not only develop a strong capstone project but also enhance your own personal and professional development as an occupational therapy practitioner.

Time management. Stay organized and plan out your project phases. Set realistic deadlines. Avoid procrastination by setting specific milestones.

Seek feedback. Regularly initiate and communicate with your capstone team for feedback and guidance. Engage with classmates or colleagues who are also working on capstone projects – they might offer fresh perspectives or constructive critiques. Early feedback helps shape your project, and periodic check-ins ensure you are on track.

Stay flexible. While structure is important, sometimes the process does not go as planned. Stay flexible, and be open to adapting your approach if new information or challenges arise. Flexibility allows you to problem-solve effectively and can lead to unexpected, rewarding outcomes. Remember that aligned with the design thinking mindsets, this is all an iterative process.

Self-care is essential. Balancing work and school can be draining, so make sure to prioritize self-care. This might mean ensuring you get enough sleep, exercising regularly, eating well, and taking time for relaxation. Create clear boundaries between your work, school, and personal life. This may mean setting specific times for studying and times for work and making sure to give yourself personal time to recharge. A fresh mind often leads to better decision-making and creativity.

Establish a support system. Talk to your employer about your capstone project and overall goals and how they align with your professional development. Be transparent with your employer about your academic commitments. You'll also need emotional and practical support from family and friends. Share your goals with them, and ask for help with things like childcare, household tasks, or just some encouragement when you are feeling overwhelmed.

Use resources wisely. Leverage services at your academic program, such as the library and writing center. Engage with the OT community whether it is being present on online discussion forums or attending conferences or workshops to get a broader view of your capstone topic. Networking with professionals in the field can offer new insights or help you refine your ideas.

Celebrate milestones. It is easy to focus on the end result and miss the small victories along the way. Celebrate milestones, whether it is completing a difficult assignment, defending your capstone proposal, finalizing your data collection, or completing your data analysis. Recognizing progress can help keep motivation high.

Keep the end goal in mind. Ensure that your project has practical applications for the field of OT, whether through direct patient care, program development, or advancing knowledge. Ask yourself: How will your project outcomes or findings help advance the profession or improve patient care?

Think beyond graduation. Your capstone project might be a stepping stone to further opportunities. Consider how you might use your findings to create a professional continuing education course, implement change in a clinical setting, or pursue additional scholarly activities.

STUDENT SECTION CHAPTER SUMMARY

As a post-professional OTD student, you are embarking on a rigorous yet exciting process. The initial development and design of the PPOTD capstone is a fast-paced timeline to ensure timely completion. Each project must be closely reviewed by faculty to avoid projects being too large for the timeline available. You need to understand what is feasible to execute during your time in the program. This process can be daunting to start but rewarding upon completion. Each piece of this process is relevant and important. Taking the time to understand how all the pieces fit together will prevent you from getting offtrack during your process.

Section 2: Educator Focus

Transformational Learning Phases and Framework for the Post-Professional OTD Educator

Through the capstone process, you, the educator, within a post-professional OTD program, will most

likely be leaning into the principles of adult learning initially described by Knowles to best meet the needs of your students. Adults are self-directed, bring a wealth of prior experience to the learning process, are goal-oriented, are motivated by practical, problem-solving needs, and have a readiness to learn (Merriam & Bierema, 2014). Applying these adult learning principles through the lens of Mezirow's (1997) transformational learning theory may help guide you as you prepare the capstone curriculum for the PP OTD student. The connection between Mezirow's transformational learning theory and the post-professional OTD capstone project is rooted in the concept of perspective transformation – how learners change their understanding of the world through new insights and experiences.

As the student initially begins the process of the capstone, you will be encouraging them to critically reflect on their existing beliefs, assumptions, and perspectives to determine a disorienting dilemma, which can lead to a starting point for their capstone project. Your students may challenge a clinical or administrative process in the workplace, social and/or occupational injustices for the patients they are treating or a population of people in which they have a connection, or a programmatic problem that may be affecting their day-to-day ability to provide the best care to their patients. Whatever the challenge, you will guide them through the capstone process to self-reflect, engage in discourse and new experiences, assist them to solve problems, question their prior assumptions, take action through the capstone project development and implementation, and disseminate their gained knowledge. Mezirow (1997) also argues that transformational learning affects not only professional practice but also personal identity. As your PP OTD students engage in transformational learning during the capstone experience and project, they often experience a shift in how they see themselves as professionals and as individuals. This growth in personal and professional identity has the ability to not just impact the setting where the capstone project takes place but the occupational therapy profession as a whole.

INTRODUCTION FOR EDUCATOR

Working with post-professional OTD students provides you as an educator an opportunity to stay connected with clinical practice beyond your own work. This connection to clinical practice creates an avenue to learn about potential trends that may be occurring in a specific area of practice or a gap in literature that may be the area of focus for the PP OTD student's capstone. The capstone project is the culminating project where you may be providing support to the student over the span of several semesters. Similarly, to the entry-level OTD capstone process, the role of the educator is to ensure the student understands the role of the project, the roles and responsibilities of the capstone team members, and the process for designing, implementing, evaluating, and disseminating the project (Kaldenberg & Delbert, 2024). As the educator, you will work with the student through this transformative process that can be viewed as the 5Ds: **discussion**, **discovery**, **design**, **drafts**, and **dissemination**.

EDUCATOR REFLECTIVE QUESTIONS

1. What areas of occupational therapy practice would the student want to examine?
2. Is there a protocol the student would want to investigate to find a more efficient way of doing things?
3. Would the student want to look at clinical outcomes based on a specific diagnosis?
4. Why is it essential to continue to improve practice scholarship or practice knowledge?
5. How will this benefit the student and others in practice?

EDUCATOR OBJECTIVES

By the end of reading this chapter, the educator will be able to design teaching methods to meet the stated student learning objectives:

1. Compare and contrast doctoral dissertation vs. entry-level OTD capstone vs. post-professional (PP OTD) capstone projects.
2. Explain the roles and responsibilities of the PP OTD capstone team members.
3. Design a post-professional capstone project.
4. Evaluate outcomes of the PP OTD capstone project.
5. Compare and contrast PP OTD project dissemination methods.

COMPARE AND CONTRAST

As educators, we commonly receive questions from students relating to the culminating project(s) within our doctoral programs. You may find a theme or reoccurring question from students wanting to understand the differences between a dissertation, a research project, and the PP OTD capstone. It may be helpful to explain to the student the differences in their association with a specific degree path. Writing a dissertation in higher education, specifically doctoral degree programming, has been a hallmark of the doctor of philosophy (PhD) degree, which is considered to be research-focused. Essentially, a *dissertation* is a long essay addressing a specific topic that is divided into chapters and sections, which can be written over the span of many months or even years, and includes original, empirical research (University of Arizona Global Campus, 2023). The entry-level OTD culminating project is primarily referred to as the doctoral capstone, which, as you now understand from the previous chapters in this text, can be a rewarding and student-focused project that is oftentimes connected to an agency, such as a clinical site or community site. Although the capstone project may have similarities, the post-professional capstone process and the project are notably different from the entry-level.

Post-professional capstones, as explained within the student section of this chapter, allow the student to address clinical problems with practical solutions through a project-based process. The capstone process allows for the PP OTD student to bring in clinical expertise and real-world knowledge from practice engagement to influence the area and type of project. As their faculty mentor, it may be beneficial to have focused conversations with the PP OTD student to help them understand the overarching benefit the PP capstone has on their current area of practice or place of employment. The project is structured in a way that meets your institution's academic requirements and the PP OTD student's scholarship goals. One activity that you may find helpful to incorporate into the capstone discovery process is asking the student to generate a purpose statement and PICO. Examples have been provided in Text Box 13-7, demonstrating how the PP OTD student's scholarship goals may be evident in their purpose statement and PICO, thus influencing the capstone project. The scholarship goals may be influential in the development of the project, as well as the individuals involved beyond the student and you as the mentor. Additionally, the variance of academic requirements has a direct influence on who is included as a member in the capstone project process.

TEXT BOX 13-7

Examples of PP OTD Student Capstone PICO or Purpose Statements

- To create a quick reference guide for increasing access of evidence-based resources for fieldwork students and entry-level clinicians.
- This survey aims to gather insights into cultural responsibility within occupational therapy educational programs. Your experiences and perspectives will contribute to the development of culturally responsible clinicians and enhance classroom practices.
- Does poor sleep hygiene in working women and/or caregivers living in underserved communities have an impact on occupational balance?
- To examine the degree to which a novel and comprehensive occupational therapy program administered to patients with first CMC OA of the hand can improve outcomes (decrease

TEXT BOX 13-7 (continued)

pain, increase occupational performance, strengthen related muscles).

- This mixed-methods research evaluated the necessity of curated ACOG-OT program development documents to write a guidebook that advocates for OT as a standard of care in hospital settings.

THE PP OTD CAPSTONE TEAM

Post-professional capstone projects are not held to specific accreditation standards or have a strong influence from the capstone site as to the project's aim. Understanding your role as the educator may have various responsibilities based on the infrastructure of the student's capstone team. The members of the team (Table 13-2) can vary based on the influence of the program's structure and type of project. At minimum, the team members include the PP OTD student and the assigned faculty mentor. The roles and responsibilities may vary based on how many members are incorporated into the capstone project team.

The primary role and majority of the responsibilities rest in the position of the PP OTD student. The responsibilities of the student resemble many of the requirements outlined for entry-level OTD capstone students as noted in Chapter 1. The PP OTD student will work collaboratively with you, as their course instructor, as well as their assigned faculty mentor, to identify their preferred direction of the project, create the scholarly question, develop the plan, implement the project, evaluate project outcomes, and disseminate as instructed.

The faculty mentor can be considered the student's primary academic support. The role of the faculty mentor ensures the student is informed and prepared for the academic requirements of the capstone project. With many similarities to the faculty role or "capstone chair," as noted in the entry-level capstone process, see Chapter 1, this role works with the student in a collaborative approach, offering guidance on the direction of the project, serve as a resource for institution-focused requirements (e.g., IRB process), and consult on content related to the area of practice while ensuring the project requirements are met.

If your institution does not have an expanded capstone team, you may also assume the roles of content expert, course instructor, and research director when applicable. Understanding these other roles and what they might include can be beneficial if your institution is interested in revising the current structure.

The content expert commonly has extensive knowledge and/or clinical experience in the desired area of the capstone project. They serve on the capstone team as someone who can provide support and/or mentorship in the area of practice or advanced skill(s). If you or PP OTD student seeks to adopt a content expert as an additional capstone team member, consideration should be given to whether or not the person could be selected from the institution's faculty or, if necessary, to choose from the industry or work setting. The content expert has a vital role that can provide the PP OTD student with additional information and feedback to incorporate into the capstone project to ensure success and mastery of knowledge/content.

The role of research director may be adopted by institutions or programs that have a group matriculating in a cohort-style model to the capstone process. A research director may be a faculty member who oversees guiding all PP OTD students through the research component of the capstone project and serving as a resource during the data collection and analysis phase of the project.

The capstone course instructor is another role that your institution may utilize as a key PP OTD capstone team member. In many PP OTD programs, the capstone project occurs across the curriculum in multiple courses and semesters. This role can be viewed as the post-professional capstone coordinator or a faculty member who has been assigned as the instructor of record for capstone coursework. The capstone course instructor may be a role fulfilled by a faculty member who holds an administrative appointment, such as the post-professional OTD program director.

It is important to remember that the structure of the capstone team can and will vary based on institutional infrastructure, programmatic needs, and project-specific outcomes. Within Table 13-2, examples are provided for you to see the variance in capstone team members from four differing institutions: two public institutions and two

Table 13-2 Examples of Potential Capstone Teams

UNIVERSITY	CAPSTONE TEAM MEMBERS				
Valparaiso University	Student	Faculty mentor	Content expert		
Indiana University, Indianapolis	Student	Faculty mentor	Content expert	Capstone course instructor	Research director
Eastern Kentucky University	Student	Faculty mentor	Faculty committee member		
Spalding University	Student	Faculty mentor			

private institutions. The examples suggest the key members for all programs would be the role of the student and faculty mentor, with emphasis also on a third person, either the content expert or an additional faculty member.

THE PP OTD CAPSTONE PROJECT

As an educator, you will identify that working with the PP OTD capstone student may differ from your experiences if you've had a role within an entry-level OTD capstone. It is beneficial to consider this mentorship as a transformative learning process between the educator and the student (Misawa & McClain, 2019). The phases, after you have been assigned to the student's capstone team, can be organized into the 5Ds: *discussion*, *discovery*, *design*, *drafts*, and *dissemination*.

The Discussion

The discussion phase often resembles the initial consultation or meeting with the PP OTD student, where you, as the course instructor or faculty mentor, take the opportunity to assist the student in exploring ideas, topics, or even areas of practice that interest them. This step in the capstone project can be structured in several different ways: (1) as a discussion forum prompt within a capstone project–related course, either synchronous or asynchronous (see Image Text Boxes 13-8 and 13-9; (2) dialogue in a one-on-one meeting; or (3) a structured worksheet that provides the student with self-reflective questions or prompts (see Text Box 13-10). When working with the PP OTD student in a one-on-one dialogue, you may consider including conversations related to program development and continuous quality improvement (CQI) options for the capstone project. If the student expresses interest in aligning their capstone project with their place of employment, it may be beneficial to provide the student with the information that the CQI process may be an option where the capstone project could help improve overall workflow and/or productivity.

TEXT BOX 13-8

Sample Discussion Forum Questions Within an Online Course

Discussion Prompt 1

Reflect on your current area of practice in occupational therapy. Identify a specific population, condition, or challenge that interests you. What are some emerging trends, unmet needs, or opportunities for innovation within this area? How could occupational therapy address these issues to improve client outcomes or community well-being? Share your thoughts, and consider how these ideas might inspire future research or program development for your capstone.

TEXT BOX 13-8 (continued)

Discussion Prompt 2

Reflect on your current place of employment and its connection to your area of practice in occupational therapy. Identify a specific population, condition, or challenge you encounter regularly. What are some emerging trends, unmet needs, or opportunities for innovation within your workplace? How could your capstone project address these? Share your insights, and consider how these ideas could inspire future improvements or initiatives in your role.

TEXT BOX 13-9

Group Discussion and Brainstorming Discussion Board Post

Instructions

- Divide the class into small groups (3–4 students per group) to discuss their findings from their personal reflection (see Text Box 13-8) and needs assessment exercises.
- In their groups, students should:
  - Share the areas of interest or challenges they identified in steps 1 and 2.
  - Brainstorm potential project ideas that address both their personal interest and the needs of their capstone setting (workplace).
  - Consider the feasibility of each idea, including resources, timeline, and potential impact.
- Each group should come up with 2–3 viable project ideas and prepare a brief summary of each.

OUTCOME

Students will benefit from peer input, which will help refine their project ideas and identify, a focus that is both meaningful and feasible.

TEXT BOX 13-10

Personal Reflection on Professional Interests Assignment

Instructions

- Begin by asking each student to reflect on the following questions:
  - What aspects of occupational therapy am I most passionate about (e.g., pediatrics, mental health, geriatrics, hand therapy, neurorehabilitation . . .)?
  - What are the clinical challenges I encourage in my current role that I feel could be addressed through a capstone project?
  - How do I envision my career in the next 5 to 10 years? What role do I want to play in shaping OT practice, education, or research?

TEXT BOX 13-10 (continued)

- Students should write down their responses and identify any reoccurring themes or areas of interest.

Outcome

Students will have a clearer understanding of their personal professional passions and career aspirations, which will serve as the foundation for their capstone project.

Discovery

After the initial discussions have occurred, the PP OTD student's area of interest will be discovered. As the educator, you will be providing support during this initial preparation phase through guiding the student to also *discover the gaps* within the literature, beginning to formulate a research question to ultimately shape the design of the capstone project. You may find the resource(s) in Chapter 5, outlining the PICO development process, to be a useful tool at this point in the discovery phase. A practical application of these worksheets found in the appendices of Chapter 5 would be for you to embed an assignment into your course, allowing the PP OTD student to strengthen their project's focus. A version of the worksheet can be utilized as a precursor assignment prior to a one-on-one meeting or incorporating the worksheet as a self-directed assignment where the student either turns in the worksheet or attaches it with a narrative in a discussion forum.

The discovery phase gives you a chance to work with the PP OTD student to narrow down the project focus. When trying to narrow the project focus, it is beneficial to advise the PP OTD student to initiate dialogue with their place of employment relating to the capstone project idea(s). These conversations are helpful as the student considers the feasibility of the project, the permissions or approvals needed, and the project's timeline before conducting a formal needs assessment. As the mentor, you may need to coach the student to identify the administration or the hierarchy for approval of projects within their place of employment in order to have initial conversations and gain approval before moving forward with the formal capstone project. Additionally, you will work closely with the student to begin to assemble the capstone team if your institution's structure allocates more than the student and faculty mentor. You may structure your course(s) to have the student identify potential team members. For example, in Table 13-2 of the student section of this chapter, two institutions have a capstone team member who is identified as the "content expert." Within this role, you may fulfill the content expert and faculty mentor. However, in situations where either your institution does not allow one person to fulfill more than one role or you are not able to fulfill the "content expert" role, you may work in conjunction with

the student to identify individuals within the area of practice that may meet this requirement.

Additional discovery of the capstone project may provide you an opportunity to consult with the student on the type of project they desire and provide direction on the steps they will need to complete within the assigned time frame. You may provide the student with an outline that gives more structure to the program-specific requirements to ensure they are well-informed before advancing to the design phase. One example might be a template (see Text Box 13-11) utilized by your program for assisting students in developing their capstone project proposal. The project proposal template provides you the opportunity to explain the minimum requirements a student must complete when designing their proposed project and demonstrate how the series of capstone courses contribute to the project's final outcomes. These requirements can be set as a standard for all capstone proposals, regardless of the nature of the project.

TEXT BOX 13-11

Outline of Program-Specific Requirements

Scholarly Project Proposal Template Example

Literature review and linkage to theoretical framework in OCTH 799.

Required assignment graded in OCCT 785.

To progress to OCCT 790 and implement their project, students must complete the proposal's requirement to the satisfaction of the OCCT 785 instructor.

I. Title Page
II. Literature Review and Theoretical Framework
III. Project Proposal
   a. Project Purpose
   b. Description of Proposed Project
      i. Population
      ii. Proposed Site/Location of the Project
      iii. Project Activities
   c. Proposed Evaluation Methods
   d. Proposed Dissemination Plans
   e. Discussion
      i. Relationship to the Distinct Value of Occupational Therapy
      ii. Project Strengths
      iii. Project Risks/Barriers
      iv. Ethical Risks, Including Plan for IRB (If Necessary)
IV. Conclusion
   a. Value of the Project
   b. Potential for Project Success
V. References
VI. Appendices
   a. PICO/Evidence Search Form
   b. Evidence Table (20–25 high-quality sources)
   c. Logic Model

Design

Within the design and implementation phases of the post-professional capstone, you will mentor the PP OTD student through the refinement of the scholarly question, complete a thorough needs assessment, identify relevant resources through an in-depth literature review process, develop the problem and purpose, complete the institutional review board (IRB) process when applicable, and then support the project's implementation process while the student gathers data. As referenced in earlier chapters, the literature search is a critical piece of the capstone project. In Chapter 5, the literature search process is identified as a way for the student, in this case, the PP OTD student, to review and utilize data from their scholarly inquiry process. At this point in the capstone process, you may find yourself providing more support and feedback to the student, ensuring they are able to utilize the resources necessary for the literature search process, and offering mentorship on identifying and refining search terms.

If the student experiences challenges in the literature search process, one way to assist them in developing these skills would be to synchronously engage in an online exercise where the mentor and student use the same database or search engine to replicate one another's search parameters. Modeling the literature search process may give the PP OTD student an opportunity to identify additional methods (e.g., use of Booleans or truncation) to expand or limit the search. If your capstone team supports the use of a content expert beyond yourself, oftentimes, you will find this is a point in the process where their expertise is beneficial. A practical application of the content experts' guidance may be generated through advisement via email or one-on-one meetings. If you structure the course assignments in a way that allows the use of the PICO worksheet, which includes the search terms, it may be beneficial to seek the feedback from the content expert before the student moves too far forward in the literature search process.

Another resource used in the literature search process is a designated research librarian who may assist the PP OTD student in refining the search terms. As the course instructor or faculty mentor, you may want to help the student locate these resources, if your institution supports designated research librarians. Another step that may be included in this phase is the development of the problem and purpose. Identifying these items may be conducted through a capstone proposal process.

The capstone proposal process may differ based on your program's structure of capstone coursework. Drafting a proposal can provide the student an initial opportunity to place their thoughts and plans in one central location. This assignment establishes a clear line of communication between the PP OTD student and faculty mentor, adding in other key members as your institution allows. At this point in the capstone design process, you will want to provide guidance to the student on the project to ensure the content meets the objectives and the required time frame.

Often, we could consider this to be a "Goldie Locks" concept, "[a] project not too big, a project not too small, but a project that is just right and obtainable in the timeframe." You may find it beneficial to provide a synchronous class where the students in the planning and design phase are provided examples of project ideas that are "too big," "too small," and "just right/obtainable" in the given time frame. Then, as a learning exercise, you can facilitate an activity where students can brainstorm their initial project ideas with peers receiving feedback, implementing strategies to consider if their initial idea is focused and relevant to meet their professional goals and the learning objectives for the capstone project.

After the project proposal has been agreed upon, you may need to guide the student through the institutional review board (IRB) process, as noted in Chapter 7. With a PP OTD capstone project, this might involve procedures both at the academic institution as well as the setting of the capstone project. Locating your institution's IRB website and resources will be a helpful strategy to ensure the student is well-informed and following the ethical procedures for their type of project. As an assignment, you may desire to incorporate a worksheet or decision tree into the course that assists the student in identifying the IRB process and path needed for their project (see Text Box 13-12, IRB Process and Path Assignment, and Text Box 13-13, Research Determination Activity). The IRB resources and webpage from your institution may be a strong resource to include in your online course, ensuring students have a resource section with a quick reference to ethical guidelines and decision-making materials. Additionally, suppose your program is not structured in a way that allows the students early exposure to the Office of Sponsored Research or a university-level representative who works in alignment with the IRB process, such as a guest lecture or workshop within the research coursework. In that case, it may be beneficial for you as the faculty mentor to develop a connection point. One option for connecting the student with university personnel who work within research parameters might be hosting a synchronous class, where students can ask questions about the IRB process.

TEXT BOX 13-12

IRB Process and Path Assignment
IRB Proposal: What Path Is Needed?

You are designing your capstone project based on your chosen topic and PICO questions. You have identified HOW the project is relevant to OT and includes some evaluation components (e.g., assessment, survey, focus groups, feedback form, patient outcomes, etc.). Familiarize yourself with the IRB website and requirements, including the flowchart and graphic describing the IRB process. You must complete CITI training before submitting this assignment.

TEXT BOX 13-12 (continued)

Complete the Research Determination and Review Level Screening Form. This form is required before submitting any IRB proposal. You will use this form to determine which type of proposal you must complete.

Complete the appropriate IRB protocol based on the Research Determination and Review Level Screening Form results. For this assignment, you will complete the IRB proposal in a Microsoft Word document.

Submit your IRB proposal and relevant attachments in Microsoft Word format via the assignment submission portal in Canvas LMS.

Similar to when you submit an IRB proposal, you should expect feedback and revisions on your proposal from the assigned faculty mentor. These revisions must be completed to receive your final grade for the assignment.

TEXT BOX 13-13

Human Research Determination Learning Activity

Supervision

Although student investigators may complete this questionnaire, all research conducted at XXX University must be supervised by a faculty member or full-time staff member who has successfully completed the human subjects' ethics training.

Purpose of the Questionnaire

In everyday language, we use the word "research" to describe a wide variety of activities. We use the same word to describe library research for a paper as research designed to test the effectiveness of a new treatment for a disease. Although both activities involve scholarly pursuits, they are very different activities and do not require the same kind of ethical oversight from the IRB. Clearly, doing library research where you read journals and books does not require ethical oversight, whereas a clinical trial designed to test the effectiveness of a new treatment would require ethical oversight. The challenge is that most projects fall somewhere between these two extremes, and knowing if your project needs ethical oversight from the IRB is not a simple question.

To determine if a project needs ethical oversight by the IRB, you need to know if the project meets the federal definition of *research*, as well as the definition of *human subjects*. The following questions will help you determine if your study meets the federal definition of "human subjects research" that requires IRB oversight. If it does not meet this definition, your project does not require IRB review. If it does meet this definition, you will answer additional questions that will help you determine what level of review is required.

TEXT BOX 13-13 (continued)

Example questions might include:

- Is the intent of the project to contribute to generalizable knowledge?
- Is this project a systematic investigation?
- Are the participants "living subjects"?

One factor to consider now would be the setting or site the student identified in their proposal for the capstone project. In many cases, we see the PP OTD student identifying their current place of employment as the capstone site. Incorporating discussions via the online forums in class may allow the student to identify possible ethical considerations that may arise when working through the IRB process. Requiring your students to complete CITI training is a must to allow the student to identify any potential ethical issues they may see given their initial proposed capstone. As a course instructor or faculty mentor, you may find it beneficial to incorporate ethical problems as a topic of discussion in your one-on-one meetings. As the PP OTD student gains approval for the proposed project to be implemented, you may identify a schedule for periodic check-ins as they carry out the project and begin data gathering. Identifying key points in your capstone curriculum will allow you, as the faculty mentor, and others on the capstone team, the opportunity to ensure the PP OTD student receives adequate support. Options for the timeline of the periodic check-ins may vary based on the project, but at minimum in the early stages, it may be beneficial to consider either weekly or biweekly meetings. As the project starts, you may find it beneficial to have less frequent meetings but remain connected with the student to ensure progress is occurring and on track. Understand that not all capstone projects are structured in the same way; therefore, the use of discussion forums with variable time frames may be beneficial for students enrolled in the capstone course(s).

After the project has been carried out, the PP OTD student will begin the data analysis portion of the project. Based upon the type of the capstone project, the analysis process and related program evaluation procedures can vary. At a minimum, as discussed in Chapter 8, the PP OTD student should engage in project evaluation, which will influence the synthesis of the results and aid in evaluating the overall outcomes of the capstone project.

A capstone project has the potential to significantly influence a PP OTD student's work setting in various ways, depending on the area of practice, the focus of the projects, the nature of the research (if conducted), and the practical applications of the findings. As the faculty mentor, some key points to discuss with the PP OTD student relate to how their capstone can impact their work setting, which may include knowledge transfer, innovation or quality improvement, enhanced professional practice, policy influence, or career advancement or change. If the capstone project involves research, it often produces new knowledge or insights that can directly inform best practices, policies, or strategies within a given work setting. For instance, the capstone project may reveal more efficient treatment methods. The dissemination of this knowledge can improve treatment practices, benefiting the healthcare environment, the consumer or client, and the overall outcomes for the profession. Regarding innovation or quality improvement, a PP OTD student's capstone project may focus on solving complex, unresolved issues or addressing gaps in existing knowledge. The project results may provide innovative solutions to ongoing challenges within the work setting. Completing a capstone project often positions an individual as a subject-matter expert. This added credibility can influence their role within the work setting, enabling them to assume greater leadership responsibilities, mentor others, or lead specialized initiatives that rely on the expertise gained through the doctoral project. For many, capstone projects often have direct applications to day-to-day practice. Project outcomes can offer new frameworks, techniques, or therapeutic approaches that enhance the effectiveness of their work. This can lead to higher-quality outcomes for clients or stakeholders and contribute to the professional development of others in the field. In some instances, doctoral research can influence organizational or governmental policies. For example, a capstone related to public health concerns can result in recommendations for policy changes that affect health initiatives or services provided. Lastly, the outcomes of the capstone project could open new career opportunities. In academia, successful projects or research may lead to publishing papers, presenting at conferences, and establishing oneself as an expert in the field. In non-academic work environments, the project outcomes can lead to scholarship advancement, promotions, new responsibilities, or even the creation of new roles within the organization. Ultimately, the influence of a capstone project on one's work setting is shaped by how the outcomes or findings are applied and how effectively they address the needs and challenges of the workplace. This process often drives both personal and organizational growth, resulting in long-term benefits.

As the course instructor or faculty mentor, you will guide the student through the examination of all components of their capstone project in preparation for dissemination. Earlier in the chapter, the PP OTD student was instructed on the importance of this step to evaluate the project, making sure it is relevant, effective, efficient, impactful, and sustainable (Kaldenberg & Delbert, 2024). You may find it helpful to refer to Chapter 8 when suggesting ways the PP OTD student can assess the sustainability and relevancy of their capstone project.

Drafts

As the faculty mentor, your role in the draft process of the PP OTD student's capstone includes providing guidance and structured feedback throughout each phase of project. From initial discovery and exploration of ideas to the design and implementation of their project, you will support the student in refining their work through multiple drafts, ensuring clarity, coherence, and alignment with the project goals and outcomes. Each draft may serve as a foundation for ongoing revisions, allowing the student to integrate feedback from you as the mentor and from other capstone team members when appropriate. In addition to incorporating feedback, drafts may provide the PP OTD student with an opportunity to strengthen their analysis and ultimately prepare for the dissemination phase of their capstone and options for their final work.

Dissemination

Methods of dissemination appear to differ within PP OTD programs. Similar to the uniqueness of the capstone team members, your institution may have specific evaluative methods that accompany the PP OTD capstone dissemination process. If you are evaluating your methods of dissemination and questioning what options are being utilized, Text Box 13-14 provides a sample of four programs for reference. Two common dissemination methods include the student developing a presentation and completing a written paper. Note that this written paper should not be labeled or identified as a dissertation, as this is not the intended product or outcome of a scholarly capstone project. Some programs may require a variation of the presentation, with options including a formal podium-style presentation, a poster presentation, a virtual presentation or a blend of these options. You may require the PP OTD student to complete a written project, which may be a tangible product of dissemination, or you may be specific in requiring the student to structure it in the form of a journal article. For example, if the student is interested in making a career change with their PP OTD and the capstone project lends itself to support the area of occupational therapy education, you, as the faculty mentor, may guide the student to write the paper as a manuscript for submission to the *Journal of Occupational Therapy Education*. You could also mentor this same student to create their presentation in a way that could be considered for a conference proposal. As an instructor, you might establish an assignment in the capstone course for the student to write up a mock conference proposal aligned with state/national conference proposal guidelines. Not only is this a good learning activity to promote professional writing abilities, it also is excellent preparation to transform this "assignment" into an actual proposal submission.

TEXT BOX 13-14

Examples of Dissemination Methods

Valparaiso University

Required: Project completion form, virtual poster presentation, written project

TEXT BOX 13-14 (continued)

Optional: Request for feedback from site/agency, and conference proposal

Indiana University Indianapolis

Required: Presentation, poster presentation, written project
Optional: Conference proposal

Eastern Kentucky University

Required: Virtual presentation, written project.

Spalding University

Required: Project completion form, virtual presentation, written project

As the faculty mentor, you will continue to learn a great deal about the PP OTD students in their capstone journey. Although your institution and post-professional program may have requirements for dissemination, you hold an important role in supporting the student on their path to dissemination. If you have the ability to expand or customize the method of dissemination for the PP OTD student, consider the following examples: in-person presentations, virtual presentations, pre-recorded presentations, papers or manuscripts, journal articles, conference proposals or presentations, and continuing education workshops or webinars. For example, a PP OTD student might be able to pitch the design of a continued education course to a CE provider that aligns with their capstone project.

Your connection to the PP OTD student and deep understanding of their project provides you the opportunity to encourage additional avenues that can contribute to their success. As the PP OTD student begins to wrap up their journey, you will have several items to address. One important factor to consider is the development of authorship guidelines or policies within your PP OTD program. If your capstone team members exceed that of the PP OTD student and faculty mentor, then you may want to have specific policies to include all relevant parties. Discussion about authorship and intellectual property should occur early during the capstone process. At the very minimum, you may want to consider having a standard approach to the designation of authorship, where the PP OTD student is the first author. Additional consideration may be given to the option of other capstone team members being listed as co-authors, but it is recommended to have a formal agreement in place prior to the start of the capstone project. As the faculty mentor and/or the course instructor, you may want to consider incorporating learning activities that allow the PP OTD student to learn about ethical considerations that may occur related to authorship. (ee Text Box 13-16.)

TEXT BOX 13-16

Ethical Considerations Discussion Forum Example

Discussion Question #4: Ethical considerations in publication – what a large topic! This can encompass

TEXT BOX 13-16 (continued)

everything from copyright to plagiarism, authorship to piecemeal publications. In the assigned reading for today's session, you read details and how it relates to publication misconduct. This is important to review as many of these acts of misconduct are related to lack of knowledge; hence, arming yourself with this knowledge will put you in a good place as you move forward with your publication.

- Which of these areas is most relevant to your capstone project? Why is that, and what are you doing to prevent problems or concerns?
- Have you included everything necessary to prevent ethical concerns within your capstone project?
- Any concerns related to authorship or intellectual property around products created during the capstone project? Is this something you have taken into consideration?

EDUCATOR CHAPTER SUMMARY

As an educator within a PP OTD program, the framework of the 5Ds, along with human-centered design and transformative learning theory, can all be useful models to guide mentorship of PP OTD students throughout the capstone. Throughout this process, you will watch the growth and development of ideas turn into action, and action turn into outcomes. The process requires a significant amount of time and dedication from the PP OTD student, and you will be a constant in the process. It is also important to understand that most likely your PP OTD students will be balancing work, school, and personal life while completing this educational journey. Acknowledgment of these roles, change of routines through the academic journey, and provide emotional support will be critical for the PP OTD student. Be sure to emphasize the "Tips for Success" with your student cohorts, which are provided in the student section of this chapter. Each component of the capstone process is important for academic success and will be rewarding for the student upon completion. Remember, your benefit may reach beyond the mentoring and editing process by including encouragement and recognizing their dedication to the capstone process.

REFERENCES

Accreditation Council for Occupational Therapy Education. (2023). *2023 Accreditation Council for Occupational Therapy Education (ACOTE®) standards and interpretive guide.* https://acoteonline.org/accreditation-explained/standards/

American Occupational Therapy Association. (2022). Academic terminal degree. *American Journal of Occupational Therapy, 76*(Suppl. 3), 7613410260. https://doi.org/10.5014/ajot.2022.76S3013

American Psychological Association. (2020). *Publication manual of the American Psychological Association 2020: The official guide to APA style* (7th ed.). American Psychological Association.

Asiello, J. D., & Winstead, S. R. (2025). Design thinking as a theoretical framework to spark innovation in post-professional occupational therapy doctoral projects. *Journal of Occupational Therapy Education, 9*(1). https://encompass.eku.edu/jote/vol9/iss1/11

Bitanga, M., & Austria, M. (2013). Climbing the clinical ladder – one rung at a time. *Nursing Management, 44*(5), 23, 24–27. https://doi.org/10.1097/01.NUMA.0000429008.93011.a3

Bouchrika, I. (2024). *How to wrist research methodology in 2024: Overview, tips, and techniques.* https://research.com/research/how-to-write-research-methodology#:~:text=Justifying%20your%20methodological%20choices%20is%20a%20critical,selected%20particular%20methods%20over%20alternatives%2C%20showing%20that

Case-Smith, J., Page, S. J., Darragh, A., Rybski, M., & Cleary, D. (2014). The professional occupational therapy doctoral degree: Why do it? *American Journal of Occupational Therapy, 68*(2), e55–e60. https://doi.org/10.5014/ajot.2014.008805

Gutman, S. A. (2017). *Journal article writing and publication: Your guide to mastering clinical health care reporting standards.* Routledge, Taylor & Francis Group.

IDEO. (2015). *The field guide to human-centered design.* Ideo.org.

Indiana University Human Research Protection Program. (n.d.). *Human subjects research, and when it needs review.* https://research.iu.edu/compliance/human-subjects/review-levels/index.html

Kaldenberg, J & Delbert, T. (2024). Occupational therapy doctoral capstone research agenda: A scoping review. *American Journal of Occupational Therapy, 78*(5), 7805205150. https://doi.org/10.5014/ajot.2024.050669

Lampe, A., Jewell, V., Dunn, R., Lawson, T., Stewart, E., & Linhart, J. (2020). Career goals and student perceptions of a post-professional occupational therapy doctoral experiential component. *Journal of Occupational Therapy Education, 4*(2). https://doi.org/10.26681/jote.2020.040211

Merriam, S. B., & Bierema, L. L. (2014). *Adult learning linking theory and practice.* Jossey-Bass.

Mezirow, J. (1997). Transformative learning: Theory to practice. *New Directions for Adult and Continuing Education,* (74), 5–12. https://doi.org/10.1002/ace.7401

Misawa, M., & McClain, A. (2019). A mentoring approach: Fostering transformative learning in adult graduate education. *Journal of Transformative Learning, 6*(2), 52–62.

Moyers, P., & Quint, N. (2025). The issue is-discovery of knowledge in practice. *American Journal of Occupational Therapy, 79,* 7901347010. https://doi.org/10.5014/ajot.2025.050880

National Library of Medicine. (n.d.). *Using PubMed in evidence-based practice.* https://www.nlm.nih.gov/oet/ed/pubmed/pubmed_in_ebp/index.html

Office for Human Protections Research. (2021). *Lesson 3: What are IRBs?.* https://www.hhs.gov/ohrp/education-and-outreach/online-education/human-research-protection-training/lesson-3-what-are-irbs/index.html

Rains, R., & Pfaff, M. (2024). The post-professional occupational therapy doctorate. *OT Practice, 29*(4), 28–30.

Sackett, D. L., Rosenberg, W. M., Gray, J. A., Haynes, R. B., & Richardson, W. S. (1996). Evidence based medicine: What it is and what it isn't. *BMJ (Clinical Research Ed.), 312*(7023), 71–72. https://doi.org/10.1136/bmj.312.7023.71

University of Arizona Global Campus. (2023). *Writing a dissertation & applied doctoral project.* https://writingcenter.uagc.edu/writing-dissertation-applied-doctoral-project

University of Queensland. (n.d.). *What is evidence-based practice?* OTseeker. https://www.otseeker.com/resources/WhatIsEvidenceBasedPractice.aspx

Whitney, R. V., & Davis, C. A. (2013). *A writer's toolkit for occupational therapy and health care professionals: An insider's guide to writing, communicating, and getting published.* AOTA Press.

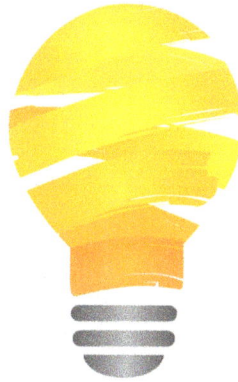

Index

Note: Page numbers in *italic* indicate a figure and page numbers in **bold** indicate a table on the corresponding page.

For Product Safety Concerns and Information please contact our EU
representative GPSR@taylorandfrancis.com
Taylor & Francis Verlag GmbH, Kaufingerstraße 24, 80331 München, Germany

www.ingramcontent.com/pod-product-compliance
Lightning Source LLC
Chambersburg PA
CBHW081047220326
41598CB00038B/7017

9 781032 892207